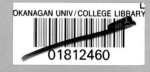
DATE DUE

Analysis and Evaluation of Nursing Theories

Analysis and Evaluation of Nursing Theories

Jacqueline Fawcett, PhD, FAAN

Professor
University of Pennsylvania
School of Nursing
Philadelphia, Pennsylvania

 F. A. DAVIS COMPANY • Philadelphia

F.A. Davis Company
1915 Arch Street
Philadelphia, PA 19103

Printed in the United States of America

Last digit indicates print number: 10 9 8 7 6 5 4 3 2 1

As new scientific information becomes available through basic and clinical research, recommended treatments and drug therapies undergo changes. The author(s) and publisher have done everything possible to make this book accurate, up to date, and in accord with accepted standards at the time of publication. The authors, editors, and publisher are not responsible for errors or omissions or for consequences from application of the book, and make no warranty, expressed or implied, in regard to the contents of the book. Any practice described in this book should be applied by the reader in accordance with professional standards of care used in regard to the unique circumstances that may apply in each situation. The reader is advised always to check product information (package inserts) for changes and new information regarding dose and contraindications before administering any drug. Caution is especially urged when using new or infrequently ordered drugs.

Library of Congress Cataloging-in-Publication Data

Fawcett, Jacqueline.
    Analysis and evaluation of nursing theories / Jacqueline Fawcett.
        p.   cm.
    Companion v. to: Analysis and evaluation of conceptual models of nursing / Jacqueline Fawcett, 1989.
    Includes bibliographical references and index.
    ISBN 0-8036-3413-7 (hard : alk. paper)
    1. Nursing—Philosophy.   I. Fawcett, Jacqueline. Analysis and evaluation of conceptual models of nursing.   II. Title.
    [DNLM: 1. Nursing Theory.   WY 86 F278a 1993]
RT84.5.F39   1993
610.73—dc20
DNLM/DLC
for Library of Congress   93-9610
                                                                      CIP

Preface

This book was written for all nurses and nursing students who are interested in the development of nursing theories and the use of those theories to guide nursing research and inform nursing practice. This book and its companion volume, *Analysis and Evaluation of Conceptual Models of Nursing* (also published by F. A. Davis Company), represent my continuing attempt to clarify the confusion about conceptual models and theories still seen in the nursing literature. This book covers the major grand and middle-range theories of contemporary nursing.

Chapter 1 presents my vision of the structure of contemporary nursing knowledge, including the metaparadigm, philosophies, conceptual models, theories, and empirical indicators. Two special features of the chapter are the discussion of alternative views of the nursing metaparadigm and a new schema of worldviews.

Chapter 2 presents an original framework for analysis and evaluation of nursing theories. The framework clearly separates questions for analysis from those for evaluation and is appliable to both grand and middle-range theories.

Chapters 3 through 8 present comprehensive and objective reviews of the most recent versions of nursing theories by Madeleine Leininger, Margaret Newman, Ida Jean Orlando, Rosemarie Parse, Hildegard Peplau, and Jean Watson. Each of those chapters is structured according to the framework for analysis and evaluation of nursing theories that is presented in Chapter 2. Each chapter also includes many direct quotes from the theorist's original works. The quotations reflect the language customs of the time of publication of the theory; pronouns used by the theorist have not been altered to reflect current nonsexist language. It is hoped that the retention of the original language will not diminish the reader's appreciation of the theorist's contributions.

Chapter 9 presents a discussion of alternative approaches to testing nursing theories. Emphasis is placed on the identification of requirements and criteria for theory-testing that are appropriate for grand theories and those that are appropriate for middle-range theories.

Each chapter of the book includes a list of key terms or key concepts that are defined and described in the chapter. Each chapter also includes an annotated bibliography of the published literature related to the content of that chapter. The bibliographies for Chapters 3 through 8 include the original works of the theorist that are directly related to the theory, critiques of the theory, and publications in which the theory clearly served as a basis for an application in research, education, practice, or administration. In addition, lists of relevant doctoral dissertations and master's theses are included in the bibliographies for Chapters 3 through 8.

Most chapters also include tables that highlight or expand certain narrative points. Chapter 1 includes several diagrams to illustrate the structural hierarchy of contemporary nursing knowledge, and Chapter 9 includes a diagram of the reciprocal relationship between theory development and theory utilization. Chapter 3 (Leininger's theory) and Chapter 7 (Peplau's theory) also include diagrams to illustrate relationships among the theory concepts and their dimensions.

The Appendix focuses on the technology available to enhance understanding of the theories and to facilitate literature reviews. Lists of audiotapes and videotapes of interviews with the theorists and presentations at conferences about nursing theories are given with distribution sources. In addition, strategies for computer-based searches of the nursing theory literature are outlined.

Chapters 1 and 2 should be read before the remainder of the book. Those first two chapters provide the background that facilitates understanding of the place of nursing theories in the structural hierarchy of nursing knowledge, as well as the schema used for the analysis and evaluation of each nursing theory. Chapter 9 may be read at any time. That chapter should be of special interest to researchers and clinical nurse specialists who are interested in diverse approaches to testing grand and middle-range nursing theories.

The writing of this book was a challenging experience that greatly enhanced my understanding of the major contemporary nursing theories. Its preparation is due to many people. First and foremost, I acknowledge Madeleine Leininger, Margaret Newman, Ida Jean Orlando, Rosemarie Parse, Hildegard Peplau, and Jean Watson. Their pioneering efforts to explicate and refine the theoretical base for the discipline of nursing made this volume possible. My conversations with them have broadened my appreciation of their hard work in overcoming the many obstacles that slowed the integration of their theories into the mainstream of nursing knowledge.

I am deeply indebted to Marie-Christine Bournaki, who provided invaluable assistance with the preparation of the annotated bibliographies. I am also indebted to my students and colleagues for the many citations of relevant publications they have shared with me. Special recognition is given to Elizabeth Hobdell, who has given me copies of theory-based publications from pediatric nursing journals for several years.

The questions about nursing knowledge raised by my colleagues and students at the University of Pennsylvania have stimulated and challenged me to refine and clarify my ideas. I have also been stimulated and challenged by the questions raised by students and faculty at the schools where I have held visiting professorships, including the University of San Diego, Vanderbilt University, the University of Alabama at Birmingham, Loyola University of Chicago, and Case Western Reserve University.

I am especially grateful to my husband, John S. Fawcett, for the love, support, and understanding he has continuously offered, no matter how distracted I have been by my writing. I am also grateful to Captains Linda J. and Douglas K. Lee, as well as Clara E. Lee and Rachel M. Lee, of the schooner *Heritage*, for the relaxed sailing along the coast of Maine and time away from telephones and mail that contributed to the completion of this book.

I also acknowledge the encouragement given to me by Robert G. Martone, Alan Sorkowitz, and Ruth De George of F. A. Davis Company. Finally, I acknowledge all the people who contributed to the production of this edition, especially Herbert J. Powell, Jr.

Jacqueline Fawcett

Credits

Quotations from Peplau, H. E. (1992) were excerpted from Interpersonal relations: A theoretical framework for application in nursing practice. *Nursing Science Quarterly, 5,* 13–18. Copyright by Chestnut House Publications. Reprinted by permission.

Quotations from Watson, J., *Nursing: Human science and human care. A theory of nursing* were excerpted with permission from the National League for Nursing. Copyright 1988 by the National League for Nursing.

Contents

The Structure of Contemporary Nursing Knowledge_____

This chapter sets the stage for the remainder of the book. Here the components of contemporary nursing knowledge are identified, defined, and placed in a structural hierarchy. In this chapter, the emphasis is on the distinctions in level of abstraction of the components of the hierarchy, including the metaparadigm of nursing, philosophies of nursing, conceptual models of nursing, nursing theories, and empirical indicators.

The key terms of the structural hierarchy of nursing knowledge are listed below. Each term is fully defined and described in this chapter.

KEY TERMS _____

Metaparadigm	Nursing Theories
Person	Concepts
Environment	Propositions
Health	Nonrelational
Nursing	Propositions
Philosophies	Existence Propositions
Reaction Worldview	Definitional Propositions
Reciprocal Interaction	Relational Propositions
Worldview	Scope
Simultaneous Action	Grand Theories
Worldview	Middle-Range Theories
Conceptual Models of Nursing	Empirical Indicators

COMPONENTS OF CONTEMPORARY NURSING KNOWLEDGE

Contemporary nursing knowledge encompasses the metaparadigm, multiple philosophies, conceptual models, theories, and empirical indicators. Although the emphasis in this book is on nursing theories, understanding of that component of nursing knowledge is enhanced by consideration of the more abstract metaparadigm, philosophies, and conceptual models of nursing, as well as the more concrete empirical indicators. The five components of contemporary nursing knowledge and their levels of abstraction form a structural hierarchy (Fig. 1–1).

The Metaparadigm of Nursing

The **metaparadigm** is the most abstract component in the structural hierarchy of contemporary nursing knowledge: it is made up of highly abstract concepts that identify the phenomena of interest to the discipline and general propositions that describe the relationships among the phenomena (Kuhn, 1977).

The phenomena of particular interest to the discipline of nursing are represented by four concepts: *person, environment, health,* and *nursing. Person* refers to the recipients of nursing, including individuals, families, communities, and other groups. *Environment* refers to the

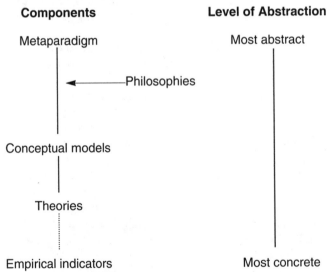

Figure 1–1. The structural hierarchy of contemporary nursing knowledge: components and levels of abstraction.

person's significant others and physical surroundings, as well as to the setting in which nursing occurs. *Health* is the person's state of well-being, which can range from high-level wellness to terminal illness. *Nursing* refers to the definition of nursing, the actions taken by nurses on behalf of or in conjunction with the person, and the goals or outcomes of nursing actions. Nursing actions typically are viewed as a systematic process of assessment, labeling, planning, intervention, and evaluation.

The relationships among the metaparadigm concepts are described in four propositions (Donaldson & Crowley, 1978; Gortner, 1980). The first proposition focuses on the person and health; it states that *the discipline of nursing is concerned with the principles and laws that govern the life-process, well-being, and optimal functioning of human beings, sick or well.*

The second proposition emphasizes the interaction between the person and the environment; it states that *the discipline of nursing is concerned with the patterning of human behavior in interaction with the environment in normal life events and critical life situations.*

The third proposition focuses on health and nursing; it declares that *the discipline of nursing is concerned with the nursing actions or processes by which positive changes in health status are effected.*

The fourth proposition links the person, the environment, and health; it asserts that *the discipline of nursing is concerned with the wholeness or health of human beings, recognizing that they are in continuous interaction with their environments.*

Proposals for Alternative Metaparadigm Concepts and Propositions

The version of the nursing metaparadigm presented above should not be regarded as premature closure on explication of phenomena of interest to the discipline of nursing. Indeed, it is anticipated that modifications in the metaparadigm concepts and propositions will be offered as the discipline of nursing evolves.

One modification that already has been suggested is that the term *client* replace *person* (Newman, 1983). Client, however, reflects a particular view of the person, and, therefore, it should not be used to represent phenomena of interest to the entire discipline of nursing.

Another modification that has been proposed is the elimination of the concept *nursing* from the metaparadigm (Conway, 1985, 1989). Conway claimed that nursing represents the discipline or the profession and is not an appropriate metaparadigm concept because it creates a tautology. Similarly, Meleis (1991) commented, "It would be an instance of tautological conceptualizing to define nursing by all the concepts and then include nursing as one of the concepts" (p. 101). Kolcaba and Kolcaba (1991), however, rejected the charge of tautology. They noted that inasmuch as the metaparadigm concept *nursing* stands for *nursing activities* or *nursing actions*, a tautology is not created.

Conway (1985) did not offer a substitute metaparadigm concept for nursing. In contrast, Meleis (1991) offered two central concepts within the overall domain of nursing knowledge as substitutes. She maintained that the concept *nursing process* focuses on and provides the purpose for interactions between the nurse and the patient. Moreover, she regarded the concept *nursing therapeutics* as the actions the nurse uses to enhance, bring about, or facilitate health. Although Meleis's proposal has merit in that it further specifies nursing, the inclusion of the two concepts creates an unnecessary redundancy at the metaparadigm level.

Other scholars view nursing as a distinct phenomenon of interest to the discipline. Kim (1987) identified nursing as a component of two domains of nursing knowledge. She regarded nursing as the central feature of the practice domain and as an essential component of the client-nurse domain. In addition, Barnum (1990) identified nursing acts as a commonplace, that is, a topic addressed by most nursing theories. Finally, King (1984) found that nursing was a central concept in the philosophies of nursing education of several nursing education programs. This finding suggests that the concept *nursing* is a discipline-wide phenomenon.

A potential modification in the metaparadigm is the exclusion of the concept *environment*. Barnum (1990) did not include environment in her list of nursing commonplaces. She did, however, point out that "a complete theory of nursing is one that contains context, content, and process [and that] context is the environment in which the nursing act takes place" (p. 59). Thus, Barnum's view of environment as a metaparadigm concept is unclear.

Another potential modification in the metaparadigm is the exclusion of the concept *health*. Kim (1987) identified four domains of nursing knowledge. The client domain is concerned with the client's development, problems, and health care experiences. The client-nurse domain focuses on encounters between client and nurse and the interactions between the two in the process of providing nursing care. The practice domain emphasizes the cognitive, behavioral, and social aspects of nurses' professional actions. The environment domain includes the time, space, and quality variations of the client's environment.

Hinshaw (1987) pointed out that Kim's work does not include the concept *health* and asked: "Is health a strand that permeates each of the ... domains ... rather than a major separate domain?" (p. 112). Kim (personal communication, October 31, 1986) has indicated that the client domain could encompass health.

Three other suggested modifications in the version of the metaparadigm presented in this chapter are more radical than rewording, adding to, or eliminating a concept. One proposal calls for a new metaparadigm proposition that would replace the four propositions given earlier in this chapter. Newman, Sime, and Corcoran-Perry (1991) claimed that the focus of the discipline of nursing is summarized in the following statement: "Nursing is the study of caring in the human health experience" (p. 3). In a later publication, they asserted that "the theme of caring is sufficiently dominant, when combined with the theme of the human health experience, to be considered as the focus of the discipline" (Newman, Sime, & Corcoran-Perry, 1992, p. vii).

Despite those authors' claims to the contrary, their proposition represents just one frame of reference for nursing and for health. In fact, Newman and her colleagues (1991) ended their initial treatise by maintaining that caring in the human health experience can be most fully elaborated only through a unitary-transformative perspective.

Moreover, although the authors offered their proposition as a single statement that integrates "concepts commonly identified with nursing at the metaparadigm level" (p. 3), and although they identified the metaparadigm concepts as person, environment, health, and nursing, their proposition does not include environment. In an attempt to clarify their position, Newman, Sime, and Corcoran-Perry (1992) later stated, "we view the concept of environment as inherent in and inseparable from the integrated focus of caring in the human health experience" (p. vii).

Another proposal comes from Malloch, Martinez, Nelson, Predeger, Speakman, Steinbinder, and Tracy (1992), who are doctoral students at the University of Colorado School of Nursing. They suggested a revision of the Newman, Sime, and Corcoran-Perry (1991) statement. Their focus statement is: "Nursing is the study and practice of caring within contexts of the human health experience" (p. vi). Malloch and her colleagues maintained that their statement extends the focus of the discipline to nursing practice and incorporates the environment by the use of the term "contexts." They noted that environment "includes, but is not limited to, culture, community, and ecology" (p. vi). Moreover, they claimed that the use of the term "caring" brings unity to the metaparadigm concepts of person, environment, health, and nursing. Apparently, they do not regard caring as a particular perspective of nursing.

Still another proposal calls for the elimination of the four metaparadigm concepts and propositions and the substitution of the concepts *human care*, *environmental contexts*, and *well-being (health)* and a proposition asserting the centrality of caring to the discipline of nursing. Leininger (1990) claimed that "human care/caring [is] the central phenomenon and essence of nursing" (p. 19) and Watson (1990) maintained that "human caring needs to be explicitly incorporated into nursing's metaparadigm" (p. 21). Even more to the point, Leininger (1991a) maintained that "Care is the essence of nursing and the central, dominant, and unifying focus of nursing" (p. 35). On the basis of that position, Leininger (1988, 1991c) rejected the nursing metaparadigm concepts of person and nursing. She commented,

> The author rejects the idea that nursing and person explain nursing, for one cannot explain nor predict the same phenomenon one is studying. Nursing is the phenomenon to be explained. Moreover, person, per se, is not sufficient to explain nursing as it fails to account for groups, families, social institutions, and cultures. (1988, p. 154)

> The concepts of person and nursing are quite inappropriate. Person is far too limited and nursing cannot be logically used to explain and predict nursing. The latter is a redundancy and a contradiction to explain the same phenomenon being studied by the same concept. (1991c, p. 152)

In another publication, Leininger (1991a) continued to reject the metaparadigm concept of person, and she apparently rejected environment and health as well. She states,

> From an anthropological and nursing perspective, the use of the term person has serious problems when used transculturally, as many non-Western cultures do not focus on or believe in the concept person, and often there is no linguistic term for person in a culture, family and institutions being more prominent. While environment is very important to nursing, I would contend it is certainly not unique to nursing, and there are very few nurses who have advanced formal study and are prepared to study a large number of different types of environments or ecological niches worldwide. [The metaparadigm] concepts had serious problems except for that of health. Again, as a concept health is not distinct to nursing although nursing plays a major role in health attainment and maintenance—many disciplines have studied health. (pp. 39–40)

In her discussions, Leininger failed to acknowledge that an earlier discussion of the metaparadigm concept person indicated that person can refer to any entity that is a recipient of nursing actions, including individuals, families and other types of groups, communities, and societies (Fawcett, 1984). Furthermore, in her 1991a publication, Leininger did not acknowledge that the point of the inclusion of the concept environment in the metaparadigm is to provide a context for the person, to indicate that the recipient of nursing actions is surrounded by and interacts with other people and the social structure (Fawcett, 1984). In fact, she neither acknowledged her own previously published statement that "Care should be central to [the] nursing metaparadigm and supported by the concepts of health and environmental contexts" (Leininger, 1988, p. 154), nor acknowledged her statement in the same book that "In the very near future, one can predict that the current concepts of person, environment, health, and nursing will no longer be upheld. Instead, human care, environmental contexts, and well-being (or health) will become of major interest to most nurse researchers and new theorists" (Leininger, 1991b, p. 406). Moreover, Leininger has not acknowledged that the inclusion of the concept nursing in the metaparadigm was not to create a tautology, but rather to serve as a single-word symbol of all nursing actions and activities taken on behalf of or in conjunction with the person, family, community, or other entity (Fawcett, 1984).

In addition, both Leininger and Watson failed to acknowledge that although the term caring is included in several conceptualizations of the discipline of nursing (Morse, Solberg, Neander, Bottorff, & Johnson, 1990), it is not a dominant theme in every conceptualization and, therefore, does not represent a discipline-wide viewpoint. In fact, caring reflects a particular view of nursing and a particular kind of nursing (Eriksson, 1989). Moreover, as Swanson (1991) pointed out, although there may be "characteristic behavior patterns that are universal expressions of nurse caring . . . caring is not uniquely a nursing phenomenon" (p. 165).

In sum, Leininger's discussions about the metaparadigm tend to be contradictory, and she fails to acknowledge that her ideas could be readily incorporated into the widely cited metaparadigm concepts person, environment, health, and nursing. More specifically, person already refers to collectives as well as to individuals, environment already is viewed as context, health already refers to a broad spectrum of states that includes well-being, and nursing actions can be viewed as directed toward human care.

Function of the Metaparadigm

The concepts and propositions of a metaparadigm are admittedly extremely global and provide no definitive direction for such activities as research and clinical practice. That is to be expected because the metaparadigm "is the broadest consensus within a discipline. It provides the general parameters of the field and gives scientists a broad orientation from which to work (Hardy, 1978, p. 38). Thus, the function of a metaparadigm is to summarize the intellectual and social missions of a discipline and place a boundary on the subject matter of that discipline (Kim, 1989). By so doing, the metaparadigm of a discipline distinguishes that discipline from others. The metaparadigm of nursing, for example, tells the nurse to focus on "the wholeness or health of humans, recognizing that humans are in continuous interaction with their environments" (Donaldson & Crowley, 1978, p. 119). The metaparadigm of medicine, in contrast, tells the physician to focus on the diagnosis and treatment of diseases.

A metaparadigm, by virtue of its global nature, "acts as an encapsulating unit, or framework, within which the more restricted ... structures develop (Eckberg & Hill, 1979, p. 927). Accordingly, the phenomena identified by nursing's metaparadigm are further developed in the other components of the structural hierarchy of contemporary nursing knowledge.

Philosophies

The **philosophy** is the next component in the structural hierarchy of contemporary nursing knowledge. A philosophy may be defined as a statement of beliefs and values about human beings and their world (Kim, 1989; Seaver & Cartwright, 1977). An example of a philosophical statement is "The individual ... behaves purposefully, not in a sequence of cause and effect" (Roy, 1988, p. 32).

Philosophies encompass ontological claims about the nature of human beings and the goal of the discipline, epistemic claims regarding how knowledge is developed, and ethical claims about what the members of a discipline should do (Salsberry, 1991). Different philosophies, (worldviews), lead to different conceptualizations of the central concepts of a discipline and to different statements about the nature of the relationships among those concepts (Altman & Rogoff, 1987).

As can be seen in Figure 1–1, the philosophy does not follow directly from the metaparadigm of the discipline, nor does it directly precede conceptual models. Rather, the metaparadigm of a discipline identifies the phenomena about which philosophical claims are made. The content and focus of each conceptual model and theory then reflect the philosophical claims. For example, a philosophy may make the claim that all people are equal. This philosophical claim would be reflected in a conceptual model that depicts the nurse and the patient as equal partners in health care (Kershaw, 1990). Furthermore, a philosophy is not empirically testable. It should, however, be defendable (Salsberry, 1991).

Nursing knowledge development is guided by philosophical claims about the nature of human beings and the human-environment relationship. The dominant philosophy is humanism (Gortner, 1990), with an emphasis on "humanistic (moral) values of caring and the promotion of individual welfare and rights" (Fry, 1981, p. 5). A review of existing conceptual models of nursing and nursing theories has revealed that although a humanistic philosophy is evident, elements of four sets of worldviews also can be discerned.

One set of worldviews is the mechanism-organicism dichotomy. The characteristics of those two philosophical approaches to the study of the human-environment relationship were described by Reese and Overton (1970), among others, and they are outlined in Table 1–1. Hall (1981) proposed another set of worldviews that reflects philosophical

TABLE 1–1.   Characteristics of the Organismic and Mechanistic Worldviews

Organicism	*Mechanism*
Metaphor is the living organism.	Metaphor is the machine.
Human beings are active.	Human beings are reactive.
Behavior is probabilistic.	Behavior is a predictable linear chain.
Holism and expansionism are assumed—focus is on wholes.	Elementarism and reductionism are assumed—focus is on parts.
Development is qualitative and quantitative.	Development is quantitative.

Source: From "From a Plethora of Paradigms to Parsimony in World Views" by J. Fawcett, 1993, *Nursing Science Quarterly*, 6, pp. 56–58. Copyright 1993 by Chestnut House Publications. Reprinted by permission.

claims about the nature of change in human beings and the human-environment relationship. The characteristics of those views, which are labeled change and persistence, are given in Table 1–2.

Parse (1987) discussed the features of still another set of philosophical claims, which she called the totality and simultaneity paradigms. The characteristics of those two paradigms are listed in Table 1–3.

TABLE 1–2.   Characteristics of the Change and Persistence Worldviews

Change	*Persistence*
Metaphor is growth.	Metaphor is stability.
Change is inherent and natural.	Stability is natural and normal.
Change is continuous.	Change occurs only for survival.
Intraindividual variance.	Intraindividual invariance.
Progress is valued.	Solidarity is valued.
Realization of potential is emphasized.	Conservation and retrenchment are emphasized.

Source: From "From a Plethora of Paradigms to Parsimony in World Views" by J. Fawcett, 1993, *Nursing Science Quarterly*, 6, pp. 56–58. Copyright 1993 by Chestnut House Publications. Reprinted by permission.

TABLE 1–3.   Characteristics of the Simultaneity and Totality Paradigms

Simultaneity	*Totality*
Human beings are more than and different from the sum of their parts.	Human beings are bio-psycho-social-spiritual organisms.
Human beings are in mutual rhythmical interchange with their environments.	Human beings interact with their environments.
Health is how humans experience personal living, a process of becoming and a set of value priorities.	Human beings strive toward an optimal level of health through manipulation of the environment.

Source: From "From a Plethora of Paradigms to Parsimony in World Views" by J. Fawcett, 1993, *Nursing Science Quarterly*, 6, pp. 56–58. Copyright 1993 by Chestnut House Publications. Reprinted by permission.

Recently, Newman (1992) identified what she claims are the three prevailing paradigms for nursing knowledge development. The characteristics of her three paradigms—the particulate-deterministic, the integrative-interactive, and the unitary-transformative—are summarized in Table 1–4. Newman (1992) explained that "the first of the paired words [in the names of the three paradigms] describes the view of the entity being studied and the second describes the notion of how change occurs" (p. 10).

An analysis of the characteristics of the four sets of worldviews

TABLE 1–4.   Characteristics of the Particulate-Deterministic, Interactive-Integrative, and Unitary-Transformative Paradigms

Particulate-Deterministic	Interactive-Integrative	Unitary-Transformative
Phenomena are isolatable, reducible entities with definable, measurable properties.	Reality is multidimensional and contextual.	Human beings are unitary and evolving as self-organizing fields.
Entities have orderly and predictable connections.	Entities are context-dependent and relative.	Human fields are identified by pattern and by interaction with the larger whole.
Change occurs as a consequence of antecedent conditions that can be predicted and controlled.	Change is a function of multiple antecedent factors and probabilistic relationships.	Change is unidirectional and unpredictable.
Relationships are linear and causal.	Moves away from linearity and addresses reciprocal relationships.	Systems move through stages of organization and disorganization to more complex organization.
Only objective, observable phenomena are studied.	Both objective and subjective phenomena are studied, with emphasis on objectivity, control, and predictability.	Emphasis is on personal knowledge and pattern recognition.

Source: From "From a Plethora of Paradigms to Parsimony in World Views" by J. Fawcett, 1993, *Nursing Science Quarterly, 6,* pp. 56–58. Copyright 1993 by Chestnut House Publications. Reprinted by permission.

TABLE 1–5.   The Reaction Worldview

Humans are bio-psycho-social-spiritual beings.
Human beings react to external environmental stimuli in a linear, causal
 manner.
Change occurs only for survival and as a consequence of predictable and
 controllable antecedent conditions.
Only objective phenomena that can be isolated, defined, observed, and
 measured are studied.

Source: From "From a Plethora of Paradigms to Parsimony in World Views" by J. Fawcett,
1993, *Nursing Science Quarterly, 6,* pp. 56–58. Copyright 1993 by Chestnut House Publications. Reprinted by permission.

revealed some similarities and yielded a single parsimonious set of
three worldviews: *reaction, reciprocal interaction,* and *simultaneous
action* (Fawcett, 1993). More specifically, the analysis revealed that the
particulate-deterministic paradigm is similar to mechanism, persistence, and totality. The combination of characteristics from those perspectives yielded the reaction worldview (Table 1–5).

Furthermore, the analysis indicated that the interactive-integrative paradigm is similar to organicism and reflects some elements of
simultaneity and some elements of totality. In addition, that paradigm
can incorporate elements of both change and persistence. Taken
together, those perspectives yielded the reciprocal interaction worldview (Table 1–6).

Finally, the analysis suggested that the unitary-transformative paradigm is similar to organicism but even more similar to simultaneity. In
addition, the elements of change are most evident in that paradigm.
Combining the characteristics of those perspectives resulted in the
simultaneous action worldview (Table 1–7).

TABLE 1–6.   The Reciprocal Interaction Worldview

Human beings are holistic.
Parts are viewed only in the context of the whole.

Human beings are active.
Interactions between human beings and their environments are reciprocal.

Reality is multidimensional, context-dependent, and relative.

Change is a function of multiple antecedent factors.
Change is probabilistic and may be continuous or may be only for survival.

Both objective and subjective phenomena are studied through quantitative
 and qualitative methods of inquiry.
Emphasis is placed on empirical observations, methodological controls, and
 inferential data analytic techniques.

Source: From "From a Plethora of Paradigms to Parsimony in World Views" by J. Fawcett,
1993, *Nursing Science Quarterly, 6,* pp. 56–58. Copyright 1993 by Chestnut House Publications. Reprinted by permission.

TABLE 1–7.   The Simultaneous Action Worldview

Unitary human beings are identified by pattern.

Human beings are in mutual rhythmical interchange with their environments.

Human beings change continuously and evolve as self-organized fields. Change is unidirectional and unpredictable as human beings move through stages of organization and disorganization to more complex organization.

Phenomena of interest are personal knowledge and pattern recognition.

Source: From "From a Plethora of Paradigms to Parsimony in World Views" by J. Fawcett, 1993, *Nursing Science Quarterly, 6,* pp. 56–58. Copyright 1993 by Chestnut House Publications. Reprinted by permission.

Conceptual Models of Nursing

The **conceptual model** is the third component in the structural hierarchy of contemporary nursing knowledge. Conceptual models, which are also called conceptual frameworks, conceptual systems, paradigms, and disciplinary matrices, are less abstract than metaparadigms but more abstract than theories.

Conceptual models are made up of concepts and propositions. The concepts of a conceptual model are quite abstract and general. Thus, they are not directly observed in the real world, nor are they limited to any specific individual, group, situation, or event. Client system stability is an example of a conceptual model concept (Neuman, 1989). It can refer to various types of systems, including individuals, families, and communities, that encounter many different situations and events.

The propositions that describe or link conceptual model concepts also are quite abstract and general; therefore, they are not amenable to direct empirical observation or test. Some propositions are general descriptions or definitions of the conceptual model concepts. Lines of defense, for example, are described as barriers to stressors (Neuman, 1989). Because conceptual model concepts are so abstract, not all of them are defined, and those that are defined typically have broad definitions. Definitional propositions for conceptual model concepts, therefore, do not state how the concepts are empirically observed or measured, and they should not be expected to do so. Indeed, conceptual models have been described as "clusters of interre*lated* but not necessarily inter*defined* concepts" (Hill & Hanson, 1960, p. 300). [Emphasis added.]

Other propositions state the relationships among conceptual model concepts in a general manner. They are exemplified by the following statement: "[The focal, contextual, and residual] stimuli determine a range of coping for the person" (Roy & Andrews, 1991, p. 11).

The conceptual models of a discipline provide different perspectives or frames of reference for the phenomena identified by the metaparadigm of that discipline. As Kuhn (1970) explained, although adherents of different models are looking at the same phenomena, "in some areas they see different things, and they see them in different relations to one another" (p. 150). Different perspectives of the phenomena identified by the nursing metaparadigm (person, environment, health, nursing) are evident in the major conceptual models of nursing, including Johnson's (1990) Behavioral System Model, King's (1990) Interacting Systems Framework, Levine's (1991) Conservation Model, Neuman's (1989) Systems Model, Orem's (1991) Self-Care Framework, Rogers's (1990) Science of Unitary Human Beings, and Roy's (Roy & Andrews, 1991) Adaptation Model. An overview of the content of each of those nursing models is given in Table 1–8. More detailed accounts of the models are available in the original works by their authors, as well as in the text *Analysis and Evaluation of Conceptual Models of Nursing* (Fawcett, 1989).

Examination of the content of various conceptual models reveals that each model reflects the philosophical stance, cognitive orientation, research tradition, and practice modalities of a particular group of scholars within a discipline, rather than the beliefs, values, thoughts, research methods, and approaches to practice of all members of that discipline. In fact, although a consensus about relevant phenomena is reflected in the single metaparadigm of each discipline, diversity is evident in multiple conceptual models (Fig. 1–2).

The abstract and general nature of the content of a conceptual model precludes definitive directives for practical activities. Each conceptual model does, however, include general guidelines or rules for research, clinical practice, education, and administration. For example, the rules for research identify the following: The phenomena that are to be studied; the distinctive nature of the problems to be studied and the purposes to be fulfilled by the research; subjects who are to provide the data and the settings in which data are to be gathered; the research designs, instruments, and procedures that are to be employed; the methods to be employed in reducing and analyzing the data; and the nature of contributions that the research will make to the advancement of knowledge (Laudan, 1981; Schlotfeldt, 1975).

Research is the vehicle for theory development. Thus, the rules for research that are associated with a conceptual model function as guidelines for the generation and testing of nursing theories, which are the next component of contemporary nursing knowledge.

Nursing Theories

The fourth component in the structural hierarchy of contemporary nursing knowledge is the **theory**. Theories are less abstract than conceptual models but more abstract than empirical indicators.

The *concepts* of a theory are more specific and concrete than those

TABLE 1–8.   Overviews of Seven Conceptual Models of Nursing

Conceptual Model	Person	Environment	Health	Nursing
Johnson's Behavioral System Model	A behavioral system with seven subsystems: Attachment Dependency Ingestion Elimination Sexual Aggression Achievement	Internal External	Behavioral system balance and stability. Efficient and effective behavioral functioning. Purposeful, orderly, and predictable behavior	Definition: A service that is complementary to that of medicine and other health professions but which makes its own distinctive contribution to the health and well-being of people Goal: Restore, maintain, or attain behavioral system balance and stability Actions: Impose external regulatory or control mechanisms. Alter set or add choices for behavior. Provide protection, nurturance, or stimulation
King's Interacting Systems Framework	Personal system: Focus on perception, self, growth and development, body image, time, space, learning	Internal External	Dynamic life experiences of a human being. Ability to function in social roles	Definition: Perceiving, thinking, relating, judging, and acting vis-a-vis the behavior of individuals who come to a nursing situation

Model				
	Interpersonal system: Focus on interaction, communication, transaction, role, stress, coping Social system: Focus on organization, authority, power, status, decision making, control			*Goal:* Help individuals maintain their health so they can function in their roles *Actions:* A process of action, reaction, interaction, and transaction directed toward establishment of goals and goal attainment
Levine's Conservation Model	A holistic being, a system of systems. Organismic responses are fight or flight, stress, basic orienting system, visual system, auditory system, haptic system, taste-smell system	Operational Perceptual Conceptual	Health and disease are patterns of adaptive change	*Definition:* A human interaction *Goal:* Promotion of wholeness for people, sick or well *Actions:* Conservation of energy, structural integrity, social integrity, personal integrity
Neuman's Systems Model	A client system composed of five variables: Physiological Psychological Sociocultural	Internal External Created	Client system stability	*Definition:* A unique profession that is concerned with all the variables affecting an individual's response to stressors

TABLE 1-8. Overviews of Seven Conceptual Models of Nursing (Continued)

Conceptual Model	Person	Environment	Health	Nursing
Neuman's Systems Model	Developmental Spiritual Central core surrounded by flexible and normal lines of defense and lines of resistance			Goal: To facilitate optimal wellness through retention, attainment, or maintenance of client system stability Actions: Primary prevention Secondary prevention Tertiary prevention
Orem's Self-Care Framework	Self-care agent Therapeutic self-care demand made up of: Universal self-care requisites Developmental self-care requisites Health deviation self-care requisites	The person's external surroundings	Soundness or wholeness of developed human structures and of bodily and mental functioning	Definition: A helping service, a creative effort to help people Goal: Help people to meet their own therapeutic self-care demands Actions: Wholly compensatory, partly compensatory, and supportive-educative nursing systems. Assist by acting for or doing, guiding, physical and/or psychological support, providing a developmental environment, teaching

	Person	Environment	Health	Nursing
Rogers's Science of Unitary Human Beings	A unitary human being, a patterned, open, pandimensional energy field	A patterned, open, pandimensional energy field	An expression of the life process	*Definition:* A learned profession that is both a science and an art *Goal:* Help people achieve maximum well-being *Actions:* Deliberative mutual patterning that involves environmental patterning to promote helicy, integrality, and resonancy
Roy's Adaptation Model	An adaptive system with four response modes: Physiological Self-Concept Role Function Interdependence Regulator and cognator coping mechanisms	Focal stimuli Contextual stimuli Residual stimuli	Being and becoming an integrated and whole person	*Definition:* A theoretical system of knowledge that prescribes a process of analysis and action related to care of the ill or potentially ill person *Goal:* Promotion of adaptation *Actions:* Management of environmental stimuli, including increasing, decreasing, maintaining, removing, altering, or changing

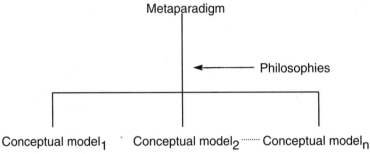

Figure 1-2. Single metaparadigm and multiple conceptual models.

of a conceptual model. They are, therefore, closely tied to particular individuals, groups, situations, or events. Examples of theory concepts are oxygen tension, Type A behavior, social support, health-related hardiness, and functional status.

The *propositions* of a theory also are more specific than those of a conceptual model. *Nonrelational propositions* define or describe the concepts of a theory. One type of nonrelational proposition states the *existence* of a concept. An example is: there is a phenomenon known as health-related hardiness (Pollock & Duffy, 1990). Another type of nonrelational proposition is the definition. *Definitional propositions* are required for all theory concepts. Indeed, although the concepts of a conceptual model may be only broadly defined, the concepts of a theory must be constitutively defined. Constitutive definitions, which are also called theoretical definitions, provide meanings for concepts by defining the concepts in terms of other concepts; they are circular in nature. An example of a constitutive definition is: health-related hardiness is defined as attitudes toward control, commitment, and challenge that buffer the negative effects of health stressors (Pollock & Duffy, 1990).

Empirical testing of a theory requires that its concepts be operationally defined. Operational definitions specify the way in which the concept is to be observed or measured; therefore, they connect constitutively defined concepts to the real world. An example of an operational definition is: health-related hardiness is measured by the Health-Related Hardiness Scale (Pollock & Duffy, 1990).

Relational propositions link two or more concepts; they express an association between concepts or identify the effect of one concept on another. An example of a relational proposition is: health-related hardiness is positively related to physiological adaptation (Pollock, Christian, & Sands, 1990).

Relational propositions can assert various characteristics of the association between concepts. Some of those characteristics are the existence of a relationship, the sign of the relationship (positive or negative); the shape of the relationship (linear, curvilinear); the strength or magnitude of the relationship (small, moderate, large); the symmetry of the relationship (asymmetrical or unidirectional, symmetrical or reciprocal); and the time sequence of the occurrence of the concepts in the relationship (concurrent or sequential) (Fawcett & Downs, 1992).

Scope of a Theory

Although theories address relatively specific and concrete phenomena, they do vary in *scope*. Scope refers to the relative level of substantive specificity of a theory and the concreteness of its concepts and propositions.

Theories that are broadest in scope are called *grand theories*. They are substantively nonspecific, being made up of relatively abstract concepts that lack operational definitions and relatively abstract propositions that are not amenable to direct empirical generation or testing. Indeed, grand theories rarely are developed by means of empirical research; rather, they are developed through thoughtful and insightful appraisal of existing ideas or creative leaps beyond existing knowledge. An example of a grand nursing theory is Newman's (1986) Theory of Health as Expanding Consciousness; it is described in detail in Chapter 4.

Theories that are more circumscribed are called *middle-range theories*. They are substantively specific, encompassing a limited number of concepts and a limited aspect of the real world. They are made up of relatively concrete concepts that are operationally defined and relatively concrete propositions that can be empirically generated or tested in a direct manner.

A middle-range theory may be a description of a particular phenomenon, an explanation of the relations between phenomena, or a prediction of the effects of one phenomenon on another. Descriptive theories describe or name specific characteristics of individuals, groups, situations, or events by summarizing the commonalities found in discrete observations into one or more concepts and their associated subconcepts or dimensions. They are generated and tested by descriptive research. For example, Aroian (1990) conducted a study to generate a descriptive naming theory of psychological adaptation to migration and resettlement. She identified six central categories or dimensions of the migration and resettlement process: loss and disruption, novelty, occupation, language, subordination, and feeling at home.

Descriptive theories may also include classification of several concepts or the dimensions of a single concept. The classification schema, which frequently is referred to as a typology or taxonomy, may propose mutually exclusive, overlapping, hierarchical, or sequential dimensions. An example of a descriptive classification theory is the taxonomy of nursing diagnoses developed by the members of the North American Nursing Diagnosis Association (Carroll-Johnston, 1988). Nine human response patterns (choosing, communicating, exchanging, feeling, knowing, moving, perceiving, relating, and valuing) are regarded as mutually exclusive categories in which the named dimensions—the actual nursing diagnoses—are classified. The human response pattern of choosing, for example, encompasses the dimensions of Family Coping, impaired; Health-Seeking Behavior; and Individual Coping, impaired.

Explanatory theories specify relationships between two or more concepts. They are developed by correlational research. One example of an explanatory theory is the theory of adaptation to chronic illness (Pollock, 1986). Pollock used correlational procedures to test relationships between health-related hardiness and physiological and psychological adaptation. Another example is Aaronson and Macnee's (1989) theory of the relationship between balanced nutrition and weight gain during pregnancy, which was also tested by means of correlational procedures.

Predictive theories move beyond explanation to the prediction of precise relationships between two or more concepts or the prediction of differences between groups. Experimental research is used to generate and test predictive theories. For example, Holtzclaw (1990) designed an experimental study to test a theory of the effects of extremity wraps on amphotericin B–induced febrile shivering.

Conceptual Models and Theories

Conceptual models influence theory development. More specifically, each conceptual model provides

> a focus which directs the questions one asks and the theories one proposes and subsequently tests. It provides a network within which questions, theories, and data fit together and makes possible the identification of needed areas of theory development. (Newman, 1979, p. 6)

Conceptual models act as guides for theory development, then, by focusing attention on certain concepts and their relationships, they place the concepts and their relationships in a distinctive context. For example, Johnson's Behavioral System Model emphasizes the person's behavior, King's Interacting Systems Framework focuses on attainment of goals, Levine's Conservation Model requires consideration of conservation of energy and integrity of the human being, Neuman's Systems Model highlights client system stability, Orem's Self-Care Framework emphasizes self-care abilities, Rogers's Science of Unitary Human Beings draws attention to the unity of human life, and Roy's Adaptation

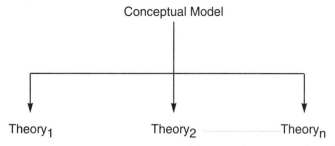

Figure 1–3. Multiple theories derived from each conceptual model.

Model focuses on the individual's ability to adapt to a constantly changing environment.

As can be seen in Figure 1–3, several theories are required to fully describe, explain, and predict all of the phenomena encompassed by a conceptual model. That is because any one theory deals with only a portion of the domain of inquiry identified by a model. Each theory is, therefore, more circumscribed than its parent conceptual model.

Both grand and middle-range theories may be derived directly from a conceptual model. Middle-range theories may also be derived from a grand theory, which previously was derived from a conceptual model (Fig. 1–4).

An example of middle-range theory derivation from a conceptual model and a grand theory is Alligood's (1991) theory of the relationships among creativity, actualization, and empathy in persons 18 to 92 years of age. That middle-range theory was derived from the grand theory of accelerating change, which was previously derived from Rogers's Science of Unitary Human Beings (Fig. 1–5).

An example of a middle-range theory that was derived directly from a conceptual model is the theory of functional status following

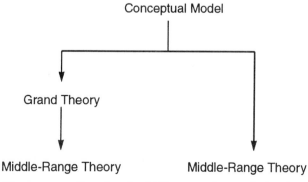

Figure 1–4. Grand and middle-range theory derivation.

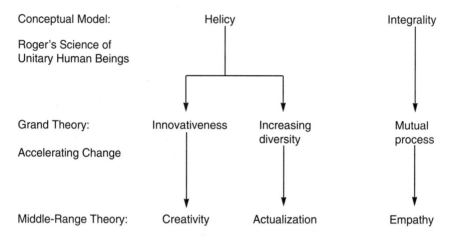

Figure 1–5.   Derivation of grand and middle-range theories from a conceptual model: the theory of creativity, actualization, and empathy. (Adapted from "Testing Rogers' Theory of Accelerating Change: The Relationships among Creativity, Actualization, and Empathy in Persons 18 to 92 years of age" by M. R. Alligood, 1991, *Western Journal of Nursing Research, 13,* p. 85. Copyright 1991 by Sage Publications, Inc. Adapted by permission.)

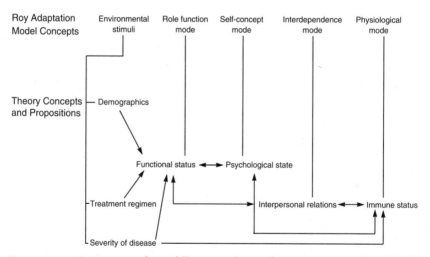

Figure 1–6.   Derivation of a middle-range theory from a conceptual model: the theory of functional status following diagnosis of breast cancer. (Adapted from "A Framework for Studying Functional Status after Diagnosis of Breast Cancer" by L. Tulman and J. Fawcett, 1990, *Cancer Nursing, 13,* p. 98. Copyright 1990 by Raven Press. Adapted by permission.)

diagnosis of breast cancer (Tulman & Fawcett, 1990). As can be seen in Figure 1–6, the theory was derived directly from concepts of the Roy Adaptation Model. The theory proposes that the functional status of women with breast cancer is influenced by psychological state, interpersonal relationships, immune status, treatment regimen, severity of disease, and demographic factors.

Empirical Indicators

The generation and testing of middle-range theories is accomplished through the use of **empirical indicators,** which are the fifth and final component in the structural hierarchy of contemporary nursing knowledge. As illustrated in Figure 1–7, empirical indicators are the very specific and concrete real-world proxies for middle-range theory concepts. More specifically, they are the actual instruments, experimental conditions, and procedures that are used to observe or measure the concepts of a middle-range theory. For example, the Health-Related Hardiness Scale (Pollock & Duffy, 1990) is the instrument that serves as the empirical indicator for the concept of health-related hardiness in the theory of adaptation to chronic illness. Similarly, the experimental condition of applying terry cloth towels to each extremity is an empirical indicator in Holtzclaw's (1990) shivering theory.

Empirical indicators are identified in operational definitions. Conjectures about empirical indicators are stated in a special type of proposition called the hypothesis. More specifically, a hypothesis is a prediction about the scores obtained from the empirical indicators. Suppose, for example, that a proposition states that health-related hardiness is positively related to psychological adaptation, that health-related hardiness is measured by the Health-Related Hardiness Scale, and that psychological adaptation is measured by the Mental Health Index (Pollock, Christian, & Sands, 1990). The hypothesis would state: as scores on the Health-Related Hardiness Scale increase, scores on the Mental Health Index will increase.

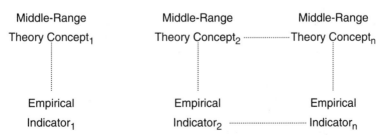

Figure 1–7. Middle-range theory concepts and their empirical indicators.

NOTES ON TERMINOLOGY

Some nurse authors do not make distinctions between conceptual models and theories (e.g., Fitzpatrick & Whall, 1989; George, 1990; Marriner-Tomey, 1989; Meleis, 1991; Riehl-Sisca, 1989). Apparently, they either do not recognize the difference between the two components of nursing knowledge or they regard the distinction as a semantic point. In contrast, the position taken in this book is that there is a discernible difference in the level of abstraction of conceptual models and theories and that that difference mandates regarding them as separate structures. The position is in keeping with earlier works by Rogers (1970) and Reilly (1975) in nursing, Reese and Overton (1970) in developmental psychology, and Nye and Berardo (1966) in sociology, all of which clearly point out the difference in level of abstraction between conceptual models and theories.

Furthermore, other authors consider conceptual models and grand theories to be synonymous (e.g., Barnum, 1990; Kim, 1983). Although it is recognized that the line between a conceptual model and a grand theory can be difficult to discern without a detailed analysis of the formulation, it is more accurate to separate the two. The distinction between a conceptual model and a grand theory is illustrated by Rogers's conceptual model of nursing and Newman's grand theory. Newman (1986) noted that her theory of health "is grounded in my own personal experience but stimulated by Martha Rogers's insistence on the unitary nature of a human being in interaction with the environment (Rogers, 1970)," (p. 4). Rogers's conceptual model provides a frame of reference for all four concepts of the nursing metaparadigm (person, environment, health, nursing), whereas Newman's grand theory emphasizes the concept of health. This example illustrates the fact that although a grand theory is quite abstract, it still is more circumscribed than a conceptual model.

CONCLUSION

This chapter presents an overview of the structural hierarchy of contemporary nursing knowledge. In summary, a metaparadigm is the most abstract component of the hierarchy; it identifies the phenomena of interest to the discipline. A philosophy, which is the next component of the hierarchy, is a statement of beliefs and values about the phenomena identified by the metaparadigm. A conceptual model, which is a set of interrelated abstract and general concepts and propositions, is the third component of the hierarchy. A theory, which is a set of relatively specific and concrete concepts and propositions that characterizes a relatively circumscribed phenomenon, is the fourth component. Finally, an empirical indicator, which is the real-world referent for a concept, is the most concrete component of the hierarchy. In this book, emphasis is placed on grand and middle-range nursing theories.

REFERENCES

Aaronson, L. S., & Macnee, C. L. (1989). The relationship between weight gain and nutrition in pregnancy. *Nursing Research, 38,* 223–227.

Alligood, M. R. (1991). Testing Rogers' theory of accelerating change. The relationships among creativity, actualization, and empathy in persons 18 to 92 years of age. *Western Journal of Nursing Research, 13,* 84–96.

Altman, I., & Rogoff, B. (1987). World views in psychology: Trait, interactional, organismic, and transactional perspectives. In D. Stokols & I. Altman (Eds.), *Handbook of environmental psychology* (pp. 7–40). New York: John Wiley & Sons.

Aroian, K. J. (1990). A model of psychological adaptation to migration and resettlement. *Nursing Research, 39,* 5–10.

Barnum, B. J. S. (1990). *Nursing theory: Analysis, application, evaluation* (3rd ed.). Glenview, IL: Scott, Foresman/Little, Brown Higher Education.

Carroll-Johnston, R. M. (Ed.). (1988). *Classification of nursing diagnoses. Proceedings of the Eighth Conference, North American Nursing Diagnosis Association.* Philadelphia: J. B. Lippincott.

Conway, M. E. (1985). Toward greater specificity in defining nursing's metaparadigm. *Advances in Nursing Science, 7*(4), 73–81.

Conway, M. E. (1989, April). *Nursing's metaparadigm: Current perspectives.* Paper presented at the Spring Doctoral Forum, Medical College of Georgia School of Nursing, Augusta.

Donaldson, S. K., & Crowley, D. M. (1978). The discipline of nursing. *Nursing Outlook, 26,* 113–120.

Eckberg, D. L., & Hill, L., Jr. (1979). The paradigm concept and sociology: A critical review. *American Sociological Review, 44,* 925–937.

Eriksson, K. (1989). Caring paradigms: A study of the origins and the development of caring paradigms among nursing students. *Scandinavian Journal of Caring Sciences, 3,* 169–176.

Fawcett, J. (1984). *Analysis and evaluation of conceptual models of nursing.* Philadelphia: F.A. Davis.

Fawcett, J. (1989). *Analysis and evaluation of conceptual models of nursing* (2nd ed.). Philadelphia: F.A. Davis.

Fawcett, J. (1993). From a plethora of paradigms to parsimony in world views. *Nursing Science Quarterly, 6,* 56–58.

Fawcett, J., & Downs, F. S. (1992). *The relationship of theory and research* (2nd ed.). Philadelphia: F.A. Davis.

Fitzpatrick, J. J., & Whall, A. L. (1989). *Conceptual models of nursing: Analysis and application* (2nd ed.). Norwalk, CT: Appleton and Lange.

Fry, S. (1981). Accountability in research: The relationship of scientific and humanistic values. *Advances in Nursing Science, 4*(1), 1–13.

George, J. B. (Ed.). (1990). *Nursing theories: The base for professional nursing practice* (3rd ed.). Norwalk, CT: Appleton and Lange.

Gortner, S. R. (1980). Nursing science in transition. *Nursing Research, 29,* 180–183.

Gortner, S. R. (1990). Nursing values and science: Toward a science philosophy. *Image: Journal of Nursing Scholarship, 22,* 101–105.

Hall, B. A. (1981). The change paradigm in nursing: Growth versus persistence. *Advances in Nursing Science, 3*(4), 1–6.

Hardy, M. E. (1978). Perspectives on nursing theory. *Advances in Nursing Science, 1*(1), 37–48.

Hill, R., & Hanson, D. A. (1960). The identification of conceptual frameworks utilized in family study. *Marriage and Family Living, 22,* 299–311.

Hinshaw, A. S. (1987). Response to "Structuring the nursing knowledge system: A typology of four domains." *Scholarly Inquiry for Nursing Practice, 1*, 111–114.

Holtzclaw, B. J. (1990). Effects of extremity wraps to control drug-induced shivering: A pilot study. *Nursing Research, 39*, 280–283.

Johnson, D. E. (1990). The behavioral system model for nursing. In M. E. Parker (Ed.), *Nursing theories in practice* (pp. 23–32). New York: National League for Nursing.

Kershaw, B. (1990). Nursing models as philosophies of care. *NursingPractice, 4*(1), 25–27.

Kim, H. S. (1983). *The nature of theoretical thinking in nursing.* Norwalk, CT: Appleton-Century-Crofts.

Kim, H. S. (1987). Structuring the nursing knowledge system: A typology of four domains. *Scholarly Inquiry for Nursing Practice, 1*, 99–110.

Kim, H. S. (1989). Theoretical thinking in nursing: Problems and prospects. *Recent Advances in Nursing, 24*, 106–122.

King, I. M. (1984). Philosophy of nursing education: A national survey. *Western Journal of Nursing Research, 6*, 387–406.

King, I. M. (1990). King's conceptual framework and theory of goal attainment. In M. E. Parker (Ed.), *Nursing theories in practice* (pp. 73–84). New York: National League for Nursing.

Kolcaba, K. Y., & Kolcaba, R. J. (1991). *In defense of the metaparadigm for nursing.* Unpublished manuscript.

Kuhn, T. S. (1970). *The structure of scientific revolutions* (2nd ed.). Chicago: University of Chicago Press.

Kuhn, T. S. (1977). Second thoughts on paradigms. In F. Suppe (Ed.), *The structure of scientific theories* (2nd ed., pp. 459–517). Chicago: University of Illinois Press.

Laudan, L. (1981). A problem-solving approach to scientific progress. In I. Hacking (Ed.), *Scientific revolutions* (pp. 144–155). Fair Lawn, NJ: Oxford University Press.

Leininger, M. M. (1988). Leininger's theory of nursing: Cultural care diversity and universality. *Nursing Science Quarterly, 1*, 152–160.

Leininger, M. M. (1990). Historic and epistemologic dimensions of care and caring with future directions. In J. S. Stevenson & T. Tripp-Reimer (Eds.), *Knowledge about care and caring: State of the art and future developments* (pp. 19–31). Kansas City, MO: American Academy of Nursing.

Leininger, M. M. (1991a). The theory of culture care diversity and universality. In M. M. Leininger (Ed.), *Culture care diversity and universality: A theory of nursing* (pp. 5–65). New York: National League for Nursing.

Leininger, M. M. (1991b). Looking to the future of nursing and the relevancy of culture care theory. In M. M. Leininger (Ed.), *Culture care diversity and universality: A theory of nursing* (pp. 391–418). New York: National League for Nursing.

Leininger, M. M. (1991c). Letter to the editor: Reflections on an international theory of nursing. *International Nursing Review, 38*, 152.

Levine, M. E. (1991). The conservation principles: A model for health. In K. M. Schaefer & J. B. Pond (Eds.), *Levine's conservation model: A framework for nursing practice* (pp. 1–11). Philadelphia: F.A. Davis.

Malloch, K., Martinez, R., Nelson, L., Predeger, B., Speakman, L., Steinbinder, A., & Tracy, J. (1992). *To the editor* [Letter] *Advances in Nursing Science, 15*(2), vi–vii.

Marriner-Tomey, A. (1989). *Nursing theorists and their work* (2nd ed.). St. Louis: C.V. Mosby.

Meleis, A. I. (1991). *Theoretical nursing: Development and progress* (2nd ed.). Philadelphia: J.B. Lippincott.

Morse, J. M., Solberg, S. M., Neander, W. L., Bottorff, J. L., & Johnson, J. L. (1990). Concepts of caring and caring as a concept. *Advances in Nursing Science, 13*(1), 1–14.

Neuman, B. (1989). *The Neuman Systems Model* (2nd ed.). Norwalk, CT: Appleton and Lange.

Newman, M. A. (1979). *Theory development in nursing.* Philadelphia: F.A. Davis.

Newman, M. A. (1983). The continuing revolution: A history of nursing science. In N. L. Chaska (Ed.), *The nursing profession: A time to speak* (pp. 385–393). New York: McGraw-Hill.

Newman, M. A. (1986). *Health as expanding consciousness.* St. Louis: C.V. Mosby.

Newman, M. A. (1992). Prevailing paradigms in nursing. *Nursing Outlook, 40*, 10–13, 32.

Newman, M. A., Sime, A. M., & Corcoran-Perry, S. A. (1991). The focus of the discipline of nursing. *Advances in Nursing Science, 14*(1), 1–6.

Newman, M. A., Sime, A. M., & Corcoran-Perry, S. A. (1992). Authors' reply [to Fawcett's Letter to the Editor]. *Advances in Nursing Science, 14*(3), vi–vii.

Nye, F. I., & Berardo, F. N. (Eds.). (1966). *Emerging conceptual frameworks in family analysis.* New York: Macmillan.

Orem, D. E. (1991). *Nursing: Concepts of practice* (4th ed.). St. Louis: Mosby Year Book.

Parse, R. R. (1987). *Nursing science: Major paradigms, theories, and critiques.* Philadelphia: W.B. Saunders.

Pollock, S. E. (1986). Human responses to chronic illness: Physiologic and psychosocial adaptation. *Nursing Research, 35,* 90–95.

Pollock, S. E., Christian, B. J., & Sands, D. (1990). Responses to chronic illness: Analysis of psychological and physiological adaptation. *Nursing Research, 39,* 300–304.

Pollock, S. E. & Duffy, M. E. (1990). The Health-Related Hardiness Scale: Development and psychometric analysis. *Nursing Research, 39,* 218–222.

Reese, H. W., & Overton, W. F. (1970). Models of development and theories of development. In L. R. Goulet & P. B. Baltes (Eds.), *Life span developmental psychology: Research and theory* (pp. 115–145). New York: Academic Press.

Reilly, D. E. (1975). Why a conceptual framework? *Nursing Outlook, 23,* 566–569.

Riehl-Sisca, J. P. (1989). *Conceptual models for nursing practice* (4th ed.). Norwalk, CT: Appleton and Lange.

Rogers, M. E. (1970). *An introduction to the theoretical basis of nursing.* Philadelphia: F.A. Davis.

Rogers, M. E. (1990). Nursing: Science of unitary, irreducible, human beings: Update 1990. In E. A. M. Barrett (Ed.), *Visions of Rogers' science-based nursing* (pp. 5–11). New York: National League for Nursing.

Roy, C. (1988). An explication of the philosophical assumptions of the Roy adaptation model. *Nursing Science Quarterly, 1,* 26–34.

Roy, C., & Andrews, H. A. (1991). *The Roy Adaptation Model: The definitive statement.* Norwalk, CT: Appleton and Lange.

Salsberry, P. (1991, May). *A philosophy of nursing: What is it? What is it not?* Paper presented at the Philosophy in the Nurse's World Conference, Banff, Alberta, Canada.

Schlotfeldt, R. M. (1975). The need for a conceptual framework. In P. J. Verhonick (Ed.), *Nursing Research I* (pp. 3–24). Boston: Little, Brown.

Seaver, J. W., & Cartwright, C. A. (1977). A pluralistic foundation for training early childhood professionals. *Curriculum Inquiry, 7,* 305–329.

Swanson, K. M. (1991). Empirical development of a middle range theory of caring. *Nursing Research, 40,* 161–165.

Tulman, L., & Fawcett, J. (1990). A framework for studying functional status after diagnosis of breast cancer. *Cancer Nursing, 13,* 95–99.

Watson, J. (1990). Caring knowledge and informed moral passion. *Advances in Nursing Science, 13*(1), 15–24.

ANNOTATED BIBLIOGRAPHY

Altman, I., & Rogoff, B. (1987). World views in psychology: Trait, interactional, organismic, and transactional perspectives. In D. Stokols & I. Altman (Eds.), *Handbook of environmental psychology* (pp. 7–40). New York: Wiley.

The authors describe the characteristics of the trait, interactional, organismic, and transactional worldviews. They maintain that worldviews are philosopical approaches that underlie research and theory development.

Barnum, B. J. S. (1990). *Nursing theory: Analysis, application, evaluation* (3rd ed.). Glenview, IL: Scott, Foresman/Little, Brown Higher Education.

Barnum states that the function of the book is to help readers learn to effectively critique nursing theory materials. She uses the following set of commonplaces for theory analysis: nursing acts, the patient, health, the relationship of nursing acts to the patient, the relationship of nursing acts to health, and the relationship of the patient to health. No attempt is made to present a comprehensive discussion or interpretation of contemporary nursing theories, although several theories and conceptual models are used to exemplify various aspects of theory analysis. No clear distinctions are made between conceptual models and theories.

Conway, M. E. (1985). Toward greater specificity in defining nursing's metaparadigm. *Advances in Nursing Science, 7*(4), 73–81.

Conway rejects the inclusion of nursing in the nursing metaparadigm, arguing that to include it creates a tautology. She notes that "nursing" represents the discipline.

Donaldson, S. K., & Crowley, D. M. (1978). The discipline of nursing. *Nursing Outlook, 26,* 113–120.

The authors of this classic paper identify the characteristics of academic and professional disciplines. They describe nursing as a professional discipline and identify recurring themes found in the nursing literature since the time of Nightingale.

Eckberg, D. L., & Hill, L., Jr. (1979). The paradigm concept and sociology: A critical review. *American Sociological Review, 44,* 925–937.

The authors review the many definitions of paradigm and draw distinctions among metaparadigm, paradigms or disciplinary matrices, and exemplars.

Fawcett, J. (1984). The metaparadigm of nursing: Present status and future refinements. *Image: The Journal of Nursing Scholarship, 16,* 84–87.

The author identifies the central concepts and themes of the nursing discipline and formalizes them as nursing's metaparadigm. She also describes the notion of paradigms or disciplinary matrices and claims that these are represented by conceptual models of nursing. In addition, she explains that exemplars are represented by programs of nursing research.

Fawcett, J. (1989). *Analysis and evaluation of conceptual models of nursing* (2nd ed.). Philadelphia: F. A. Davis.

This book contains detailed analyses and evaluations of seven major conceptual models of nursing, including works by Johnson, King, Levine, Neuman, Orem, Rogers, and Roy. The book serves as a companion volume to the present book.

Fawcett, J. (1992). To the editor [Letter]. *Advances in Nursing Science, 14*(3), vi.

The author points out that the statement offered by Newman, Sime, and Corcoran-Perry (1991) to describe the focus of the discipline of nursing fails to account for the metaparadigm concept of environment and to acknowledge that caring is just one perspective of nursing.

Fawcett, J. (1993). From a plethora of paradigms to parsimony in world views. *Nursing Science Quarterly, 6,* 56–58.

The article presents a discussion of various worldviews in nursing and offers a parsimonious approach to the philosophical foundations of nursing knowledge. The characteristics of three newly conceptualized worldviews are given: reaction, reciprocal interaction, and simultaneous action.

Fitzpatrick, J. J., & Whall, A. L. (1989). *Conceptual models of nursing. Analysis and application* (2nd ed.). Norwalk, CT: Appleton and Lange.

This edited book consists of reviews of many nursing formulations, including those by Peplau, Orlando, Leininger, Newman, Watson, and Parse. The works of Nightingale; Wiedenbach; Henderson; Abdellah; Levine; Johnson; Orem; Roy; Paterson and Zderad; Schlotfeldt; Newman; King; Rogers; Allen; Erickson, Tomlin, and Swain; and Fitzpatrick are also included. No distinctions are made between nursing theories and conceptual models of nursing.

Forchuk, C. (1991). Reconceptualizing the environment of the individual with a chronic mental illness. *Issues in Mental Health Nursing, 12,* 159–170.

Forchuk argues that the continuity of environments experienced by clients with chronic mental illness must be taken into account. She noted the influence of Orlando and Peplau on viewing the environment within an interpersonal context.

George, J. B. (Ed.). (1990). *Nursing theories: The base for professional nursing practice* (3rd ed.). Norwalk, CT: Appleton and Lange.

This edited book contains reviews of several nursing formulations. Full chapters are devoted to the works of Peplau, Orlando, Watson, Parse, and Leininger, as well as those by Nightingale, Henderson, Hall, Orem, Johnson, Abdellah, Wiedenbach, Levine, King, Rogers, Roy, Newman, and Paterson and Zderad. Brief overviews of Newman's theory, as well as of the works by Adam, Hadley, and Fitzpatrick, are included in a chapter on other extant theories. No distinctions are made between nursing theories and conceptual models of nursing.

Hall, B. A. (1981). The change paradigm in nursing: Growth versus persistence. *Advances in Nursing Science, 3*(4), 1–6.
Hall describes the characteristics of the change and persistence paradigms as they are used in nursing.

Hardy, M. E. (1978). Perspectives on nursing theory. *Advances in Nursing Science, 1*(1): 37–48.
Hardy identifies the stages of scientific development, using Kuhn's notions of metaparadigm, paradigm, and exemplar. She also discusses the development of theory.

Ingram, R. (1991). Why does nursing need theory? *Journal of Advanced Nursing, 16,* 350–353.
The author claims that nursing needs theory to enhance professional autonomy and the power of nursing, improve the coherence of purpose for practice, and enhance communication in nursing.

Kleffel, D. (1991). Rethinking the environment as a domain of nursing knowledge. *Advances in Nursing Science, 14*(1), 40–51.
Kleffel maintains that the relevant nursing environment is typically limited to the client and to psychosocial phenomena. She argues for a broader, multidimensional perspective that incorporates epidemiological and ecologic approaches, with an emphasis on society, rather than the individual, as the locus of change.

Kim, H. S. (1987). Structuring the nursing knowledge system: A typology of four domains. *Scholarly Inquiry for Nursing Practice, 1,* 99–110.
Kim identifies four domains of nursing knowledge: client, client-nurse, practice, and environment.

Kim, H. S. (1989). Theoretical thinking in nursing: Problems and prospects. *Recent Advances in Nursing, 24,* 106–122.
Kim presents a five-level framework for analysis of theoretical thinking in nursing that is similar to the one used in this book. The levels are: level I, philosophy of science; level II, metaparadigm; level II, nursing philosophy; level IV, paradigm, and level V, theory.

King, I. M. (1984). Philosophy of nursing education: A national survey. *Western Journal of Nursing Research, 6,* 387–406.
King reports the results of a survey of the commonalities in terms used in philosophy statements of the National League for Nursing accredited basic nursing education programs. Common terms are man, health, environment, social systems, role, perception, interpersonal relations, nursing, and God.

Kuhn, T. S. (1977). Second thoughts on paradigms. In F. Suppe (Ed.), *The structure of scientific theories* (2nd ed., pp. 459–517). Chicago: University of Illinois Press.
Kuhn reviews his earlier multiple uses of the term paradigm and introduces the notions of the disciplinary matrix and the exemplar, which he regards as more accurate terms.

Leininger, M. M. (1991). Looking to the future of nursing and the relevancy of culture care theory. In M. M. Leininger (Ed.), *Culture care diversity and universality: A theory of nursing* (pp. 391–418). New York: National League for Nursing.
Leininger offers the concepts of human care, environmental contexts, and well-being (or health) as substitutes for the metaparadigm concepts of person, environment, health, and nursing. She maintains that human care/caring is the central phenomenon and essence of nursing.

Leininger, M. M. (1991). Nursing theories to guide differentiated nursing practices. In I. E. Goertzen (Ed.), *Differentiating nursing practice into the twenty-first century* (pp. 27–29). Kansas City, MO: American Academy of Nursing.
Leininger identifies the contributions made by conceptual models of nursing and nursing theories to the differentiation of nursing practice. She points out that Canada leads the United States in the use of theory-directed nursing practices. The paper was

presented at a conference sponsored by the American Academy of Nursing, the American Nurses Association, and the American Organization of Nurse Executives held in 1990 in Charleston, South Carolina.

Madden, B. P. (1990). The hybrid model for concept development: Its value for the study of therapeutic alliance. *Advances in Nursing Science, 12*(3), 75–87.

Madden noted that the definition of therapeutic alliance as "a process that emerges within a provider-client interaction in which both the client and the provider are (1) actively working toward the goal of developing client health behaviors chosen for consistency with the client's current health status and life style, (2) focusing on mutual negotiation to determine activities to be carried out toward that goal, and (3) using a supportive and equitable therapeutic relationship to facilitate that goal" (p. 85) is consistent with Peplau's and Travelbee's perspectives, as well as with Orlando's notion of the primacy of the nurse-client relationship.

Malloch, K., Martinez, R., Nelson, L., Predeger, B., Speakman, L., Steinbinder, A., & Tracy, J. (1992). To the editor [Letter]. *Advances in Nursing Science, 15*(2), vi–vii.

Malloch and her colleagues suggest the following revision of the Newman, Sime, and Corcoran-Perry (1991) statement: Nursing is the study and practice of caring within contexts of the human health experience. They maintain that their statement extends the focus to nursing practice and incorporates the environment by the use of the term "contexts." The authors claim that the use of the term "caring" brings unity to the metaparadigm concepts of person, environment, health, and nursing.

Marriner-Tomey, A. (1989). *Nursing theorists and their work* (2nd ed.). St. Louis: C.V. Mosby.

This edited book consists of reviews of various nursing formulations. Theorists' works are clustered into four categories—the art and science of humanistic nursing (Nightingale, Henderson, Abdellah, Hall, Orem, Adam, Leininger, Watson, Parse, Benner); interpersonal relationships (Peplau; Travelbee; Orlando; Wiedenbach; Riehl-Sisca; Erickson, Tomlin, and Swain; Bernard; Mercer); systems (Johnson, Roy, King, Neuman); and energy fields (Levine, Rogers, Fitzpatrick, Newman). No distinctions are made between conceptual models and theories.

Meleis, A. I. (1991). *Theoretical nursing: Development and progress* (2nd ed.). Philadelphia: J.B. Lippincott.

Meleis presents a comprehensive historical review of the development of nursing knowledge and identifies the concepts that are central to the domain of nursing as nursing client, transitions, interaction, nursing process, environment, nursing therapeutics, and health. She notes that nursing per se is not a central concept of the nursing domain because its inclusion would create a tautology. Meleis regards all nursing formulations as theories and classifies them in the categories of nursing clients (Johnson, Neuman); human being-environment interactions (Rogers); interactions (King, Orlando, Paterson and Zderad, Travelbee, Wiedenbach); and nursing therapeutics (Levine, Orem). Meleis includes a comprehensive analysis of the theoretical literature in nursing and an extensive bibliography.

Mitchell, G. J., & Cody, W. K. (1992). Nursing knowledge and human science: Ontological and epistemological considerations. *Nursing Science Quarterly, 5,* 54–61.

Mitchell and Cody define and describe human science within the context of Dilthey's perspective. They also examine the extent to which works by Paterson and Zderad, Newman, Watson, and Parse meet ontological and epistemological criteria for human science.

Moody, L. E., & Hutchinson, S. A. (1989). Relating your study to a theoretical context. In H. S. Wilson, *Research in nursing* (2nd ed., pp. 275–332). Redwood City, CA: Addison-Wesley.

Moody and Hutchinson define and describe the components of nursing knowledge, including the metaparadigm; paradigms, models, or philosophies; grand theories; middle-range theories; and practice theories. They also describe the relationship of theory and research and explain how theories are linked with the research process. Very brief overviews of some nursing formulations are given, including Nightingale, Hall, Henderson, Peplau, Abdellah, Orem, Rogers, Levine, Roy, King, Neuman, and Parse.

Morse, J. M., Solberg, S. M., Neander, W. L., Bottorff, J. L., & Johnson, J. L. (1990). Concepts of caring and caring as a concept. *Advances in Nursing Science, 13*(1), 1–14.

Morse, J. M., Bottorff, J., Neander, W., & Solberg, S. (1991). Comparative analysis of conceptualizations and theories of caring. *Image: Journal of Nursing Scholarship, 23*, 119–126.

The authors argue that various perspectives of caring must be clarified. They identified five epistemological perspectives of caring: caring as a human state, caring as a moral imperative or ideal, caring as an affect, caring as an interpersonal relationship, and caring as a nursing intervention. Identified outcomes of caring are the subjective experience and physiological responses. In the 1990 article, the authors concluded that knowledge development related to caring in nursing is limited by the lack of refinement of caring theory, lack of definitions of caring attributes, failure to examine caring from a dialectic perspective, and a focus on the nurse rather than the patient. In the 1991 article, the authors identify the implications of the five perspectives of caring for nursing practice and conclude that the concept of caring often lacks relevance for nursing practice.

Newman, M. A. (1983). The continuing revolution: A history of nursing science. In N. L. Chaska (Ed.), *The nursing profession. A time to speak* (pp. 385–393). New York: McGraw Hill.

Newman comments that the domain of nursing has always included the nurse, the patient, the situation in which they find themselves, and the purpose of their being together, or the health of the patient. She goes on to say that the major components of the nursing [meta]paradigm are nursing (as an action); client (human being); environment (of the client and of the nurse-client); and health.

Newman, M. A. (1992). Prevailing paradigms in nursing. *Nursing Outlook, 40*, 10–13, 32.

Newman outlines the characteristics of what she considers to be the three major paradigms in contemporary nursing: particulate-deterministic, interactive-integrative, and unitary-transformative.

Newman, M. A., Sime, A. M., & Corcoran-Perry, S. A. (1991). The focus of the discipline of nursing. *Advances in Nursing Science, 14*(1), 1–6.

Newman and her colleagues argue that the statement that best summarizes the focus of contemporary nursing is: nursing is the study of caring in the human health perspective.

Newman, M. A., Sime, A. M., & Corcoran-Perry, S. A. (1992). Authors' reply [Letter to the editor]. *Advances in Nursing Science, 14*(3), vi–vii.

Newman and her co-authors reply to Fawcett's (1992) critique of their 1991 publication on a new focus statement for nursing. They agree with Fawcett that caring is not a theme of every conceptualization of nursing, but they claim that caring is sufficiently dominant, in combination with the theme of the human health experience, to be considered the focus of the discipline. They acknowledge that person, environment, health, and nursing are relevant to the discipline and explain that they regard the concept of environment as inherent in and inseparable from the integrated focus of caring in the human health experience. Furthermore, although they acknowledge the need for multiple perspectives of knowledge development, they regard the unitary-transformative perspective as particularly important for the study of nursing phenomena.

O'Toole, M. (Ed.). (1992). *Miller-Keane encyclopedia and dictionary of medicine, nursing, and allied health* (5th ed.). Philadelphia: W. B. Saunders.

The encyclopedia includes definitions for metaparadigm, conceptual model, and nursing theory. Very brief overviews are given of works by Johnson, King, Levine, Neuman, Newman, Orem, Parse, Rogers, Roy, and Watson.

Parker, M. E. (Ed.). (1990). *Nursing theories in practice.* New York: National League for Nursing.

This book includes papers presented at two nursing theorist conferences sponsored by Cedars Medical Center in Miami, Florida in 1989 and 1990. Papers by Johnson, Orem, King, Rogers, Newman, Levine, Neuman, and Watson are included, along with papers by others who describe the use of those nursing models and theories in clinical practice.

Parse, R. R. (1987). *Nursing science. Major paradigms, theories, and critiques.* Philadelphia: W.B. Saunders.
Parse outlines the characteristics of what she considers to be the two predominant paradigms in contemporary nursing: totality and simultaneity. The book also includes papers presented by Peplau (an historical overview of nursing science), Roy, Orem, King, Rogers, and Parse at a conference held in Pittsburgh, Pennsylvania in 1985, as well as critiques of the theorists' works.

Reese, H. W., & Overton, W. F. (1970). Models of development and theories of development. In L. R. Goulet & P. B. Baltes (Eds.), *Life span developmental psychology: Research and theory* (pp. 115–145). New York: Academic Press.
The authors identify the relationship between models and theories. They also describe the characteristics of the mechanistic and organismic worldviews.

Reilly, D. E. (1975). Why a conceptual framework? *Nursing Outlook, 23,* 566–569.
Reilly presents one of the earliest and most lucid discussions of the differences between conceptual models and theories.

Riehl-Sisca, J. P. (1989). *Conceptual models for nursing practice* (4th ed.). Norwalk, CT: Appleton and Lange.
This edited book presents original works by several nurse theorists, critiques of the works, and examples of the use of the works in nursing practice. Works are classified as systems (Neuman, Roy, King); developmental (Rogers, Watson, Parse, Chrisman, and Riehl-Sisca); or interaction models (Levine, Orem, Riehl-Sisca). No distinctions are made between conceptual models and theories.

Sarter, B. (1988). Philosophical sources of nursing theory. *Nursing Science Quarterly, 1,* 52–59.
Sarter presents the results of her analysis of the philosophical origins of works by Rogers, Newman, Watson, and Parse. She suggests that an appropriate philosophical foundation for the discipline of nursing should include several themes, including process, evolution of consciousness, self-transcendence, open systems, harmony, relativity of space-time, pattern, and holism.

Smith, M. C. (1992). Metaphor in nursing theory. *Nursing Science Quarterly, 5,* 48–49.
The author describes the meaning of metaphors in theory and identifies the metaphors in various conceptual models of nursing and nursing theories. The nursing formulations and their metaphors are:
> Neuman's Systems Model: militaristic (lines of resistance and defense)
> Watson's Theory of Human Caring: holding up the arc, the roar of silence, and the argonauta
> Rogers's Science of Unitary Human Beings: a symphony
> Parse's Theory of Human Becoming: illuminating meaning in the light of true presence

Thomas, C. L. (Ed.). (1993) *Taber's cyclopedic medical dictionary* (17th ed.). Philadelphia: F. A. Davis.
The 17th edition of the dictionary includes overviews of the major conceptual models of nursing (Johnson, King, Levine, Neuman, Orem, Rogers, Roy) and nursing theories (Leininger, Newman, Orlando, Parse, Peplau, Watson). Overviews of works by Nightingale, Henderson, and Rubin also are included. Each overview includes a description of the model or theory and its implications for nursing education and nursing practice.

Torres, G. (1986). *Theoretical foundations of nursing.* Norwalk, CT: Appleton-Century-Crofts.
Torres presents reviews of several nursing formulations, which she classifies in the categories of environmental (Nightingale); need-oriented (Henderson, Abdellah, Orlando, Wiedenbach, Orem, Kinlein); systems-oriented (Johnson, Rogers, King, Neuman, Roy); and interaction process (Peplau, Hall, Levine, Travelbee, Watson) theories. She makes no distinctions between conceptual models and theories.

Watson, J. (1990). Caring knowledge and informed moral passion. *Advances in Nursing Science, 13*(1), 15–24.
Watson discusses the notion of human caring and states that the concept should be incorporated into the nursing metaparadigm.

Winstead-Fry, P. (Ed.). (1986). *Case studies in nursing theory.* New York: National League for Nursing.
This book contains chapters dealing with works by Orlando, Orem, Rogers, Roy, Neuman, Paterson and Zderad, King, and Newman. Two chapters were written by the original authors of the work (King, Orem). Other chapters were prepared by nurses who have used the conceptual model or theory extensively. An attempt is made to distinguish between conceptual models and theories.

2

Analysis and Evaluation
of Nursing Theories———

This chapter presents a framework for analysis and evaluation of nursing theories. The framework emphasizes the most important features of grand and middle-range nursing theories and is appropriate to their level of abstraction. Furthermore, it continues the emphasis on the distinctions between conceptual models and theories that is found in Chapter 1.

The major components of analysis and evaluation of nursing theories are identified in the following key terms. Each component is discussed in detail in this chapter.

KEY TERMS ———

Analysis	Internal Consistency
Theory Scope	Parsimony
Theory Context	Testability
Theory Content	Empirical Adequacy
Evaluation	Pragmatic Adequacy
Significance	

A FRAMEWORK FOR ANALYSIS AND EVALUATION
OF NURSING THEORIES

The framework that is used in this book for analysis and evaluation of nursing theories separates questions dealing with analysis from those

TABLE 2–1. A Framework for Analysis and Evaluation of Nursing Theories

Questions for Analysis

1. What is the scope of theory?
2. How is the theory related to nursing's metaparadigm?
   - Which metaparadigm concepts are addressed by the theory?
   Does the theory deal with the person?
   Does the theory deal with the environment?
   Does the theory deal with health?
   Does the theory deal with nursing processes or goals?
   - Which metaparadigm propositions are addressed by the theory?
   Does the theory deal with life processes?
   Does the theory deal with patterns of human-environment interaction?
   Does the theory deal with processes that affect health?
   Does the theory deal with the health or wholeness of the human being in interaction with the environment?
3. What philosophical claims are reflected in the theory?
   - On what values and beliefs about nursing is the theory based?
   - What worldview of the person-environment relationship is reflected in the theory?
4. From what conceptual model was the theory derived?
5. What knowledge from adjunctive disciplines was used in the development of the theory?
6. What are the concepts of the theory?
7. What are the propositions of the theory?
   - Which propositions are nonrelational?
   - Which propositions are relational?

Questions for Evaluation

1. Is the theory significant?
   - Are the metaparadigm concepts and propositions addressed by the theory explicit?
   - Are the philosophical claims on which the theory is based explicit?
   - Is the conceptual model from which the theory was derived explicit?
   - Are the authors of knowledge from adjunctive disciplines acknowledged and are bibliographical citations given?
2. Is the theory internally consistent?
   - Are all elements of the work (philosophical claims, conceptual model, theory) congruent?
   - Do the concepts reflect semantic clarity and consistency?
   - Are there any redundant concepts?
   - Do the propositions reflect structural consistency?
3. Is the theory parsimonious?
   - Is the theory stated clearly and concisely?
4. Is the theory testable?
   - Can the concepts be observed empirically?
   - Can the propositions be measured?
5. Is the theory empirically adequate?
   - Are theoretical assertions congruent with empirical evidence?
6. Is the theory pragmatically adequate?
   - Are education and special-skill training required prior to application of the theory in clinical practice?
   - For what clinical problems is the theory appropriate?
   - Is it feasible to implement clinical protocols derived from the theory?
   - Are the nursing actions compatible with expectations for nursing practice?
   - Does the clinician have the legal ability to implement the nursing actions?
   - Do the nursing actions lead to favorable outcomes?

more appropriate to evaluation (Table 2–1). The questions for analysis follow directly from the discussion of the structure of contemporary nursing knowledge that was presented in Chapter 1. Accordingly, the analysis involves an objective breakdown of the structural hierarchy of nursing knowledge containing the theory into its component parts. The questions for evaluation focus on the content and coherence of the theory, as well as on the evidence about the theory's empirical and practical aspects. The evaluation permits judgments to be made about the extent to which the theory satisfies certain criteria.

ANALYSIS OF NURSING THEORIES

Analysis of a nursing theory, using the framework presented in this chapter, is accomplished by a systematic examination of exactly what the author has written about her theory, rather than by relying on inferences about what might have been meant or by referring to other authors' interpretations of the theory. When the author of the theory has not been clear about a point or has not presented certain information, it may be necessary to make inferences or to turn to other reviews of the theory. That, however, must be noted explicitly so the distinction between the words of the theory author and those of others is clear. Theory analysis, therefore, involves a nonjudgmental, detailed examination of the theory, including its *scope, context,* and *content.*

Theory Scope

The first step in theory analysis is to classify the theory according to its *scope.* As explained in Chapter 1, grand theories are broad in scope; their concepts and propositions are relatively abstract and general. In contrast, middle-range theories are more circumscribed; their concepts and propositions are relatively specific and concrete. Middle-range theories are further classified as descriptive, explanatory, or predictive. The question to ask is:

- What is the scope of the theory?

Theory Context

The second step in theory analysis is examination of the *context* of the theory. Barnum (1990) regarded the context of a nursing theory to be "the environment in which the nursing act takes place. It tells the nature of the world of nursing and, in some cases, describes the nature of the patient's world" (p. 59). Context, as used in this book, goes beyond Barnum's description to encompass identification of the concepts and propositions of the nursing metaparadigm addressed by the theory; the philosophical claims on which the theory is based; the conceptual model, or paradigm, from which the theory was derived; and the contributions of knowledge from adjunctive disciplines to the theory development effort.

The metaparadigm of nursing, as explained in Chapter 1, is made up of four global concepts and four general propositions. The questions about the metaparadigm concepts and propositions are:

- Which metaparadigm concepts are addressed by the theory?
    Does the theory deal with the person?
    Does the theory deal with the environment?
    Does the theory deal with health?
    Does the theory deal with nursing processes or goals?
- Which metaparadigm propositions are addressed by the theory?
    Does the theory deal with life processes?
    Does the theory deal with patterns of human-environment interaction?
    Does the theory deal with processes that affect health?
    Does the theory deal with the health or wholeness of the human being in interaction with the environment?

Other questions about context focus on the philosophical claims on which the theory is based. Philosophical statements, as noted in Chapter 1, explicate values and beliefs about nursing, as well as the worldview of the relationship between the person and the environment. The questions are:

- On what values and beliefs about nursing is the theory based?
- What worldview of the person-environment relationship is reflected in the theory?

Another question dealing with the context of a theory focuses on the conceptual model from which the theory was derived. As explained in Chapter 1, a conceptual model is more abstract than a theory and serves as a guide for theory development. The question is:

- From what conceptual model was the theory derived?

The final question dealing with theory context highlights the knowledge from other disciplines used by the theorist. This question reflects recognition that "nursing theories do not spring forth fully formed" (Levine, 1988, p. 16). Instead, most nursing theorists draw on existing knowledge from adjunctive disciplines as they construct and refine their theories. The question is:

- What knowledge from adjunctive disciplines was used in the development of the theory?

Theory Content

The third step in theory analysis is examination of *content*. The content, or subject matter, of a theory is articulated through the theory's concepts and propositions. Those elements are the "building bricks that give the theory form" (Barnum, 1990, p. 61).

The concepts of a theory are words or groups of words that express a mental image of some phenomenon. They represent the special vocabulary of a theory. Furthermore, concepts give meaning to what can be imagined or observed through the senses. Thus they enable us to categorize, interpret, and structure the phenomena encompassed by the theory. Concepts can be unidimensional, or they can have more than one dimension.

The propositions of a theory are declarative statements about one or more concepts, statements that assert what is thought to be the case. As explained in Chapter 1, some nonrelational propositions state the existence of certain phenomena. Other nonrelational propositions state the constitutive and operational definitions of concepts. Relational propositions express the associations or linkages between two or more concepts, as well as the characteristics of those linkages.

Analysis of the content of a theory requires systematic examination of all descriptions of the development of the theory. The questions are:

- What are the concepts of the theory?
- What are the propositions of the theory?
    Which propositions are nonrelational?
    Which propositions are relational?

EVALUATION OF NURSING THEORIES

Evaluation of a theory requires judgments to be made about the theory's *significance, internal consistency, parsimony, testability, empirical adequacy, and pragmatic adequacy.* The evaluation is based on the results of the analysis, as well as on a review of previously published critiques, research reports, and reports of practical applications of the theory.

Evaluation of Theory Context

The first step in theory evaluation focuses on the context of the theory. The criterion is *significance*.

The significance criterion requires justification of the importance of the theory to the discipline of nursing. That criterion is met when the metaparadigmatic, philosophical, and paradigmatic origins of the theory are explicit; when the adjunctive knowledge is cited; and when the special contributions made by the theory are identified. The questions to ask when evaluating the significance of the theory are:

- Are the metaparadigm concepts and propositions addressed by the theory explicit?
- Are the philosophical claims on which the theory is based explicit?
- Is the conceptual model from which the theory was derived explicit?
- Are the authors of knowledge from adjunctive disciplines acknowledged and are bibliographical citations given? (Levine, 1992).

Evaluation of Theory Content

The second step in theory evaluation focuses on the content of the theory. The criteria are *internal consistency, parsimony,* and *testability*.

Internal Consistency

The criterion of *internal consistency* requires all elements of the theorist's work, including the philosophical claims, conceptual model, and theory, to be congruent. Furthermore, the internal consistency criterion requires concepts to reflect semantic clarity and consistency. The semantic clarity requirement is more likely to be met when a constitutive definition is given for each concept making up the theory than when no explicit definitions are given. The requirement is also more likely to be met when concepts are not redundant, that is, when only one term is used to represent each phenomenon encompassed by the theory.

The requirement of semantic consistency is met when the same term and the same definition are used for each phenomenon throughout the theory. Conversely, semantic inconsistency occurs when different terms are used for a phenomenon or different meanings are attached to the same phenomenon.

The internal consistency criterion also requires that propositions reflect structural consistency, which means that the propositions should be related to each other in a logical manner, that linkages between all concepts are specified, and that no contradictions are evident.

The questions to ask when evaluating the internal consistency of a theory are:

- Are all elements of the work (philosophical claims, conceptual model, theory) congruent?
- Do the concepts reflect semantic clarity and consistency?
- Are there any redundant concepts?
- Do the propositions reflect structural consistency?

Parsimony

The criterion of *parsimony* requires a theory to be stated in the most economical way possible without oversimplifying the phenomenon. That means that the fewer the concepts and propositions needed to fully explicate the phenomena of interest the better. The parsimony criterion is met when the most parsimonious statement clarifies rather than obscures the phenomenon. The question to ask when evaluating the parsimony of a theory is:

- Is the theory stated clearly and concisely?

Testability

A theory is *testable* if its concepts can be observed and its propositions can be measured. Concepts are empirically observable if they are connected to empirical indicators by operational definitions. Propositions are measurable when empirical indicators are substituted for concept names in the propositions and when statistical procedures can provide evidence regarding the assertions made. Thus the criterion of testability is met when specific instruments or practice protocols have been developed to observe the theory concepts and statistical techniques are available to measure the assertions made by the propositions. The assessment of testability is, therefore, facilitated by a thorough review of the research methodology literature associated with the theory, including descriptions of instruments designed to measure the concepts, research designs that will elicit the required data, and statistical or other data management techniques that will yield evidence about the theory.

Testability is frequently regarded as the primary characteristic of a scientifically useful theory. Marx (1976) maintained, "If there is no way of testing a theory it is scientifically worthless, no matter how plausible, imaginative, or innovative it may be" (p. 249).

An alternative to direct empirical testability of a theory is the criterion requiring that theories should be potentially testable. That alternative is particularly appropriate for middle-range theories that are generated by means of qualitative methods, such as grounded theory, ethnography, and phenomenology, because the empirical indicators needed to test the theory may not be available although it is believed that they can be developed.

Another alternative is indirect empirical testing, which is appropriate for grand theories. A grand theory is not amenable to direct empirical testing because of its abstract nature. Consequently, the middle-range theory–generating capacity of a grand theory should be judged, as should the testability of the middle-range theories that were derived from the grand theory.

The questions to ask when evaluating the testability of a theory are:

- Can the concepts be empirically observed?
- Can the propositions be measured?

Evaluation of Empirical Adequacy

The third step in theory evaluation deals with an assessment of the theory's validity. The criterion is *empirical adequacy*.

The empirical adequacy criterion requires the assertions made by the theory to be congruent with empirical evidence derived from research. The extent to which a theory meets this criterion is determined by means of a systematic review of the findings of all studies that have been based on the theory.

The logic of scientific inference dictates that if the empirical data conform to the theoretical assertions, it may be appropriate to tentatively accept the assertions as reasonable or valid. Conversely, if the empirical data do not conform to the assertions, it is appropriate to conclude that the assertions are false.

It is unlikely that any one test of a theory will provide the definitive evidence needed to establish empirical adequacy. Thus, decisions about empirical adequacy should take the findings of all related studies into account. Meta-analysis and other formal procedures can be used to integrate the results of related studies. Readers are referred to other texts for comprehensive discussions of those procedures (Cooper, 1989; Fawcett & Downs, 1992; Rosenthal, 1991). Suffice it to say here that the more tests of a theory that yield supporting evidence the more adequate the theory.

It is important to point out that a theory should not be regarded as the truth or an ideology that cannot be modified. Indeed, no theory should be considered final or absolute, for it is always possible that subsequent studies will yield different findings or that other theories will provide a better fit with the data. Thus the aim of evaluation of empirical adequacy is to determine the degree of confidence warranted by the best empirical evidence, rather than to determine the absolute truth of the theory. The outcome of evaluation of empirical adequacy is a judgment regarding the need to modify or refine the concepts and propositions of the theory.

The question to be asked when evaluating empirical adequacy is:

• Are theoretical assertions congruent with empirical evidence?

Evaluation of Pragmatic Adequacy

The fourth step in evaluation of a theory focuses on the theory's utility for practice. The criterion is *pragmatic adequacy*. The extent to which a theory meets this criterion is determined by reviewing all descriptions of the use of the theory in clinical practice.

The pragmatic adequacy criterion requires that nurses have a full understanding of the content of the theory as well as the interpersonal and psychomotor skills necessary to apply it (Magee, 1991). Although that may seem self-evident, it is important to acknowledge the need for education and special-skill training prior to theory application. The criterion also requires the theory to be appropriate to the clinical problems for which a theory is sought. This too may seem to be self-evident, but nursing actions are sometimes based on a theory that is unrelated to the specific problem of interest.

The criterion further requires that the application of the theory is feasible, which means that the requisite human and material resources for application are available (Magee, 1991). Feasibility is determined by an evaluation of the resources needed to establish the nursing actions as customary practice, including the time needed to learn and implement the protocols for nursing actions; the number, type, and expertise of personnel required for their implementation; and the cost of in-service education, salaries, equipment, and protocol-testing procedures. Moreover, the willingness of those who control financial resources to pay for the nursing actions, such as health care administrators and third-party payers, must be determined. In sum, the nurse must be in a setting that is conducive to application of the theory and have the time and training necessary to do it.

Furthermore, the pragmatic adequacy criterion requires that theory-based nursing actions be compatible with expectations for practice

(Magee, 1991). Compatibility should be evaluated in relation to expectations held by the health care system, the community, and the individual recipient of nursing actions. If the actions do not meet existing expectations, they should be abandoned or people should be helped to develop new expectations. Johnson (1974) commented, "Current [nursing] practice is not entirely what it might become and [thus people] might come to expect a different form of practice, given the opportunity to experience it" (p. 376).

In addition, the pragmatic adequacy criterion requires the clinician to have the legal ability to control the application and to measure the effectiveness of the theory-based nursing actions. Such control may be problematic in that clinicians are not always able to carry out legally sanctioned responsibilities because of resistance from others. Sources of resistance against implementation of theory-based nursing actions include attempts by physicians to control nursing practice, financial barriers imposed by clinical agencies and third-party payers, and skepticism by other health professionals about the ability of nurses to carry out the proposed actions (Edwardson, 1984). The cooperation and collaboration of others may, therefore, have to be secured.

Finally, this criterion requires the nursing actions to be socially meaningful by leading to favorable outcomes for recipients of the actions. Examples of favorable outcomes include a reduction in complications, improved health status, and increased satisfaction with the theory-based actions on the part of both the recipients and the clinicians.

The questions to ask when evaluating pragmatic adequacy are:

- Are education and special-skill training required prior to application of the theory in clinical practice?
- For what clinical problems is the theory appropriate?
- Is it feasible to implement clinical protocols derived from the theory?
- Are the nursing actions compatible with expectations for nursing practice?
- Does the clinician have the legal ability to implement the nursing actions?
- Do the nursing actions lead to favorable outcomes?

CONCLUSION

This chapter presents a framework for analysis and evaluation of grand and middle-range nursing theories. The framework will be applied in the next six chapters, each of which will present a comprehensive examination of a nursing theory.

The framework for analysis and evaluation of nursing theories presented in this chapter is *not* appropriate for examination of conceptual models of nursing. Readers who are interested in that component of nursing knowledge are referred to the text *Analysis and Evaluation of Conceptual Models of Nursing* (Fawcett, 1989).

REFERENCES

Barnum, B. J. S. (1990). *Nursing theory: Analysis, application, evaluation* (3rd ed.). Glenview, IL: Scott, Foresman/Little, Brown Higher Education.

Cooper, H. M. (1989). *Integrating research: A guide for literature reviews* (2nd ed.). Newbury Park, CA: Sage.

Edwardson, S. R. (1984). Using research in practice: Factors associated with the adoption of a nursing innovation. *Western Journal of Nursing Research, 6*, 141–143.

Fawcett, J. (1989). *Analysis and evaluation of conceptual models of nursing* (2nd ed.). Philadelphia: F.A. Davis.

Fawcett, J., & Downs, F. S. (1992). *The relationship of theory and research* (2nd ed). Philadelphia: F.A. Davis.

Johnson, D. E. (1974). Development of theory: A requisite for nursing as a primary health profession. *Nursing Research, 23*, 372–377.

Levine, M. E. (1988). Antecedents from adjunctive disciplines: Creation of nursing theory. *Nursing Science Quarterly, 1*, 16–21.

Levine, M. E. (1992, February). *Nursing knowledge: Improving education and practice through theory.* Paper presented at the Sigma Theta Tau Theory Conference, Chicago, IL.

Magee, M. (1991, May). *Eclecticism in nursing philosophy: Problem or solution?* Paper presented at the Philosophy in the Nurse's World Conference, Banff, Alberta, Canada.

Marx, M. H. (1976). Formal theory. In M. H. Marx & F. E. Goodson (Eds.), *Theories in contemporary psychology* (2nd ed., pp. 234–260). New York: Macmillan.

Rosenthal, R. (1991). *Meta-analytic procedures for social research* (rev. ed.). Newbury Park, CA: Sage.

Annotated Bibliography

Barnum, B. J. S. (1990). *Nursing theory: Analysis, application, evaluation* (3rd ed.). Glenview, IL: Scott, Foresman/Little Brown Higher Education.
Barnum offers criteria for evaluation of nursing theories. Criteria for internal criticism are clarity, consistency, adequacy, and logical development. Criteria for external criticism are reality convergence, utility, significance, discrimination, scope, and complexity.

Cooper, H. M. (1989). *Integrating research: A guide for literature reviews* (2nd ed.). Newbury Park, CA: Sage.
Cooper presents strategies for integrative literature reviews, with an emphasis on systematic, objective appraisals of research reports. Techniques of meta-analysis are placed in the context of the entire integrative review, from selection of the literature to preparation of the report.

Chinn, P. L., & Kramer, M. K. (1991). *Theory and nursing: A systematic approach* (3rd ed.). St. Louis: Mosby Year Book.
This book contains a scheme for analyzing and evaluating theories. Questions for analysis ask about the purpose, concepts, definitions, relationships, structure, and underlying assumptions of the theory. Evaluation criteria include clarity, simplicity, generality, accessibility, and importance.

Crossley, D. J., & Wilson, P. A. (1979). *How to argue: An introduction to logical thinking.* New York: Random House.
The authors present a cogent discussion of the logic of inductive and deductive reasoning.

Duffy, M., & Muhlenkamp, A. F. (1974). A framework for theory analysis. *Nursing Outlook, 22*, 570–574.
Duffy and Muhlenkamp identify a framework for analysis of theories that focuses on the origins of the problems with which the theory is concerned, the methods used, the character of the subject matter dealt with by the theory, and the expected outcomes of testing propositions generated by the theory. The framework is used to analyze Peplau's and Rogers's work, thereby implying that it can be used for both conceptual models (Rogers) and theories (Peplau).

Ellis, R. (1968). Characteristics of significant theories. *Nursing Research, 17*, 217–222.
Ellis identifies criteria for evaluation of theories, including scope, complexity, testability, usefulness, values, hypotheses, and terminology.

Fawcett, J., & Downs, F. S. (1992). *The relationship of theory and research* (2nd ed). Philadelphia: F. A. Davis.
The authors present a detailed framework for the analysis and evaluation of middle-range theories presented in research reports. They note that such theories often are not presented formally and, therefore, their components (concepts and propositions) must be extracted from the published reports.

Hardy, M. E. (1978). Perspectives on nursing theory. *Advances in Nursing Science, 1*(1), 37–48.
Hardy discusses the stages of scientific development, the nature of theory, and criteria for theory evaluation, including logical adequacy, empirical adequacy, usefulness, and significance.

Levine, M. E. (1988). Antecedents from adjunctive disciplines: Creation of nursing theory. *Nursing Science Quarterly, 1*, 16–21.
Levine argues that nursing must acknowledge the fact that it shares a body of knowledge with other disciplines that are concerned with health care. She claims that inasmuch as so-called adjunctive knowledge is antecedent to all nursing theory, analysis of nursing theories should identify the adjunctive sources and determine whether the use of those sources is warranted and correct.

Marriner-Tomey, A. (1989). Introduction to analysis of nursing theories. In A. Marriner-Tomey, *Nursing theorists and their work* (2nd ed., pp. 3–14). St. Louis: C. V. Mosby.
Drawing heavily from other authors' frameworks, Marriner-Tomey identifies the following criteria for evaluation of theory: clarity, simplicity, generality, empirical precision, and derivable consequences.

Meleis, A. I. (1991). *Theoretical nursing: Development and progress* (2nd ed.). Philadelphia: J.B. Lippincott.
Meleis's framework for theory evaluation encompasses description, analysis, critique, and testing. Description of the theory focuses on identification of its structural components (assumptions, concepts, propositions) and functional components (focus, client, nursing, health, nurse-patient interactions, environment, nursing problem, nursing therapeutics). Analysis deals with analysis of the concepts (definitions, antecedents, consequences, exemplars) and the theory (theorist's educational and experiential background, professional network, and sociocultural context); the theory's paradigmatic origins (references, citations, assumptions, concepts, propositions, hypotheses, laws); and its internal dimensions (rationale, system of relations, content, beginnings, scope, goal, context, abstractness, method). Critique encompasses clarity; consistency; simplicity/complexity; tautology; teleology; visual and graphic presentation; logical representation; geographical origin and spread; influence of the theorist versus the theory; usefulness for practice, research, education, and administration; and the external components of personal values, congruence with other professional values, congruence with social values, and social significance. Various forms of theory testing include testing utility in practice, teaching, or administration; testing propositions from other disciplines; testing propositions from other disciplines as they relate to nursing; testing nursing concepts; and testing nursing propositions.

Rosenthal, R. (1984). *Meta-analytic procedures for social research.* Beverly Hills: Sage.
Rosenthal presents a comprehensible discussion of various techniques of meta-analysis, including combining probabilities and calculation and combining of effect sizes. A technique for calculating the practical importance of effect sizes is also included.

Shearing, C. D. (1973). How to make theories untestable: A guide to theorists. *The American Sociologist, 8,* 33–37.
In this masterpiece of satire, Shearing claims that because theories are so frequently presented in an untestable form, scholars might as well follow his guidelines for making theories untestable. The guidelines stipulate that no operational definitions should be provided, no relational propositions should be stated, or if stated, should state unclear associations between concepts, and that the theory should be presented in an internally inconsistent manner. The converse of those guidelines is, of course, needed to meet the criterion of testability.

Torres, G. (1990). The place of concepts and theories within nursing. In J. B. George (Ed.), *Nursing theories. The base for professional nursing practice* (3rd ed., pp. 1–12). Norwalk, CT: Appleton and Lange.
Torres identifies the following basic characteristics of theories: (1) Theories can interrelate concepts in such a way as to create a different way of looking at a particular phenomenon; (2) Theories must be logical in nature; (3) Theories should be relatively simple yet generalizable; (4) Theories can be the bases for hypotheses that can be tested; (5) Theories contribute to and assist in increasing the general body of knowledge within the discipline through the research implemented to validate them; (6) Theories can be utilized by practitioners to guide and improve their practice; (7) Theories must be consistent with other validated theories, laws, and principles but will leave open unanswered questions that need to be investigated.

3

Leininger's Theory of Culture Care Diversity and Universality

Madeleine Leininger is the founder of transcultural nursing and leads the systematic study of human caring within a transcultural context. In addition, she initiated the Transcultural Nursing Society, a worldwide organization devoted to the study and practice of transcultural nursing care.

"The idea of transcultural nursing, the theory of Culture Care, and preserving care as the essence of nursing," Leininger (1991a) explained, "developed together in the mid-1950s and early 1960s" (p. 14). Leininger (1988, 1991a) noted that her early clinical work with disturbed children was the catalyst for her idea of transcultural nursing. Elaborating, she stated:

> The idea for the theory began while studying the role of the clinical specialist in child psychiatric nursing in 1954 and while documenting the ways that care and nursing practice could accurately describe and reflect nursing knowledge. (1988, p. 152)

> The behavior and nursing care needs of African, Jewish, Appalachian, German, and Anglo-American children were clearly different except for some physical care needs. In a way, I experienced cultural shock and I felt helpless to assist children who so clearly expressed different cultural patterns and ways they wanted care. These cultural differences were related to playing, eating, sleeping, interaction, and many

other areas of their daily care. The children were so expressive and persistent in what they wanted or needed, yet I was unable to respond appropriately to them—I did not understand their behavior. Later, I came to learn that their behavior was culturally constituted and influenced their mental health. (1991a, p. 14)

Leininger (1991a) also explained that her theory is based on her predictions that although diverse cultural phenomena exist worldwide, some phenomena are universal. Moreover, she proposed that "human care practices existed in all human cultures since the beginning of Homo sapiens, but their manifestations and uses remained undiscovered" (p. 36). She further proposed that the knowledge of human care practices is discovered by studying the local, insider, generic folk, or *emic*, knowledge that is "derived from the *people*" (p. 36). Viewed from that perspective, the nurse's knowledge is outsider, or *etic*, knowledge.

Although Leininger began to publish her ideas regarding culture and care many years ago, one of the earliest formal presentations of the theory, then called Transcultural Care Diversity and Universality, was in a 1985 journal article. Another formal presentation of the theory was in a 1988 journal article under the title "Cultural Care Diversity and Universality." In a recent (1991a) definitive work on it, the theory is titled "Culture Care Diversity and Universality."

The concepts of the Theory of Culture Care Diversity and Universality are listed below. Each concept is defined and described later in this chapter.

KEY CONCEPTS

Care	Worldview
Caring	Cultural Care
Culture	Cultural Care Diversity
Cultural and Social Structure	Cultural Care Universality
Dimensions	Care Systems
Technological Factors	Generic Lay Care System
Religious and	Professional Health Care
Philosophical Factors	System
Kinship and Social Factors	Cultural-Congruent Nursing
Political and Legal Factors	Care
Economic Factors	Cultural Care Preservation
Educational Factors	or Maintenance
Cultural Values and	Cultural Care
Lifeways	Accommodation or
Language	Negotiation
Ethnohistory	Cultural Care Repatterning
Environmental Context	or Restructuring
Holistic Health (Well-Being)	

ANALYSIS OF THE THEORY OF CULTURE CARE DIVERSITY AND UNIVERSALITY

This section presents an analysis of Leininger's theory. The analysis is based on Leininger's publications about her theory, drawing primarily from her 1991 book chapter, "The Theory of Culture Care Diversity and Universality," as well as from her 1985 journal article, "Transcultural Care Diversity and Universality: A Theory of Nursing" and her 1988 journal article, "Leininger's Theory of Nursing: Cultural Care Diversity and Universality."

Scope of the Theory

The purpose of the Theory of Culture Care Diversity and Universality is, as Leininger (1991a) explained, "to discover human care diversities and universalities . . . and then to discover ways to provide culturally congruent care to people of different or similar cultures in order to maintain or regain their well-being, health, or face death in a culturally appropriate way" (p. 39). The central thesis of the theory is that "different cultures perceive, know, and practice care in different ways, yet there are some commonalities about care among all cultures in the world" (Leininger, 1985, p. 210).

The Theory of Culture Care Diversity and Universality is classified as a grand theory. That classification is supported by the stated purpose of the theory, which indicates that the theory is a guide for the generation of more specific middle-range theories of various cultures. The classification of grand theory is further supported by Leininger's (1991a) comments that her theory was "conceptualized to be used in the discovery of all cultures over time" (p. 41) and that the theory meets the need "to know and explain nursing worldwide" (p. 41).

Context of the Theory

Metaparadigm Concepts and Proposition

Leininger (1988, 1991a, 1991e) explicitly rejected the widely cited metaparadigm concepts of person, environment, health, and nursing and the associated propositions as the central focus of the discipline of nursing. Rather, she proposed a metaparadigm comprising the concepts "human care, environmental contexts, and well-being (or health)" (1991e, p. 406) and the proposition asserting that "Care is the essence of nursing and the central, dominant, and unifying focus of nursing" (1991a, p. 35).

Philosophical Claims

Leininger (1991a) claims allegiance to a holistic nursing perspective. She commented:

> I did not conceptualize culture care as a compartmentalized or fragmented idea with separate physical, biological, psychological, social, or cultural perspectives. Instead, I theorized culture and human care as a holistic and unified perspective to reflect individuals or groups of total caring lifeways or influencers on their well-being or illness. (p. 23)

The foundational philosophical claims undergirding the Theory of Culture Care Diversity and Universality are Leininger's (1991a) beliefs about nursing and culture care. She stated,

> Grounded in anthropological insights and the nature of nursing, I believed that nursing was a transcultural care phenomenon and a lived experience. (p. 40)

Culture care, Leininger (1991a) believes,

> provides a distinctive feature by which to know, interpret, and explain nursing as a discipline and profession . . . [as well as] the substantive knowledge to know, explain, interpret, predict, and legitimize nursing as a discipline and profession. (p. 35)

Specific philosophical claims undergirding the Theory of Culture Care Diversity and Universality are evident in some of Leininger's (1985) "philosophical and epistemological assumptions, [which were] largely derived from anthropology, but with new and reformulated statements to describe, interpret, and predict nursing" (p. 210). Those claims are:

1. Care has been essential for human survival, development, and to face critical or recurrent life events such as illness, disability, and death.
2. Humans are caring beings capable of being concerned about, holding interest in, or having regard for other people's needs, well-being, [and] survival.
3. Humans are cultural beings who have survived through time and place because of their ability to care for infants, young, and older adults in a variety of environments and ways.
4. Human care is universal; yet there are diverse expressions, meanings, patterns (or lifestyles), and action modalities.
5. Nursing is essentially a transcultural care profession in that nurses provide nursing care to people of different cultures; yet nurses do not fully value or practice this perspective.
6. Nursing must be based upon transcultural care knowledge and skill to be effective, legitimate, and relevant to people of diverse cultures in the world.
7. Culturally based nursing care is the critical factor for determining

health promotion and maintenance, and recovery from illness and disability.

8. There can be no effective cure without care, but there may be care without cure.
9. Human care patterns, conditions, and actions are largely based upon cultural care values, beliefs, and practices of particular cultures, and of the universal nature of humans as caring beings.
10. Care expressions, patterns, and lifestyles take on different meanings in different cultural contexts.
11. All human cultures have folk and professional health care practices. (p. 210)

In a later publication, Leininger (1991a) made several statements, which she labeled "assumptive premises," that can be used to "guide nurses in their discovery of Culture Care phenomena" (p. 44). Several of those statements represent additional philosophical claims undergirding the Theory of Culture Care Diversity and Universality. Other "assumptive premises" represent theoretical propositions and will, therefore, be presented in the theory content section of this chapter. The assumptive premises that represent philosophical claims are:

1. Care (caring) is essential for well-being, health, healing, growth, survival, and to face handicaps or death.
2. Culture care is the broadest holistic means to know, explain, interpret, and predict nursing care phenomena to guide nursing care practices.
3. Nursing is a transcultural humanistic and scientific care discipline and profession with the central purpose to serve human beings worldwide.
4. Care (caring) is essential to curing and healing, for there can be no curing without caring.
5. Culturally congruent or beneficial nursing care can only occur when the individual, group, family, community, or culture care values, expressions, or patterns are known and used appropriately and in meaningful ways by the nurse with the people.
6. Culture care differences and similarities between professional caregiver(s) and client (generic) care-receiver(s) exist in any human culture worldwide. (pp. 44–45)

Another philosophical claim was extracted from one of Leininger's publications: "People are born, live, become ill, and die within a cultural belief and practice system, but are dependent upon human care for growth and survival" (1988, p. 155).

Two additional statements represent the philosophical claims on which the research methodology associated with the Theory of Culture Care Diversity and Universality rests:

1. The qualitative paradigm provides new ways of knowing and different ways to discover epistemic and ontological dimensions of human care transculturally. (Leininger, 1991a, p. 45)

2. Care phenomen[a] can be discovered by examining social structure, language, and the world view of cultural groups. (Leininger,
1985, p. 210)

Examination reveals that Leininger's philosophical claims reflect
the *reciprocal interaction* worldview. That classification is supported by
Leininger's (1991a) statements that her work does not reflect "causal,
linear, or logical positivistic relationships, or a rigid social structure system perspective" (p. 50), and that "all care modalities require *coparticipation of nurse and clients (consumers) working together* to identify,
plan, implement, and evaluate each caring mode for culturally congruent nursing care" (p. 44).

Conceptual Model

Although Leininger (1991a) rejected the metaparadigm concepts of
person, environment, health, and nursing, she has formulated descriptions of those terms that, taken together, represent the conceptual
model on which the Theory of Culture Care Diversity and Universality
is based. The person is viewed as an individual human caring and cultural being, as well as a family, a group, a social institution, or a culture
(Leininger, 1985, 1988, 1991a).

The environment is, according to Leininger (1991a), "very important to nursing" (p. 40). She has referred to the environment as physical
or ecological and views it as a context "in which individuals and cultural groups live" (personal communication cited in Luna & Cameron,
1989, p. 230). Health, for Leininger (1985, 1991a), encompasses a broad
spectrum of conditions, including well-being, illness, disability, and
handicap.

Leininger (1991a) conceptualizes nursing "as a transcultural
human care discipline and profession," and caring as "a universal feature of nursing in all nursing cultures" (p. 26). Nursing is explicitly
defined as

> a learned humanistic and scientific profession and discipline which is
> focused on human care phenomena and activities in order to assist,
> support, facilitate, or enable individuals or groups to maintain or
> regain their well-being (or health) in culturally meaningful and bene-
> ficial ways, or to help people face handicaps or death. (p. 47)

Antecedent Knowledge

Leininger's early clinical experiences as a child psychiatric mental
health nurse, her formal study of anthropology, and her own ethnographic and ethnonursing studies were the major influences on the
development of the Theory of Culture Care Diversity and Universality.

No one person or existing theory served as antecedent knowledge. In her explanation of influences on the theory, Leininger (1991a) commented:

> I am frequently asked what nurses, persons, or ideologies influenced my thinking. I would have to answer, rather candidly, that there was no one person or philosophic school of thought, or ideology *per se* that directly influenced my thinking. I developed the theory by working on the potential interrelationships of culture and care through creative thinking, and by philosophizing from my past professional nursing experiences and anthropological insights. (p. 20)

Furthermore, Leininger (1991a) pointed out that she avoided "choosing a particular school of thought from psychobiology, anthropology, or nursing" (p. 23). Instead, she selectively drew on theoretical ideas about culture from anthropology and about care from nursing.

Leininger (1991a) did, however, acknowledge several scholars whose "critical thinking was helpful" (p. 20), including Professors Fogelson, Spiro, Read, Watson, and Jacobs of the University of Washington Department of Anthropology. She also acknowledged the contributions of Margaret Mead to her thinking, as well as her "frequent scholarly dialogues" (p. 21) with students and faculty of the University of Washington School of Nursing, especially with Dorothy Crowley, Oliver Osborne, Delores Little, and Beverly Horn.

Moreover, in her 1970 book, Leininger noted that "most anthropological theories, concepts, and research findings about man have direct or indirect relevance to nursing" (p. 27). She identified the following specific contributions that anthropology could make to nursing:

1. The concept of man's existence and development from a longitudinal perspective.
2. The cross-cultural and comparative perspective of man.
3. The culture concept.
4. The holistic and cultural context approach in the understanding of man.
5. The realization that health and illness states are strongly influenced and often primarily determined by the cultural background of an individual.
6. The cross-cultural anthropological insights into child-rearing and socialization processes of cultural groups.
7. The participant-observation field-study method.
8. Linguistic knowledge about comparative and descriptive language forms and their meanings. (pp. 18–26)

In addition, Leininger (1991b) acknowledged and cited Pike's notion of emic and etic. She commented, "In the late 1950s, I learned by chance about Pike's (1954) use of the terms 'emic' and 'etic' in linguistic studies and thought that they would be most helpful to explicate and understand human care transculturally" (p. 77).

The specific content of the Theory of Culture Care Diversity and Universality was induced not only from Leininger's knowledge of anthropology and her perspective of nursing, but also from her own research findings. She commented, "From several mini studies . . . I had discovered that culture care phenomena were largely embedded in the worldview, religious (or spiritual), kinship, and other areas of the social structure" (1991a, p. 35).

Content of the Theory

Analysis of Leininger's publications revealed that the concepts of the Theory of Culture Care Diversity and Universality are *care, caring, culture, language, ethnohistory, environmental context, holistic health (well-being), worldview, cultural care, care systems,* and *cultural-congruent nursing care.* Leininger has continued to refine the definitions of those concepts over the years. Unless otherwise noted, the definitions given here were taken from her 1991a book chapter.

Care, which Leininger uses as a noun, "refers to abstract and concrete phenomena related to assisting, supporting, or enabling experiences or behaviors toward or for others with evident or anticipated needs to ameliorate or improve a human condition or lifeway" (p. 46).

Caring, which Leininger (1988, 1991a) has referred to as a verb and a gerund, "refers to the actions and activities directed toward assisting, supporting, or enabling another individual or group with evident or anticipated needs to ameliorate or improve a human condition or lifeway or to face death" (1991a, p. 46).

Culture "refers to the learned, shared, and transmitted values, beliefs, norms, and lifeways of a particular group that guides thinking, decisions, and actions in patterned ways" (p. 47). The concept culture encompasses several *cultural and social structure dimensions.* Collectively, the dimensions refer to "the dynamic patterns and features of interrelated structural and organizational factors of a particular culture (subculture or society) . . . and how these factors may be interrelated and function to influence human behavior in different environmental contexts" (p. 47). Leininger identified the specific dimensions as *technological factors, religious and philosophical factors, kinship and social factors, political and legal factors, economic factors, educational,* and *cultural values and lifeways.* The definitions for those dimensions were not given.

Language is mentioned by Leininger (1991a, p. 45) but is not explicitly defined. She has also referred to a "linguistic context" (1985, p. 209) and "language usages, symbols, and meanings about care" (1988, p. 155).

Ethnohistory "refers to those past facts, events, instances, experiences of individuals, groups, cultures, and institutions that are primarily people-centered (ethno) and which describe, explain, and interpret human lifeways within particular cultural contexts and over short or long periods of time" (p. 48).

Environmental context "refers to the totality of an event, situation, or particular experiences that give meaning to human expressions, interpretations, and social interactions in particular physical, ecological, sociopolitical and/or cultural settings" (p. 48).

Holistic health (well-being) is not explicitly defined. Health "refers to a state of well-being that is culturally defined, valued, and practiced, and which reflects the ability of individuals (or groups) to perform their daily role activities in culturally expressed, beneficial, and patterned lifeways" (1991a, p. 48).

Worldview "refers to the way people tend to look out on the world or their universe to form a picture of or a value stance about their life or world around them" (p. 47).

Cultural care "refers to the subjectively and objectively transmitted values, beliefs, and patterned lifeways that assist, support, or enable another individual or group to maintain their well-being, health, to improve their human condition and lifeway, to deal with illness, handicaps, or death" (p. 47). The two dimensions of culture care are *cultural care diversity* and *cultural care universality*.

Cultural care diversity "refers to the variabilities and/or differences in meanings, patterns, values, lifeways, or symbols of care within or between collectivities that are related to assistive, supportive, or enabling human care expressions" (p. 47).

Cultural care universality "refers to the common, similar, or dominant uniform care meanings, patterns, values, lifeways or symbols that are manifest among many cultures and reflect assistive, supportive, facilitative, or enabling ways to help people" (p. 47).

Care systems, per se, is not defined. Leininger (1985) did, however, provide a definition for health systems. She stated, "Health system(s) refers to the values, norms, and structural features of an organization designed for serving people's health needs, concerns, or conditions" (p. 209). There are two dimensions of the concept care systems: *generic lay care* and *professional health care system.*

The *generic lay care system,* also called a folk, indigenous, or naturalistic lay care system "refers to traditional or local indigenous health care or cure practices that have special meanings and uses to heal or assist people, which are generally offered in familiar home or community environmental contexts with their local practitioners" (1988, p. 156). Generic care (caring) "refers to culturally learned and transmitted lay, indigenous (traditional) or folk (home care) knowledge and skills used to provide assistive, supportive, enabling, facilitative acts (or phenomena) toward or for another individual, group or institution with evident or anticipated needs to ameliorate or improve a human health condition (or well-being), disability, lifeway, or to face death" (1991a, p. 38).

The *professional health care system* "refers to professional care or cure services offered by diverse health personnel who have been prepared through formal professional programs of study in special educational institutions" (1988, p. 156). Professional *nursing care (caring)* "refers to formal and cognitively learned professional care knowledge and practice skills obtained through educational institutions that are used to provide assistive, supportive, enabling or facilitative acts to or for another individual or group in order to improve a human health condition (or well being), disability, lifeway, or to work with dying clients" (1991a, p. 38).

Cultural-congruent nursing care "refers to those cognitively based assistive, supportive, facilitative, or enabling acts or decisions that are tailor-made to fit with individual, group, or institutional cultural values, beliefs, and lifeways in order to provide or support meaningful, beneficial, and satisfying health care, or well-being services" (p. 49). The three modes of cultural congruent nursing care, which are the dimensions of the concept, are *cultural care preservation or maintenance, cultural care accommodation or negotiation,* and *cultural care repatterning or restructuring.*

Cultural care preservation or maintenance "refers to those assistive, supportive, facilitative, or enabling professional actions and decisions that help people of a particular culture to retain and/or preserve relevant care values so that they can maintain their well being, recover from illness, or face handicaps and/or death" (p. 48).

Cultural care accommodation or negotiation "refers to those assistive, supportive, facilitative, or enabling creative professional actions and decisions that help people of a designated culture to adapt to, or to negotiate with, others for a beneficial or satisfying health outcome with professional care providers" (p. 48).

Cultural care repatterning or restructuring "refers to those assistive, supportive, facilitative, or enabling professional actions and decisions that help a client(s) reorder, change, or greatly modify their lifeways for a new, different and beneficial health care pattern while respecting the client(s) cultural values and beliefs and still providing a beneficial or healthier lifeway than before the changes were coestablished with the client(s)" (p. 49).

Nonrelational Propositions

The definitions of the concepts of the Theory of Culture Care Diversity and Universality are the primary nonrelational propositions of the theory. Other nonrelational propositions, which provide additional descriptive content to the concepts, were extracted from Leininger's 1991a book chapter. One proposition focuses on *cultural care*, asserting:

> The primacy of people relying on culture care, (generic or professional care expectations) was crucial to help people remain well, function, or survive each day. (p. 38)

Another proposition makes an assertion regarding the cultural care dimensions of *cultural care diversity* and *cultural care universality*. That proposition states:

> Culture care concepts, meanings, expressions, patterns, processes, and structural forms of care are different (diversity) and similar (towards commonalities or universalities) among all cultures of the world. (p. 45)

Two other propositions provide descriptions of the two dimensions of the concept *care systems*:

> Every human culture has generic (lay, folk, or indigenous) care knowledge and practices and usually professional care knowledge and practices which vary transculturally. (p. 45)

> The folk and professional health care systems were predicated to influence greatly the individual['s] or group['s] access to and quality of care rendered to people in favorable or less favorable ways. These two major types of health systems were capable of providing human care that was healthy, satisfying, beneficial and congruent with the clients' culture care values and needs. (p. 37)

Still another proposition focuses on *cultural-congruent nursing care*:

> Clients who experience nursing care that fails to be reasonably congruent with the client's beliefs, values, and caring lifeways will show signs of cultural conflicts, noncompliance, stresses, and ethical or moral concerns. (p. 45)

Relational Propositions

Relational propositions are depicted in the Sunrise Model (Fig. 3–1). Leininger (1985) explained that the model symbolizes "rising of the sun (care)" (p. 210). The upper portion of the circle displays the worldview and cultural and social dimensions "that influence care and health through language and environment[al] context" (p. 210). The lower part of the diagram shows the care systems and the dimensions or modalities of cultural-congruent nursing care. Together, "the upper and lower parts of the model depict a full sun—or the universe that nurses must consider to know human care and health" (p. 210).

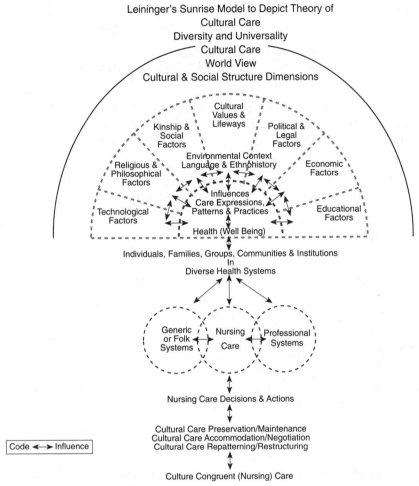

Leininger's Sunrise Model to Depict Theory of
Cultural Care
Diversity and Universality

Figure 3–1. Leininger's Sunrise Model. (From *Culture Care Diversity and Universality: A Theory of Nursing* (p. 43) by M. M. Leininger, 1991, New York: National League for Nursing. Copyright 1991 by the National League for Nursing. Reprinted by permission.)

The double-headed arrows in the diagram (↔) symbolize "influencers, but are not causal or linear relationships. The arrows flow in different areas and across major factors to depict the interrelatedness of factors and the fluidity of influencers" (Leininger, 1991a, p. 53). The broken lines (— — —) "indicate an open world or an open system of living reflective of the natural world of most humans" (p. 53).

The Sunrise Model illustrates the many reciprocal relationships among the concepts of the Theory of Culture Care Diversity and Universality. More specifically, the diagram depicts the whole of *cultural* care and illustrates that the *worldview* that people use to form a picture or value stance about their lives and the world about them influences and is influenced by the *cultural and social structure dimensions (technological, religious and philosophical, kinship and social, political and legal, economic, and educational factors; cultural values and lifeways)*. The cultural and social structure dimensions, along with *environmental context, language,* and *ethnohistory,* influence and are influenced by care expressions, patterns, and practices, which influence and are influenced by the *holistic health* or well-being of individuals, families, groups, communities and institutions, which influence and are influenced by the *generic lay* and *professional care systems,* which in turn influence and are influenced by nursing care decisions and actions, which influence and are influenced by the three dimensions or modes of *cultural-congruent nursing care.* The Sunrise Model also depicts the influences that the cultural and social structure dimensions have on one another.

Other relational propositions were extracted from Leininger's (1991a) book chapter. Links between *cultural care,* the *cultural and social structure dimensions* of the concept culture, and *environmental context* are evident in one relational proposition:

> To fully understand and predict culture caring, the nurse would need to use care data as influenced by religion, kinship, language, technology, economics, education (formal and informal), cultural values and beliefs, and the physical (ecological) environment. (p. 38)

Another relational proposition describes the linkage of *cultural care* with *worldview, language,* the *cultural and social structure dimensions* of the concept culture, *ethnohistory,* and *environmental context:*

> Cultural care values, beliefs, and practices are influenced by and tend to be embedded in the worldview, language, religious (or spiritual), kinship (social), political (or legal), educational, economic, technological, ethnohistorical, and environmental context of a particular culture. (p. 45)

The link between *care systems* and *cultural-congruent* care is evident in the following relational proposition:

> Combining generic and professional care could lead to people seeking health care services to receiving culturally congruent care. (p. 37)

Still another relational proposition links *cultural-congruent nursing care* with *health (well-being)* and *environmental context* by asserting:

> Beneficial, healthy, and satisfying culturally based nursing care contributes to the well being of individuals, families, groups, and communities within their environmental context. (p. 45)

EVALUATION OF THE THEORY OF CULTURE CARE DIVERSITY AND UNIVERSALITY

This section presents an evaluation of Leininger's Theory of Culture Care Diversity and Universality. The evaluation is based on the results of the analysis of the theory as well as on publications by others who have used or commented on this nursing theory.

Significance

Leininger (1988, 1991a) explicitly cited the metaparadigmatic origins of the Theory of Culture Care Diversity and Universality as human care, environmental context, and well-being. Moreover, she identified the philosophical basis for the theory in a series of philosophical and epistemological assumptions and assumptive premises. The analysis revealed, however, that some statements labeled by Leininger as assumptive premises were, in fact, propositions of the theory. Additional philosophical claims dealing with Leininger's beliefs about holistic nursing, culture care, and the research methodology associated with the theory were easily extracted from her publications.

Leininger did not explicitly describe the conceptual basis for the Theory of Culture Care Diversity and Universality as a conceptual model of nursing. She did, however, provide descriptions of the components of conceptual models of nursing, including person, environment, health, and nursing.

The Theory of Culture Care Diversity and Universality is a distinctive nursing theory. The theory was not, as Leininger (1991a) pointed out, "'borrowed' from anthropology, but developed anew and had to be studied within nursing views to discover the epistemic and ontological dimensions of knowledge predicted to influence well-being and health" (p. 24). With the exception of Pike (1954), Leininger did not cite specific sources of antecedent knowledge in the form of publications by scholars in anthropology and nursing, but she did acknowledge the influence of several scholars, by name, on her thinking.

Leininger's many publications about culture and her theory have had a substantial impact on nursing. Leininger (1991a) claims she realized many years ago that "When brought into teaching, curriculum, administration, clinical community practices, consultation, and nursing research, transcultural care knowledge would lead to near revolutionary changes" (p. 41). Certainly, interest in international nursing and attention to multiculturalism have expanded greatly since Leininger began to publish her ideas about the importance of culture in the 1960s (Leininger, 1991f; Mandelbaum, 1991; Meleis, 1989).

Speaking to the significance of Leininger's theory, Cohen (1991) stated:

Leininger utilized her anthropological roots to provide nursing with a way to study caring that takes into account people's culture, values, beliefs, patterns and lifeways and to provide culturally congruent care. This is especially noteworthy in a time when the world is growing smaller and our own society is comprised of many diverse cultures. . . . [Her theory has] increased awareness of cultural diversity as well as universality and [has] decreased ethnocentricity in the delivery of care within agencies and within the community. (pp. 907–908)

The special significance of the Theory of Culture Care Diversity and Universality, then, lies in the theory's contributions to understanding the influence of culture on people's experiences of health. Leininger (1991a) views her work as "the major theory to explain much of the phenomena related to transcultural nursing, accounting for diverse and similar cultures in the world" (p. 29). A special feature of the theory is the distinction between generic (indigenous or folk) care and professional nursing care.

Internal Consistency

The Theory of Culture Care Diversity and Universality is congruent with the philosophical claims and conceptual model on which it is based. Semantic clarity is evident in the explicit definitions that Leininger provided for most of the concepts of the Theory of Culture Care Diversity and Universality and their dimensions. Language is not defined, although the definition seems self-evident. Moreover, none of the cultural and social structure dimensions of the concept of culture are defined, although again those definitions seem self-evident. In addition, holistic health is not defined, but a clear definition of health is provided.

Semantic consistency is evident within each major publication of the theory (Leininger, 1985, 1988, 1991a). Some inconsistencies are, however, evident from publication to publication. The term care systems was used in the 1991a publication, but it was health systems in the 1985 and 1988 publications. Furthermore, the concept care (health) systems had three dimensions in the 1985 publication—folk system, professional system, and nursing system—but just two dimensions in the 1988 publications—folk health (well-being) system and professional health system. Moreover, the folk health system was labeled the folk, indigenous, generic, or naturalistic lay care system in the 1991a publication.

There are no concept redundancies. Each concept refers to a distinct, albeit related, phenomenon.

The analysis of the Theory of Culture Care Diversity and Universality revealed structural consistency in the form of adequate linkages among the concepts of the theory. The Sunrise Model clearly depicts linkages among the theory concepts. Indeed, the Sunrise Model achieves its stated purpose, which is "to depict a total view of the different but very closely related dimensions of the theory [and] to orient and depict the influencing dimensions, components, facets, or major concepts of the theory with an integrated total view of these dimensions" (Leininger, 1991a, p. 49). Leininger has not, however, explicated the relational propositions depicted in the Sunrise Model in narrative form. Other linkages between theory concepts were specified in relational propositions that were extracted from Leininger's publications.

Parsimony

The Theory of Culture Care Diversity and Universality is relatively parsimonious. The theory encompasses many concepts, but each one is necessary to convey Leininger's ideas effectively. The analysis of the theory yielded a more parsimonious presentation of the theory than might be expected from the list of 18 terms that Leininger (1991a) defined. The more parsimonious presentation was accomplished by categorizing some terms as dimensions of others. In particular, the definition given for cultural and social structure dimensions clearly identifies those dimensions as components of the concept culture. Similarly, it was clear that cultural care preservation or maintenance, cultural care accommodation or negotiation, and cultural care repatterning or restructuring are dimensions of the concept cultural-congruent nursing care. Finally, the definitions for generic and professional care systems clearly indicated that the two are dimensions of the concept care systems.

Testability

The Theory of Culture Care Diversity and Universality is not testable in the usual deductive meaning denoted by the term. Rather, use of a qualitative inductive research methodology that is based on the Sunrise Model of the theory yields empirical knowledge of culture care. Leininger (1991a) explained, "I envisioned the discovery of culture care knowledge as an evolutionary process largely from an inductive qualitative approach to obtain the people's viewpoints and experiences" (p. 31). More specifically, the theory "is used primarily to generate new knowledge or to gain different insights about care of diverse cultures" (p. 158). Consequently, middle-range theories of culture care are generated by means of a qualitative research method, called ethnonursing research, that is congruent with the Theory of Culture Care Diversity and Universality. Theory testing occurs as the findings of research are used in practice.

Accordingly, the purposes of research for Leininger (1991a) are to "explicate, detail, and get meanings of culture care, patterns, expressions, and practices" (p. 34), and "to discover how people cognitively knew, described, and interpreted care within their total culture lifeways, beliefs, and environment" (p. 34). The specific purpose of the ethnonursing research method is "to establish a naturalistic and largely emic open inquiry discovery method to explicate and study nursing phenomena especially related to the Theory of Culture Care Diversity and Universality" (Leininger, 1991b, p. 75).

The phenomena of interest are "emic people-based (inside culture) knowledge" (1991a, p. 34), including "human care, well-being, and health and environmental influencers" (1991b, p. 75). Leininger explained, "Getting to the people's emic views was extremely important, more important than emphasizing the researcher's etic or externally derived presumed and pre-set specific ideas" (1991a, p. 34). Use of the ethnonursing research method, then, enables the investigator "to learn from informants in their natural environmental contexts about their known or covert aspects of human care" (1991a, p. 35).

The Sunrise Model (Fig. 3–1) provides a general structure for research. Leininger (1991a) explained:

> The researcher begins with the worldview and works from the top to the bottom of the Sunrise Model. But it is possible that the nurse researcher may want to begin the exploration by focusing on care and nursing in the professional system (lower part of the model). The nurse, therefore, would study care of individuals or groups in the hospitals or homes, and gradually move the exploration to worldview, cultural, and social structural dimensions, and cover kinship, religion, and other areas depicted in the model. At the same time, the researcher remains focused on the domain of study and moves within a rough research plan influenced by how the research unfolds to obtain *emic* data from the informants and culture context. Frequently, the researcher starts at the top of the model with the worldview and social structure features and then gradually explores the professional and generic health care systems as well as possible modes of nursing actions and decisions. (pp. 50–51)

Data are collected by means of "enablers." Leininger (1991b) uses that term in preference to "instruments," which she regards as "too impersonal, mechanistic, and [fitting] with objectification, experimentation, and other methods and logical features of the quantitative paradigm" (p. 91). Specific enablers developed by Leininger (1991b) are the Stranger-Friend Model, the Observation-Participation-Reflection Model, the Phases of Ethnonursing Data Analysis Guide, the Acculturation Enabler Guide, the Life History Health Care Enabler, the Cultural Care Values and Meanings Enabler, the Culturalogical Care Assessment Guide, an audio-visual guide, and the Generic and Professional Care Enabler Guide. Leininger (1991b) noted that researchers may use one or more of those enablers or develop other enablers for in-depth studies based on the Theory of Culture Care Diversity and Universality. Data collection, processing, and analysis are facilitated by use of the Leininger-Templin-Thompson Ethnoscript Qualitative Software program (Leininger, 1990, 1991b).

The ethnonursing research method requires "a keen sense of ethical rights of informants" (1991a, p. 56). The method also requires certain skills that are learned by working with a research mentor and participating in seminars that emphasize the methodological and ethical aspects of qualitative research. Leininger (1991b) pointed out that "The challenge is to be an interested friend of the people and to participate with them in discovering their past and current cultural beliefs, values, and ideas about human care, health, well being, and other nursing dimensions" (p. 85). Another challenge is to be "able to tolerate highly ambiguous, uncertain, subjective, or vaguely known complex sets of ideas" (p. 86). Most of all, the researcher must have "patience, time, and a genuine interest in others" (p. 86). In addition, the researcher must adhere to the following requirements:

1. The researcher should seek a mentor who has experience with the ethnonursing research method.
2. The researcher must move into familiar and naturalistic people settings.
3. The researcher must have the appropriate language skills to communicate with the people in the culture and to interpret ideas and written documents.
4. The researcher must use unstructured open-ended inquiries and must be an astute observer, listener, reflector, and accuract interpreter by taking a learner's role in the most natural way possible. More specifically,
   a. The researcher must maintain an open discovery, active listening, and a genuine learning attitude in working with informants.
   b. The researcher must maintain an active and curious posture about the "why" of whatever is seen, heard, or experienced, and with appreciation of whatever informants share.
   c. The researcher must record whatever is shared by informants in a careful and conscientious way for full meanings, explanations, or interpretations to preserve informant ideas.
5. The researcher must withhold, suspend, or control personal biases, prejudices, opinions, and preprofessional interpretations.
6. The researcher must focus on the cultural context of the phenomena being studied. (Leininger, 1991b, pp. 85–87, 106–108, 111)

Leininger (1991b) noted that other qualitative research methods can be combined with ethnonursing if absolutely necessary. She claimed that compatible methods include life histories, ethnography, phenomenology, and ethnoscience.

Leininger (1991a) maintained that "specific theoretical hypotheses, positions, or tightly constructed theoretical formulations were not used [because they] would be incongruent with the inductive open discovery process" (p. 46). Despite that claim, she did offer several statements that represent testable hypotheses derived from the Theory of Culture Care Diversity and Universality. The central testable hypothesis of the theory is "While there would be diverse culture care patterns, processes, meanings, attributes, functions, and structure[s] of care worldwide, some universals also would exist." (Leininger, 1991a, p. 36)

More specifically, Leininger (1985) hypothesized that

> There are fewer universal care patterns, processes, and acts than care diversities because of human variabilities, conditions, and changing lifestyles of people. However, with rapid worldwide diffusion of information, acculturation processes, and human choices, it is predicted there will be more universal patterns than diversity care patterns by the next century. (p. 210)

Interestingly, if Leininger's prediction of more universal care patterns in the future holds true, the need for a theory focused on both universals and diversities might be eliminated.

Other statements, which Leininger (1985) labeled relational propositions, are also testable hypotheses. Those statements are:

- There is an identifiable, positive relationship between the way people of different cultures define, interpret, and know care with their recurrent patterns of thinking and living.
- The emic (inside views) of cultural care values, beliefs, and practices of cultures will show a close relationship to their daily life care patterns.
- The meaning and use of cultural care concepts varies cross-culturally and influences nursing caregiver and carereceiver practices.
- There is a meaningful relationship between social structure factors and worldview with folk and professional care practices.
- Nursing care subsubsystems [sic] are closely related to professional health care systems but differ markedly from folk health care systems.
- Nursing care decisions or actions that reflect the use of the client's cultural care values, beliefs, and practices will be positively related to [the] client's satisfactions with nursing care.
- Nursing care actions or decisions that are based on the use of cultural care preservation, accommodation, and/or repatterning in client care will be positively related to beneficial nursing care.
- Signs of intercultural care conflicts and stresses will be evident if caregivers fail to use cultural care values and beliefs of clients.
- Marked difference between the meanings and expressions of caregivers and carerecipients leads to dissatisfactions for both.

- High dependency of the clients on technological nursing care activities will be closely related to cultural care that reflects decreased personalized care actions.
- Religion and kinship care factors will be more resilient to change than technological factors.
- Western views of cultural care values will be markedly different from non-Western care values.
- Self-care practices will be evident in cultures that value individualism and independence; other-care practices will be evident in cultures that support human interdependence.
- Anglo-American nurse-client teaching methods will be dysfunctional with clients of non-Western cultural value orientations. (pp. 210, 212)

Empirical Adequacy

Inasmuch as the Theory of Culture Care Diversity and Universality is a grand theory, the evaluation of empirical adequacy focuses not on generalization of research findings but rather on the middle-range theory-generating capabilities of the grand theory. From that perspective, the theory can be said to be empirically adequate.

More specifically, a review of research derived from the Theory of Culture Care Diversity and Universality and conducted between 1960 and 1991 revealed considerable empirical support in the form of middle-range theories that are descriptions of the culture care values, linguistic meanings, and action modes from 54 Western and non-Western cultures, as well as a taxonomy of 175 care constructs identified in the study of those cultures (Leininger, 1991d). Summaries of the findings from studies of 23 cultures conducted by Leininger, her students, and other researchers were prepared by Leininger (1991d). Two of those summaries are presented in Table 3–1. The findings regarding the Gadsup Akuna of the Eastern Highlands of New Guinea were taken from the first transcultural care study, which was conducted by Leininger in the early 1960s with subsequent visits in later years. A detailed description of the study findings, presented within the context of the Theory of Culture Care Diversity and Universality, is available in Leininger (1991c). The findings regarding the Philippine-American culture are from studies by Spangler (1991, 1992) and other transcultural nurse researchers. Informants had lived in the United States for at least two decades. The other cultures represented in the summaries are middle- and upper-class Anglo-American, old-order Amish-American, Appalachian, North American Indian, southeast American Indian, Mexican-American, Haitian-American, African-American, Japanese-American, Vietnamese-American, Chinese-American, Arab-American Muslim, Polish-American, German-American, Italian-American, Greek-American, Jewish-American, Lithuanian-American, Swedish-American,

TABLE 3–1.   Summaries of the Findings of Two Studies Based on the Theory of Culture Care Diversity and Universality

Cultural Values Are:	*Culture Care Meanings and Action Modes Are:*
Gadsup Akuna of the Eastern Highlands of New Guinea	
1. Egalitarianism	1. Surveillance (to prevent sorcery)
2. Marked sex role differences	—nearby surveillance
3. Patriarchal descent recognized	—watch at a distance
4. Communal unity ("one vine"/ "line")	2. Protection (protective male caring) —of Gadsups through lifecycle
5. Prevent social accusations (sorcery)	—obeying cultural taboos and rules
6. Maintain ancestor "life-essence" and obligations	3. Nurturance —ways to help people grow and survive
7. Have "good women, children, pigs, and gardens"	—know what they need (anticipate needs) through lifecycle —eat safe foods
	4. Prevention (avoid breaking cultural taboos) to: —prevent illness and death —prevent intervillage fights and conflicts
	5. Touching
Philippine-American Culture	
1. Family unity and closeness	1. Maintain smooth relationships (Pakikisama)
2. Respect for elder/authority	
3. "Leave one-self to God" (Bahala na)	2. Save face and self-esteem (Amor propio); (Hiya—avoid shame)
4. Obligations to sociocultural ties	3. Respect for and deference to authority
5. Hot-cold beliefs	4. Being quiet; privacy
6. Use of folk foods and practices	5. Mutual reciprocity (Utang Na Loob) "the give and take" in relationships
7. Religion valued (mainly Roman Catholic)	6. Giving comfort to others
	7. Tenderness
	8. Being pleasant as possible

Source: From Leininger, 1991d, p. 358, with permission.

Finnish-American, and Danish-American. Descriptions of all published studies based on the theory are given in the annotated bibliography at the end of this chapter.

The 175 care constructs, which are listed in Table 3–2, represent care and/or caring meanings and action modes from the 54 cultures studied. Leininger (1991d) explained that "The cultural informants [from each culture] identified four or five dominant care constructs with their key meanings and action modes. None of the cultures identified more than eight major constructs" (p. 368)

TABLE 3–2. Care/Caring Constructs Derived from Studies Based on the Theory of Culture Care Diversity of Universality

Care and/or Caring Meanings and Action Modes

1. Acceptance
2. Accommodating
3. Accountability
4. Action(ing) for/about/with
5. Adapting to
6. Affection for
7. Alleviation (pain/suffering)
8. Anticipation (ing)
9. Assist (ing) others
10. Attention to/toward
11. Attitude toward
12. Being nonassertive
13. Being aware of others
14. Being authentic (real)
15. Being clean
16. Being genuine
17. Being involved
18. Being kind/pleasant
19. Being orderly
20. Being present
21. Being watchful
22. Bribing
23. Care (caring)
24. *Caritas* (charity)
25. Cleanliness
26. Closeness to
27. Cognitively knowing
28. Comfort (ing)
29. Commitment to/for
30. Communication (ing)
31. Community awareness
32. Compassion (ate)
33. Compliance with
34. Concern for/about/with
35. Congruence with
36. Connectedness
37. Consideration of
38. Consultation (ing)
39. Controlling
40. Communion with another
41. Cooperation
42. Coordination (ing)
43. Coping with/for
44. Creative thinking/acts
45. Cultural care (ing)
46. Cure (ing)
47. Dependence
48. Direct help to others
49. Discernment
50. Doing for/with
51. Eating right foods
52. Enduring
53. Embodiment
54. Emotional support
55. Empathy
56. Enabling
57. Engrossment in/about
58. Establishing harmony
59. Engrossment in/about [sic]
60. Experiencing with
61. Expressing feelings
62. Faith (in others)
63. Family involvement
64. Family support
65. Feeling for/about
66. Filial love
67. Generosity toward others
68. Gentle (ness) and firmness
69. Giving to others in need
70. Giving comfort to
71. Group assistance
72. Group awareness
73. Growth promoting
74. Hands on
75. Harmony with
76. Healing
77. Health instruction
78. Health (well being)
79. Health maintenance
80. Helping self/others
81. Helping kin/group
82. Honor (ing)
83. Hope (fullness)
84. Hospitality
85. Improving conditions
86. Inclined toward
87. Indulgence from
88. Instruction (ing)
89. Integrity
90. Interest in/about
91. Intimacy/intimate
92. Involvement with/for
93. Kindness (being kind)
94. Knowing of culture
95. Knowing (another's reality)
96. Know cultural values/taboos
97. Limiting (set limits)
98. Listening to/about

TABLE 3–2.   Care/Caring Constructs Derived from Studies Based on the Theory of Culture Care Diversity of Universality (*Continued*)

Care and/or Caring Meanings and Action Modes

99. Loving (love others)	137. Responding to context
—Christian love	138. Responsible for others
100. Maintaining harmony	139. Restoration (ing)
101. Maintaining reciprocity	140. Sacrificing
102. Maintaining privacy	141. Saving face
103. Ministering to others	142. Self-reliant (reliance)
—filial love	143. Self-responsibility
104. Need fulfillment	144. Sensitivity to others' needs
105. Nurturance (nurture)	145. Serving others (*caritas*)
106. Obedience to	146. Sharing with others
107. Obligation to	147. Silence (use of)
108. Orderliness	148. Speaking the language
109. Other-care (ing) non-self-care	149. Spiritual healing
110. Patience	150. Spiritual relatedness
111. Performing rituals	151. Stimulation (ing)
112. Permitting expressions	152. Stress alleviation
113. Personalized acts	153. Succorance
114. Physical acts	154. Suffering with/for
115. Praying with	155. Support (ing)
116. Presence (being with)	156. Surveillance (watch for)
117. Preserving (preservation)	157. Symbols (ing)
118. Prevention (ing)	158. Sympathy
119. Promoting	159. Taking care of environment
120. Promoting independence	160. Technical skills
121. Protecting (other/self)	161. Techniques
122. Purging	162. Tenderness
123. Quietness	163. Timing actions/decisions
124. Reassurance	164. Touch (ing)
125. Receiving	165. Trust (ing)
126. Reciprocity	166. Understanding
127. Reflecting goodness	167. Use of folk foods/practices
128. Reflecting with/about	168. Use of limit setting
129. Rehabilitate	169. Using nursing knowledge
130. Regard for	170. Valuing another's ways
131. Relatedness to	171. Watchfulness
132. Respecting	172. Well-being (health)
133. Respect for/about lifeways	173. Well-being (family)
134. Respecting privacy/wishes	174. Wholeness approach
135. Respecting sex differences	175. Working hard
136. Responding appropriately	

Source: From Leininger, 1991d, pp. 368–370, with permission.

The research findings also revealed that:

1. There are more signs of diversities than universalities among the 54 cultures, especially between Western and non-Western cultures.
2. Culture care meanings and practices are difficult to tease out largely because they are embedded in the social structure, in non-

Western cultures especially in kinship, religious beliefs, and political factors; whereas in Western cultures care is viewed largely as high-tech tasks, cost factors, political decisions, and problems with language to understand clients' care needs.

3. The cultural context and care values make a major difference in how care is expressed and how care takes on meanings to clients and especially families or cultures.

4. Care meanings and their uses often require knowledge of the culture and local language.

5. High-technology nursing practices in Western cultures tend to increase the distance between the client and the nurse (or professional staff), and especially within hospital or clinic institutionalized settings which frequently use high-technology nursing practices.

6. While generic (lay or folk) practices of a culture provide valuable care knowledge to guide professional nursing practices, generic care is still very little understood and valued by nurses and other health professionals.

7. Clients who have been involved as key or general informants with nurse researchers using Culture Care theory with the ethnonursing research method generally have expressed highly positive feelings, pride, and hope that more nurses will "get close to clients" and enter their broader life worldview.

8. Clients see that "their cultural ideas, beliefs, and lifeways must be fully considered by professional health personnel to help them appropriately." (Leininger, 1991a, pp. 57–58)

Leininger (1991d) noted that her question regarding what is universal and what is diverse about human care and caring "has only been partially answered with the care constructs listed in [Table 3–1]" (p. 354). She further commented:

> Currently, I am in process of doing a comparative synthesis of the care knowledge drawing on data from the care constructs of different cultures in light of the tenets of my theory. Hopefully, this synthesis will lead to the identification of universal and diverse care meanings, practices, and structure[s] of care so that this knowledge can ultimately be used both for clinical practices and for curricular and teaching purposes. (p. 355)

The generalizability of the Theory of Culture Care Diversity and Universality to all cultures has, however, been questioned. Bruni (1988) pointed out that the "formative source of the theory" [is] the American school of culture anthropology" (p. 28). Elaborating, she explained:

> Following this approach, Western societies are conceptualized principally as multicultural systems, composed of a variety of discrete ethnic or cultural groups. Functional problems are hence analysed along ethnic or cultural lines since these are perceived to constitute the

main lines of division in the society. Difficulties due to acculturation (the change process whereby one group internalizes the culture of another) and cultural shock (where a lack of congruence in beliefs and practices causes conflict) are identified as major areas of study. Transcultural nursing theorists are thus concerned with the analysis of such problems as they relate to the delivery of health care in multicultural societies. (p. 28)

Bruni (1988) maintained that the anthropological basis for Leininger's theory is static and leads to stereotyping of cultures. Bruni also pointed out that an anthropological framework is limited by "the assumption that the country of origin of a person (or his/her parents) identifies the most significant dimension of his/her experience" (p. 29). That assumption leads to a restricted analysis of people's health-related experiences because it excludes "pertinent structural variables such as class and gender" (p. 26). However, the cultural and social structure dimensions of economic factors and educational factors of the Theory of Culture Care Diversity and Universality do provide a basis for consideration of class, and gender has been addressed in at least one application of the theory (Roth, Riley, & Cohen, 1992).

Bruni's critique raises the questions of whether the Theory of Culture Care Diversity and Universality is appropriately applied in other than Western multicultural societies and whether culture is the central variable in determining people's health-related experiences. Leininger has, however, consistently claimed that the theory "is not culture-bound and can be used in any culture worldwide" (Leininger, 1991f, p. 152) and that culture is the dominant context for health and care.

Although a great deal of research based on the Theory of Culture Care Diversity and Universality has been conducted, much more is needed. In particular, studies are needed to provide empirical evidence for the hypotheses proposed by Leininger that were listed in the testability section of this chapter. In addition, despite Leininger's claims, systematic studies are needed to determine the worldwide applicability of the theory.

Pragmatic Adequacy

Nursing Education

Leininger has repeatedly pointed out that nurses must be firmly grounded in culture care knowledge. Indeed, they must master an extensive culture knowledge base and learn to make creative use of that knowledge. Furthermore, nurses must learn to be very attentive and sensitive to the client's lifeways and learn how to work with the client in a coparticipant way. Finally, nurses must learn to focus on care constructs (Table 3–2), rather than on "medical symptoms, diseases, or tasks" (Leininger, 1991a, p. 57).

The knowledge required to apply the Theory of Culture Care Diversity and Universality can be obtained in transcultural nursing education programs. As a formal area of study and practice, transcultural nursing focuses on "the cultural beliefs, values, and lifeways of diverse cultures and on the use of this knowledge to provide cultural specific or cultural universal care to individuals, families, and groups of particular cultures" (Leininger, 1989b, p. 252). Course work includes anthropology, social sciences, humanities, and liberal arts. Knowledge of those fields, combined with nursing insights, is needed to "tease out and understand areas of vital importance to a culture and caring ways" (Leininger, 1991a, p. 54).

Transcultural nursing education programs prepare both generalists and specialists (Leininger, 1989b). Transcultural nurse generalists are prepared at the baccalaureate level for "the general use of transcultural nursing concepts, principles, and practices that mostly have been generated by transcultural nurse specialists" (p. 253). Specialists, who are prepared at the doctoral level, have in-depth understanding of a few cultures and can function as field practitioners, teachers, researchers, or consultants. Certification is awarded by the Transcultural Nursing Society to nurses who have educational preparation in transcultural nursing or the equivalent and who demonstrate basic clinical competence in transcultural nursing.

Nursing Practice

The ultimate goal of the theory is to provide culturally congruent nursing care. More specifically, the goal of the theory is "to improve and to provide culturally congruent care to people that is beneficial, will fit with, and be useful to the client, family, or culture group healthy lifeways" (Leininger, 1991a, p. 39).

Leininger (1967, 1985, 1988, 1991a) has repeatedly claimed that the Theory of Culture Care Diversity and Universality can be used to guide the nursing care of individuals, groups, and institutions in all cultures of the world. The theory can also be used by nurse administrators in both education and service to more effectively deal with students, faculty, staff, and clients from various cultures (Leininger, 1989a).

Specific nursing practices or clinical protocols are derived from the findings of research based on the Theory of Culture Care Diversity and Universality. Leininger (1991a) explained that the findings are used to provide "care that blends with culture values, beliefs, and lifeways of people, and is assessed to be beneficial, satisfying, and meaningful to people of designated cultures" (p. 39).

More specifically, nursing judgments, decisions, and actions are guided by the three dimensions or modes of cultural-congruent nursing care (cultural care preservation or maintenance, cultural care accommodation or negotiation, and cultural care repatterning or restructuring). Leininger (1991a) indicated that "the nurse grounded in culture care knowledge would plan and make decisions with clients with respect to these three modes" (p. 42). She also indicated that, at times, just one mode of cultural care is needed.

Leininger (1991a) uses such terms as "judgments," "decisions," and "actions" to denote nursing practice activities. She rejects the use of the term "nursing interventions" because it "is a term that is often culture bound to Western professional nursing ideologies. Interventions tend to communicate to some cultural informants ideas of cultural interferences and imposition practices" (p. 55). She also rejects the term "nursing problems" because "all too often the client may not have a problem, or the problem may not be seen as relevant to the people by the nurse. Indeed, nursing problems may not be the people's problems" (p. 55).

Leininger (1991a) emphasized the importance of the coparticipation of nurses and clients in all phases of nursing care. She stated, "All care modalities require coparticipation of nurse and clients (consumers) working together to identify, plan, implement, and evaluate each caring mode for culturally congruent nursing care" (p. 44).

The Theory of Culture Care Diversity and Universality demonstrates pragmatic adequacy. The feasibility of implementing clinical protocols that reflect the theory is evident, and clinicians have the legal ability to implement those protocols. The extent to which nursing practice based on the Theory of Culture Care Diversity and Universality is compatible with expectations for nursing practice and the actual effects of its use have begun to be explored. For example, Roth and her colleagues (1992) developed a comprehensive nursing care plan for a pregnant Middle Eastern woman with ascending and descending aortic aneurysms that took into account her Muslim cultural beliefs and care practices related to pregnancy and childbirth. The woman was hospitalized in the cardiovascular intensive care unit of a medical center in Houston, Texas. The authors noted that "identifying the cross-cultural differences helped staff to focus on the patient as a woman and a person" (p. 316). Furthermore, Chmielarczyk (1991) reported his experiences caring for the Hausa people of Northwest Africa. He noted, "Leininger's Theory of Culture Care was highly relevant to plan and provide culturally congruent care to Hausa clients. Moreover, transcultural nursing . . . becomes a complete necessity requiring sincere effort when the cultures are antipode, and the health-care giver is the foreigner" (p. 19). Other reports of the use of the Theory of Culture Care Diversity and Universality are listed in the annotated bibliography at the end of this chapter.

CONCLUSION

Leininger has made a significant contribution to nursing knowledge development by explicating a theory that focuses on nursing care within the context of culture. Continued documentation of outcomes of the use of the Theory of Culture Care Diversity and Universality is needed, with special attention to determining whether cultural congruent nursing care will result in "fewer cultural stresses and conflicts between caregivers and clients" (Leininger, 1985, p. 210).

REFERENCES

Bruni, N. (1988). A critical analysis of transcultural theory. *Australian Journal of Advanced Nursing, 5*(3), 26–32.

Chmielarczyk, V. (1991). Transcultural nursing: Providing culturally congruent care to the Hausa of Northwest Africa. *Journal of Transcultural Nursing, 3*(1), 15–19.

Cohen, J. A. (1991). Two portraits of caring: A comparison of the artists, Leininger and Watson. *Journal of Advanced Nursing, 16*, 899–909.

Leininger, M. M. (1967). The culture concept and its relevance to nursing. *Journal of Nursing Education, 6*(2), 27–39.

Leininger, M. M. (1970). *Nursing and anthropology: Two worlds to blend.* New York: John Wiley & Sons.

Leininger, M. M. (1985). Transcultural care diversity and universality: A theory of nursing. *Nursing and Health Care, 6*, 208–212.

Leininger, M. M. (1988). Leininger's theory of nursing: Cultural care diversity and universality. *Nursing Science Quarterly, 1*, 152–160.

Leininger, M. M. (1989a). Cultural care theory and nursing administration. In B. Henry, C. Arndt, M. DiVincenti, & A. Marriner-Tomey (Eds.), *Dimensions of nursing administration: Theory, research, education, practice* (pp. 19–34). Boston: Blackwell Scientific Publications.

Leininger, M. M. (1989b). The transcultural nurse specialist: Imperative in today's world. *Nursing and Health Care, 10*, 250–256.

Leininger, M. M. (1990). *Leininger-Templin-Thompson ethnoscript qualitative software program: User's handbook.* Detroit: Wayne State University.

Leininger, M. M. (1991a). The theory of culture care diversity and universality. In M. M. Leininger (Ed.), *Culture care diversity and universality: A theory of nursing* (pp. 5–65). New York: National League for Nursing.

Leininger, M. M. (1991b). Ethnonursing: A research method with enablers to study the theory of culture care. In M. M. Leininger (Ed.), *Culture care diversity and universality: A theory of nursing* (pp. 73–117). New York: National League for Nursing.

Leininger, M. M. (1991c). Culture care of the Gadsup Akuna of the Eastern Highlands of New Guinea. In M. M. Leininger (Ed.), *Culture care diversity and universality: A theory of nursing* (pp. 231–280). New York: National League for Nursing.

Leininger, M. M. (1991d). Selected culture care findings of diverse cultures using culture care theory and ethnomethods. In M. M. Leininger (Ed.), *Culture care diversity and universality: A theory of nursing* (pp. 345–371). New York: National League for Nursing.

Leininger, M. M. (1991e). Looking to the future of nursing and the relevancy of culture care theory. In M. M. Leininger (Ed.), *Culture care diversity and universality: A theory of nursing* (pp. 391–418). New York: National League for Nursing.

Leininger, M. M. (1991f). Letter to the editor: Reflections on an international theory of nursing. *International Nursing Review, 38*, 152.

Luna, L., & Cameron, C. (1989). Leininger's transcultural nursing. In J. J. Fitzpatrick & A. L. Whall, *Conceptual models of nursing: Analysis and application* (2nd ed., pp. 227–239). Norwalk, CT: Appleton and Lange.

Mandelbaum, J. (1991). Why there cannot be an international theory of nursing. *International Nursing Review, 38*, 48, 53–55.

Meleis, A. I. (1989). International nursing: A need or a luxury? *Nursing Outlook, 37*, 138–142.

Pike, K. (1954). *Language in relation to a unified theory of the structure of human behavior.* Glendale, CA: Summer Institute of Linguistics.

Roth, C. K., Riley, B., & Cohen, S. M. (1992). Intrapartum care of a woman with aortic aneurysms. *Journal of Obstetric, Gynecologic, and Neonatal Nursing, 21*, 310–317.

Spangler, Z. (1991). Culture care of Philippine and Anglo-American nurses in a hospital context. In M. M. Leininger (Ed.), *Culture care diversity and universality: A theory of nursing* (pp. 119–146). New York: National League for Nursing.

Spangler, Z. (1992). Transcultural care values and nursing practices of Philippine-American nurses. *Journal of Transcultural Nursing, 4*(2), 28–37.

ANNOTATED BIBLIOGRAPHY

Primary Sources

Leininger, M. M. (1978). *Transcultural nursing: Concepts, theories, and practices.* New York: Wiley.
In this book, Leininger introduces the subfield of transcultural nursing and explains the relevance of the culture concept to nursing. Reprints of articles reporting studies of many cultures in the United States and in other countries are included. The use of cultural concepts in nursing curricula and practice is discussed. The second edition of this book will be published by F. A. Davis Company in December 1994.

Leininger, M. M. (1983). Cultural care: An essential goal for nursing and health care. *American Association of Nephrology Nurses and Technicians Journal, 10*(5), 11–17.
Leininger presents the central concepts, principles, and research findings on cultural care. Examples from specific cultures, especially Mexican-Americans and Anglo-Americans, are provided.

Leininger, M. M. (1985). Transcultural care diversity and universality: A theory of nursing. *Nursing and Health Care, 6*, 208–212.
Leininger presents an overview of her theory, including concept definitions and theoretical assumptions. She describes the Sunrise Model and provides examples of propositions that assert the existence of relationships between several concepts. These relationships are illustrated by the author's research findings.

Leininger, M. M. (1988). Leininger's theory of nursing: Cultural care diversity and universality. *Nursing Science Quarterly, 1*, 152–160.
Leininger presents a detailed description of her theory.

Leininger, M. M. (Ed.) (1991). *Culture care diversity and universality: A theory of nursing.* New York: National League for Nursing.
Leininger describes the historical development of her theory, presents refinements in the theory, describes appropriate research methods, and discusses the future of the theory. In addition, Leininger and several other investigators present the findings of studies derived from Leininger's theory.

Commentary by Leininger and Others

Alexander, J., Beagle, C. J., Butler, P., Dougherty, D. A., & Robards, K. D. A. (1986). Madeleine Leininger: Transcultural care theory. In A. Marriner, *Nursing theorists and their work* (pp. 144–159). St. Louis: C. V. Mosby.

Alexander, J., Beagle, C. J., Butler, P., Dougherty, D. A., Robards, K. D. A., & Velotta, C. (1989). Madeleine Leininger: Transcultural care theory. In A. Marriner-Tomey, *Nursing theorists and their work* (2nd ed., pp. 146–163). St. Louis: C. V. Mosby.
The authors describe Leininger's academic and experiential credentials and present a rudimentary analysis of her theory. They also include a cursory critique of the theory.

Bruni, N. (1988). A critical analysis of transcultural theory. *Australian Journal of Advanced Nursing, 5*(3), 26–32.
Bruni explores several areas of concern with transcultural theory that relate to the nature of its underlying theoretical framework and the analytical and explanatory power of the concept of culture. Criticisms of transcultural theory include the limited applicability of a static culture framework, lack of attention to the structural context in which health care issues arise and must be addressed, and the consequent inappropriateness of many health care strategies based on the culturalist framework.

Cohen, J. A. (1991). Two portraits of caring: A comparison of the artists, Leininger and Watson. *Journal of Advanced Nursing, 16,* 899–909.
Cohen explores the themes of caring presented by Watson and Leininger, along with their views of the nature of nursing, use of theory development strategies, and their contributions to nursing knowledge development.

Cohen, J. A. (1992). JANforum: Leininger's culture care theory of nursing. *Journal of Advanced Nursing, 17,* 1149.
Cohen clarifies and corrects the content of her 1991 article, "Two portraits of caring: A comparison of the artists, Leininger and Watson," with regard to Leininger's work. She notes that the corrections are based on personal communication with Leininger.

Davis, L. H., Dumas, R., Ferketich, S., Flaherty, M. J., Isenberg, M., Koerner, J. E., Lacey, B., Stern, P. N., Valente, S., & Meleis, A. I. (1992). AAN expert panel report: Culturally competent health care. *Nursing Outlook, 40,* 277–283.
The expert panel of the American Academy of Nursing reports their recommendations for culturally competent nursing care. Leininger's theory and related work are discussed.

Gaut, D. A., & Leininger, M. M. (1991). *Caring: The compassionate healer.* New York: National League for Nursing.
This edited book contains the papers presented at the International Association for Human Caring Research Conference held in Houston, Texas in 1990, as well as independently submitted papers on caring. The conference theme, Caring: The compassionate healer—a call to consciousness, is clearly reflected in the papers.

George, J. B. (1990). Madeleine Leininger. In J. B. George (Ed.), *Nursing theories: The base for professional nursing practice* (3rd ed., pp. 333–349). Norwalk, CT: Appleton and Lange.
George identifies Leininger's academic and experiential credentials and describes and analyzes her theory.

Greipp, M. E. (1992). Undermedication for pain: An ethical model. *Advances in Nursing Science, 15*(1), 44–53.
Greipp describes a model of ethical decision making for clients experiencing pain. The model is based on general systems theory and is compatible with Leininger's theory.

Hagell, E. I. (1989). Nursing knowledge: Women's knowledge. A sociological perspective. *Journal of Advanced Nursing, 14,* 226–233.
Hagell describes Leininger's contribution to the current perspectives on nursing and Watson's description of nursing knowledge. Several suggestions for change and improvement in nursing education are outlined.

Leininger, M. M. (1967). The culture concept and its relevance to nursing. *Journal of Nursing Education, 6*(2), 27–39. [Reprinted in Auld, M. E., & Birum, L. H. (Eds.) (1973). *The challenge of nursing: A book of readings* (pp. 39–46). St. Louis: C. V. Mosby.]
Leininger emphasizes the need for nursing to account for the culture of an individual seeking health care. Drawing from the writings of anthropologists, Leininger presents definitions of culture. A description of the Gadsup people mode of living supports the need for nurses to acknowledge cultural beliefs in providing health care services.

Leininger, M. M. (1970). *Nursing and anthropology: Two worlds to blend.* New York: Wiley.
Leininger discusses the disciplines of nursing and anthropology and the contributions that each makes to the other.

Leininger, M. M. (1971). Anthropological approach to adaptation: Case studies from nursing. In J. Murphy (Ed.), *Theoretical issues in professional nursing* (pp. 77–102). New York: Appleton-Century-Crofts.

Leininger discusses cultural and biological adaptation from an anthropological perspective. She then explains how anthropological concepts can be applied to nursing and illustrates her points with case studies from nursing situations.

Leininger, M. M. (1973). Nursing in the context of social and cultural systems. In P. Mitchell (Ed.), *Concepts basic to nursing* (pp. 34–45). New York: McGraw-Hill.

Leininger defines and discusses the basic ideas of cultural and social systems. The major components that the nurse needs to observe, study, and evaluate are described. Understanding system behavior is identified as one of the most essential areas of study and is viewed as a significant factor in changing health-care practices and maintaining effective health practices.

Leininger, M. M. and Buck, G. (Eds.). (1974). *Health care issues: Health care dimensions.* Philadelphia, F. A. Davis.

Leininger, M. M. (Ed.). (1975). *Barriers and facilitators to quality health care: Health care dimensions.* Philadelphia: F. A. Davis.

Leininger, M. M. (Ed.). (1976). *Transcultural health care issues and conditions: Health care dimensions.* Philadelphia: F. A. Davis.

The three issues of *Health Care Dimensions* include papers by many noted scholars in nursing and other disciplines addressing a broad range of health-related topics.

Leininger, M. M. (1980). Caring: A central focus of nursing and health care services. *Nursing and Health Care, 1,* 135–143, 176.

In the first part of this article, Leininger presents caring as the most critical and essential ingredient for health, human development and relatedness, well-being, and survival. Drawing from humanistic and scientific perspectives, Leininger provides definitions and uses of caring. Preliminary findings of a study of 30 cultures regarding nurses' perceptions and knowledge about caring behaviors and processes of care recipients are reported. In the next section of the article, Leininger discusses general epistemological, philosophical, and theoretical statements that permit an exploration of caring and the development of the science of caring.

Leininger, M. M. (Ed.). (1981). *Caring: An essential human need.* Thorofare, NJ: Slack. Reprinted 1988. Detroit: Wayne State University Press.

Leininger maintains that this is the first major book dealing with care. Original works by Leininger are included, along with chapters by several other scholars whose work focuses on care and caring. The papers are drawn from presentations at the First, Second, and Third National Caring Conferences held in Salt Lake City, Utah, in 1978, 1979, and 1980.

Leininger, M. M. (1981). Transcultural nursing issues for the 1980s. In J. McCloskey & H. Grace (Eds.), *Current issues in nursing* (pp. 682–692). Boston: Blackwell Scientific Publications.

Leininger identifies and discusses six major issues in transcultural nursing. She envisions transcultural nursing as the primary framework and scientific knowledge base for all of nursing education, practice, and research.

Leininger, M. M. (1981). Transcultural nursing: Its progress and its future. *Nursing and Health Care, 2,* 365–371.

Leininger discusses the importance of cultural factors as influential on the quality of health and nursing care rendered to people. She believes that knowledge about transcultural health should be integrated in the philosophical and practice base of nursing. The progress in establishing transcultural nursing academically and the problems related to nursing education and research are reported. Finally, the author presents common transcultural nursing concepts and the differences between folk and professional health system beliefs and practices.

Leininger, M. M. (Ed.). (1984). *Care: The essence of nursing and health.* Thorofare, NJ: Slack. Reprinted 1988. Detroit: Wayne State University Press.

This book is a sequel to Leininger's 1981 book, *Caring: An essential human need.* The text contains chapters addressing philosophical, theoretical, and general conceptualizations of care, as well as several reports of research dealing with caring.

Leininger, M. M. (1984). *Reference sources for transcultural health and nursing.* Thorofare, NJ: Slack.

This book contains a list of resources and references for transcultural nursing.

Leininger, M. M. (1984). Transcultural nursing: An essential knowledge and practice field for today. *The Canadian Nurse, 80*(11), 41–45.
Leininger reviews the progress of transcultural nursing since the 1950s. In discussing the cultural biases nurses may have in their practice, she emphasizes the significance of transcultural nursing and the concept of care. Finally, recent developments in nursing education, practice, and research, and in the establishment of the Transcultural Nursing Society are addressed.

Leininger, M. M. (1984). Transcultural nursing: An overview. *Nursing Outlook, 32,* 72–73.
Leininger reviews the progress of transcultural nursing since the early 1970s. The development of special programs in transcultural nursing and the relevancy of incorporating cultural concepts in nursing education and practice are discussed.

Leininger, M. M. (1987). A new generation of nurses discover transcultural nursing [Guest editorial]. *Nursing and Health Care, 8,* 263.
Leininger discusses the increasing need to integrate transcultural nursing in nursing education, practice, and research.

Leininger, M. M. (Ed.). (1988). *Care: Discovery and uses in clinical and community nursing.* Detroit: Wayne State University Press.
This edited book contains chapters addressing care values of various cultural groups, the way care is embedded and expressed through social structures, the caring needs of diverse client populations and cultural groups, the concept of the caring community, and different models of care. The book is a sequel to *Caring: An essential human need* (1981) and *Care: The essence of nursing and health* (1984).

Leininger, M. M. (1988). Madeleine M. Leininger. In T. M. Schorr & A. Zimmerman, *Making choices. Taking chances: Nurse leaders tell their stories* (pp. 187–192). St. Louis: C. V. Mosby.
Leininger discusses the influences of her family, colleagues, and academic experiences on the development of her thinking about nursing and the establishment of the subfield of transcultural nursing. A particularly interesting feature is her discussion of contacts with Margaret Mead.

Leininger, M. M. (1989). The Journal of Transcultural Nursing has become a reality [Editorial]. *Journal of Transcultural Nursing, 1*(1), 1–2.
Leininger reflects on the development of the *Journal of Transcultural Nursing* and shares the difficulties encountered in launching the new journal. Serving as the official publication of the Transcultural Nursing Society, the journal's objectives are described.

Leininger, M. M. (1989). Transcultural nursing: Quo vadis (Where goeth the field?). *Journal of Transcultural Nursing, 1*(1), 33–45.
Leininger presents an overview of transcultural nursing. The author traces specific developments of the transcultural nursing field within three major historical eras: the era of establishing the field of transcultural nursing (1955–1975); the era of program and research expansion (1975–1983); and the era of establishing transcultural nursing worldwide (1983 into the 21st century). Lastly, Leininger envisions some predictions for the future of transcultural nursing.

Leininger, M. M. (1990). A new and changing decade ahead: Are nurses prepared? [Editorial]. *Journal of Transcultural Nursing, 1*(2), 1.
Given the changes in the political, economical, and social structures of Eastern cultures, Leininger predicts transcultural migrations and experiences for nurses in the eastern European countries. Implications for transcultural nursing are addressed.

Leininger, M. (1990). Historic and epistemologic dimensions of care and caring with future directions. In J. S. Stevenson & T. Tripp-Reimer (Eds.), *Knowledge about care and caring: State of the art and future developments* (pp. 19–31). Kansas City, MO: American Academy of Nursing.
Leininger provides an overview of the history of the development of care knowledge in nursing from 1950 to the present. She identifies her own role in the development of care knowledge and discusses the need to extend and apply that knowledge worldwide.

Leininger, M. M. (Ed.). (1990). *Ethical and moral dimensions of care*. Detroit: Wayne State University Press.
This edited book contains chapters dealing with philosophical, ethical, and moral issues related to care. A chapter by Leininger focuses on the role of culture in understanding ethical and moral dimensions of human care. The book is the fourth in a series on human care and health and follows *Caring: An essential human need* (1981), *Care: The essence of nursing and health* (1984), and *Care: Discovery and uses in clinical and community nursing* (1988).

Leininger, M. M. (1991). Transcultural nursing: The study and practice field. *Imprint, 38*(2), 55, 57, 59–61, 63, 65–66.
Leininger illustrates the need to understand people's cultural values and health beliefs with a case study. She discusses the definition of transcultural nursing and explains its influence on nursing practice.

Leininger, M. M. (1992). Reflections on Nightingale with a focus on human care theory and leadership. In F. Nightingale, *Notes on nursing: What it is, and what it is not* (Commemorative edition, pp. 28–38). Philadelphia: J. B. Lippincott. (Original work published in 1859).
Leininger analyzes Nightingale's perspectives on human care and contrasts them with her theory of culture care. She also compares and contrasts Nightingale's leadership attributes with her own.

Luna, L., & Cameron, C. (1989). Leininger's transcultural nursing. In J. J. Fitzpatrick & A. L. Whall, *Conceptual models of nursing: Analysis and application* (2nd ed., pp. 227–239). Norwalk, CT: Appleton and Lange.
Luna and Cameron describe Leininger's theory, present an analysis of the theory, and briefly discuss its relation to nursing research, education, and practice.

Rosenbaum, J. (1986). Comparison of two theorists on care: Orem and Leininger. *Journal of Advanced Nursing, 11*, 409–419.
Rosenbaum compares Orem's and Leininger's use of the concepts of care and self-care.

Smith, M. J. (1988). Perspectives on nursing science. *Nursing Science Quarterly, 1*, 80–85.
This article is the transcription of a panel discussion at the Nurse Theorist Conference sponsored by Discovery International and held in Pittsburgh in May 1987. The panel was moderated by Mary Jane Smith; participants were Imogene King, Madeleine Leininger, Rosemarie Parse, Hildegard Peplau, Martha Rogers, Callista Roy, and Rozella Schlotfeldt. Questions focused on the issues of the uniqueness of theoretical frameworks, the phenomenon central to theoretical frameworks, and nursing diagnoses.

Smerke, J. M. (1990). Ethical components of caring. *Critical Care Nursing Clinics of North America, 2*, 509–513.
Consistent with Watson's and Leininger's works on caring, Smerke posits that caring is the ethical foundation for nursing. Factors such as specialization and the development of science and technology have eroded the meaning and notion of caring. Using the critical care context, Smerke describes the ethical dilemmas that critical care nurses face and maintains that nursing must bridge advancing technology with human caring.

Valentine, K. (1989). Caring is more than kindness: Modeling its complexities. *Journal of Nursing Administration, 19*(11), 28–34.
Valentine describes a conceptual model of caring derived from measures of caring obtained from nurses, patients, managers, and nursing theorists. Drawing from Leininger's conceptualization of care, the author discusses ways in which the model of caring can be applied in nursing.

Washington, R. A. (1991). A broader view [Editorial]. *Imprint, 38*(2), 4.
Washington discusses her experiences in learning the importance of transcultural nursing concepts.

Wenger, A. F. Z. (1991). The role of context in culture-specific care. In P. L. Chinn (Ed.), *Anthology on caring* (pp. 95–110). New York: National League for Nursing.

Wenger discusses the relationship between culture context and care, using a framework that incorporates Leininger's theory and a concept of high and low cultural context. She illustrates her theoretical points with findings from her earlier study of the old order Amish (see Wenger, A. F. Z. (1989). The phenomenon of care in a high context culture: The old order Amish. *Dissertation Abstracts International, 50,* 500B).

Practice

Campinha-Bacote, J. (1991). Community mental health services for the underserved: A culturally specific model. *Archives of Psychiatric Nursing, 5,* 229–235.
    The author discusses the need for culturally relevant services for African-American clients with the dual diagnoses of substance abuse and mental illness. She describes her use of Leininger's theory and a model of service delivery and outcome as the framework for a mental health clinic-based program.

Campinha-Bacote, J., & Ferguson, S. (1991). Cultural considerations in child-rearing practices: A transcultural perspective. *Journal of the National Black Nurses' Association, 5*(1), 11–17.
    The authors discuss the importance of accounting for the parental figure's belief system and cultural values when intervening with the parent-child subsystem. They provide a framework based on Leininger's theory that can be used to guide interventions focused on the issue of discipline for families of diverse cultural backgrounds.

Chmielarczyk, V. (1991). Transcultural nursing: Providing culturally congruent care to the Hausa of northwest Africa. *Journal of Transcultural Nursing, 3*(1), 15–19.
    Chmielarczyk reexamines his past experiences in providing nursing care to the Hausa people of northwest Africa within the context of Leininger's theory.

Giger, J., & Davidhizar, R. (1990). *Transcultural nursing: Assessment and intervention.* St. Louis: C. V. Mosby.
    The authors provide a detailed explanation of a format for transcultural assessment that encompasses communication, space, social organization, time, environmental control, and biological variations. The assessment format is not directly derived from Leininger's theory (c.f. Leininger, M. M. (1990). Leininger clarifies transcultural nursing [Letter to the editor]. *International Nursing Review, 37,* 356, in this section).

Good, M. E. (1992). The clinical nurse specialist in the school setting: Case management of migrant children with dental disease. *Clinical Nurse Specialist, 6,* 72–76.
    Good describes the application of Leininger's theory for clinical nurse specialist (CNS) practice with migrant children having dental disease. She also describes the role of the CNS in the Children's Dental Project of Santa Cruz County, California.

Joyner, M. (1988). Hair care for the black patient. *Journal of Pediatric Health Care, 2,* 281–287.
    Joyner maintains that Leininger's theory provides a framework in which cultural understanding can enhance the patient-provider relationship. She points out that hair care practices among black patients are deeply embedded in the cultural beliefs and practices of black people.

Kloosterman, N. D. (1991). Cultural care: The missing link in severe sensory alteration. *Nursing Science Quarterly, 4,* 119–122.
    Kloosterman maintains that Leininger's theory can provide new insights into the phenomenon of severe sensory alteration. She notes that patients who experience sensory overload, sensory deprivation, and sleep deprivation in intensive care units are actually experiencing cultural care deprivation.

Leininger, M. M. (1967). Nursing care of a patient from another culture: Japanese-American patient. *Nursing Clinics of North America, 2,* 747–762.
    Leininger describes the importance of taking culture into account in nursing practice. She illustrates her points with a case study of a Japanese-American patient.

Leininger, M. M. (1971). Some anthropological issues related to community mental health programs in the United States. *Community Mental Health Journal, 7,* 50–62.
    Leininger presents some major anthropological issues related to community mental health programs and centers in the United States. She identifies reasons why a truly community-centered approach has not been fully developed and implemented in

many centers. Emphasis is placed on the importance of understanding current cultural and social forces affecting the patient's illness and the need to incorporate these sociocultural data into existing mental health programs. The paper is based on the author's practice and consultant role with several community mental health programs.

Leininger, M. M (1973). Witchcraft practices and psychocultural therapy with urban United States families. *Human Organization, 32,* 73–83.

According to Leininger, witchcraft behavior is viewed as the psychocultural struggle of certain groups to adjust to rural-urban acculturation situations. Based on research with Spanish and Mexican-American families, the author developed a theoretical framework with three major phases aimed at guiding the psychocultural therapy of the bewitched and his or her family. An application of the framework in providing psychocultural nursing therapy to six families is presented.

Leininger, M. M. (1977). Cultural diversities of health and nursing care. *Nursing Clinics of North America, 12,* 5–18.

Leininger defines transcultural nursing and cultural diversity. She explains how cultural differences between nurses and clients influence client care. Situations involving clients and nurses from diverse cultures are used to illustrate her points.

Leininger, M. M. (1977). Transcultural nursing: A promising subfield of study for nurse educators and practitioners. In A. Reinhardt (Ed.), *Current practice in family centered community nursing* (pp. 36–50). St. Louis: C. V. Mosby.

Leininger defines transcultural nursing and shares her ideas about that new subfield of nursing. She discusses guidelines, expectations, and caveats related to transcultural nursing.

Leininger, M. M. (1986). Care facilitation and resistance factors in the culture of nursing. *Topics in Clinical Nursing, 8*(2), 1–12. [Reprinted in Wolf, Z. (Ed.). (1986). *Clinical care in nursing* (pp. 1–23). Rockville, MD: Aspen.]

Leininger identifies facilitation and resistance factors to the practice of care and presents ways to advance the profession of nursing based on humanistic and scientific care practices. Leininger discusses the impact of high technology, cost benefits, diagnostic related groups, the cult of efficiency, and the decline in nurses' altruistic attitudes and practices on the significance of care in nursing.

Leininger, M. M. (1989). The transcultural nurse specialist: Imperative in today's world. *Nursing and Health Care, 10,* 250–256.

Leininger contends that as the nurse's role is becoming increasingly multicultural, the development of transcultural nurse specialists, as experts in selected cultures, is needed in areas of nursing practice, education, and research. Characteristics and roles of transcultural nurse specialists are presented.

Leininger, M. M. (1989). Transcultural nurse specialists and generalists: New practitioners in nursing. *Journal of Transcultural Nursing, 1*(1), 4–16.

Leininger presents the nature, characteristics, educational preparation, and practice role of the transcultural nurse specialist and generalist. She addresses the growing pluralism in the world and the need for transcultural nursing to become a formal area of study and practice as well as a societal imperative for the future.

Leininger, M. M. (1990). Leininger clarifies transcultural nursing [Letter to the editor]. *International Nursing Review, 37,* 356.

Leininger critiques an article by Giger and Davidhizar that describes a format for transcultural nursing assessment (c.f. Giger, J., & Davidhizar, R. (1990). *Transcultural nursing: Assessment and intervention.* St. Louis: C. V. Mosby, in this section.) She maintains that their format is not discussed within the perspective of her view of transcultural nursing and that her Sunrise Model is the appropriate format for assessment when nursing is based on the theory of cultural care diversity and universality.

Norris, C. M. (1989). To care or not care. Questions! Questions! *Nursing and Health Care, 10,* 545–550.

Norris explains how the stereotyping of nurses as not caring parallels the increasingly technologic orientation of patient care. The author reflects on the recent care initiative as a defense against the rigor of scientific practice. The human caring value within the context of health care raises social and economical issues. The author expresses concerns about the conceptual and operational definition of care and challenges Leininger's and Watson's assertions that caring is a central focus of the discipline. The marketability of caring and implications for research are presented.

Rosenbaum, J. N. (1989). Depression: Viewed from a transcultural nursing theoretical perspective. *Journal of Advanced Nursing, 14,* 7–12.

Rosenbaum discusses phenomena related to depression transculturally and examines depression within the context of Leininger's theory of transcultural diversity and universality. Mental health and mental illness are viewed within the social structure and worldview in order to derive culturally congruent nursing care.

Roth, C. K., Riley, B., & Cohen, S. M. (1992). Intrapaturm care of a woman with aortic aneurysms. *Journal of Obstetric, Gynecologic, and Neonatal Nursing, 21,* 310–317.

The authors present a comprehensive plan of nursing care for a Muslim woman who had two aortic aneurysms. Citing Leininger, they pointed out the need for nursing care during labor and delivery to take a woman's cultural values and beliefs into account.

Symanski, M. E. (1991). Use of nursing theories in the care of families with high-risk infants: Challenges for the future. *Journal of Perinatal and Neonatal Nursing, 4*(4), 71–77.

Symanski discusses the contributions of Leininger's theory of cultural care diversity and universality and King's theory of goal attainment to the nursing care of families with high-risk infants.

Administration

Brenner, P., Boyd, C., Thompson, T. C., Marz, M. S., Buerhaus, P., & Leininger, M. (1986). The care symposium: Considerations for nursing administrators. *Journal of Nursing Administration, 16*(1), 25–30.

Boyd, C. (1986). Nursing journal recruitment advertisements: Symbolic indicators of care, pp. 27–28.

Boyd explains that the purpose of this study was to identify care symbols and picture patterns in two nursing journals' advertisements for recruitment. Consistent with Leininger's notion of cross-cultural care, 10 randomly selected pictures were analyzed for implicit and explicit symbolic meanings of care. Concerned by the misfit between the type of nurse and nursing care symbolized in the advertisements, the author expresses the need for nurse administrators to better understand the meaning and practice of the nursing care given in their institutions.

Brenner, P. (1986). Disseminating care research literature, pp. 26–27.

Concerned with nursing service administrators' involvement in care research, Brenner examined key nursing reports published in a leading nursing administration journal. Based on Watson's and Leininger's works, a content analysis of 63 articles and two reports reviewed revealed that care was never used as the major independent or dependent variable but rather appeared as an intervening variable related to job satisfaction and/or job stability. The need for research on care is addressed.

Buerhaus, P. (1986). The economics of care, p 30.

Buerhaus comments that when faced with the increasing competition with health maintenance organizations, hospital administrators are challenged to market professional nursing care. He addresses the need for administrators to articulate the value, meaning, and attributes of nursing care as the essential hospital product.

Leininger, M. (1986). (Introduction), p. 25.

Leininger introduces a series of essays by doctoral nursing students on nursing service administrators' interests, knowledge of, and use of the concept of care.

Marz, M. S. (1986). Conceptual care model for reducing stress of newly employed nurses, pp. 28–29.

Marz describes a conceptual basis for assessing employee care. Based on several studies on support, care, the environment, and stress, this author presents a creative effort to discover the use of care as an intervention to help new nurse employees reduce stress and grow in their work.

Thompson, T. C. (1986). Discovering the meaning and expressions of care by nursing service directors, p 28.
To study the philosophical views about care among nursing service administrators, Thompson interviewed and observed nursing directors from different clinical areas. Consistent with Leininger's work, care was identified as an important part of the administrators' thinking and actions.

Leininger, M. M. (1989). Cultural care theory and nursing administration. In B. Henry, C. Arndt, M. Di Vincenti, & A. Marriner-Tomey (Eds.), *Dimensions of nursing administration. Theory, research, education, practice* (pp. 19–34). Boston: Blackwell Scientific Publications.
Leininger presents her theory and discusses its relevance and usefulness to academic and clinical nursing administration. Areas of inquiry and research for nursing service and education administrators are outlined.

Education

Holtz, C., & Bairan, A. (1990). Personal contact: A method of teaching cultural empathy. *Nurse Educator, 15*, 13, 24, 28.
Holtz and Bairan propose a cultural empathy model that could serve as a guide for nursing faculty to influence student nurses' contacts with clients from a variety of cultural, socioeconomic, and geographic backgrounds. Positive sanctions as a means to reduce students' ethnocentrism and enhance nursing care and client satisfaction are presented.

Leininger, M. M. (1978). Changing foci in nursing education: Primary and transcultural care. *Journal of Advanced Nursing, 3*, 155–166.
Leininger presents the factors that have led to changes in nursing education and practice in the United States. Moreover, the author discusses two major interrelated movements, transcultural nursing and primary nursing, as promising developments to advance nursing education and practice. It is argued that these movements need to be part of local, national, and international health education and care systems. Implications for nursing education programs are discussed.

Leininger, M. M. (1978). Professional, political, and ethnocentric role behaviors and their influence in multidisciplinary health education. In M. Hardy & M. Conway (Eds.), *Role theory: Perspectives for health professionals*, (pp. 251–271). New York: Appleton-Century-Crofts.
In her discussion of multidisciplinary health education, Leininger highlights the importance of ethnocentrism as a factor that facilitates understanding of interdisciplinary behavior.

Leininger, M., & Watson, J. (Eds.). (1990). *The caring imperative in education*. New York: National League for Nursing.
This edited book contains the papers presented at the 11th National/International Caring Conference held in Denver, Colorado in 1989. The conference themes of education about caring and caring in the educational process are well represented in the 26 chapters.

Research

Beck, C. T. (1991). How students perceive faculty caring: A phenomenological study. *Nurse Educator, 16*(5), 18–22.
Beck reports the findings of her study of student perceptions of caring nursing student-faculty experiences. Themes identified were attentive presence, sharing of selves, and consequences. Caring behaviors included compassion, competence, confidence, conscience, and commitment. Beck notes that Leininger believes that nursing students need to be taught from the first day in their programs about the concept of care and how it is used in nursing practice.

Gates, M. F. (1991). Transcultural comparison of hospital and hospice as caring environments for dying patients. *Journal of Transcultural Nursing, 2*(2), 3–15.

Gates reports the results of a comparative study, guided by Leininger's theory, of a hospital oncology unit and freestanding hospice unit. She found that both environments provided a caring atmosphere/ambience.

Higgins, P. G., & Dicharry, E. K. (1990). Measurement issues in the use of the Coopersmith Self-Esteem Inventory with Navajo women. *Health Care for Women International, 11*, 251–262.
Using an ethnonursing framework, these authors examined the content validity of the widely used Coopersmith Self-Esteem Inventory with 29 Navajo women. The results indicated that cultural values influenced Navajo women's responses to the self-esteem measure as well as the meaning of self-esteem within their culture. Inasmuch as the instrument has not been used with Hispanic or Indian populations, more research is needed on the appropriateness of this measure with various cultural and racial groups.

Horsburgh, M. E. C., & Foley, D. M. (1990). The phenomena of care in Sicilian-Canadian culture: An ethnonursing case study. *Nursing Forum, 25*(3), 14–22.
Horsburgh and Foley report the findings of their study of the caring beliefs and behaviors of first- and second-generation Sicilians who immigrated to Canada. The study was based on Leininger's theory.

Leininger, M. M. (1969). Ethnoscience: A promising research approach to improve nursing practice. *Image, 3*, 2–8.
In this article, Leininger discusses an anthropological research method, ethnoscience, as a new approach for the study of health-illness systems of behavior of people with different cultural and subcultural background. Leininger defines the major concepts, principles, and theoretical views on which the ethnoscience method rests. From her research on the health practitioner roles of the Gadsup people, the author illustrates the ethnoscientific research method.

Leininger, M. M. (1976). Two strange health tribes: Gnisrun and Enicidem in the United States. *Human Organization, 35*, 253–261.
Leininger describes the most dominant cultural features of two subcultures of the health care system, the Gnisrun and the Enicidem tribes. Using an ethnographic approach, the author offers the reader a transcultural experience to gain some intriguing perspectives about the disciplines of nursing and medicine.

Leininger, M. M. (1984). Qualitative research methods—to document and discover nursing knowledge [Editorial]. *Western Journal of Nursing Research, 6*, 151–152.
Leininger maintains that although both quantitative and qualitative methods of nursing research are needed, qualitative methods have not been valued and have not received sufficient recognition in the nursing research community.

Leininger, M. M. (Ed.). (1985). *Qualitative research methods in nursing.* New York: Grune and Stratton.
This edited book contains chapters addressing several qualitative methods of research, including ethnography and ethnonursing, philosophical analysis, phenomenology, and historical inquiry.

Leininger, M. M. (1987). Importance and uses of ethnomethods: Ethnography and ethnonursing research. *Recent Advances in Nursing, 17*, 12–36.
Leininger describes the characteristics, purposes, and uses of ethnomethods as an important means to discover nursing knowledge and improve nursing care practices. She also describes ethnography and ethnonursing methods and highlights the features of ethnoscience, phenomenology, and grounded theory.

Leininger, M. M. (1987). Response to "Infant feeding practices of Vietnamese immigrants to the northwest United States." *Scholarly Inquiry for Nursing Practice, 1*, 171–174.
Leininger critiques Henderson and Brown's study of infant feeding practices of Vietnamese immigrants. She shares the findings of her own studies of the Vietnamese.

Leininger, M. M. (1990). Ethnomethods: The philosophic and epistemic bases to explicate transcultural nursing knowledge. *Journal of Transcultural Nursing, 1*(2), 40–51.
Ethnomethods of the qualitative paradigm are described by Leininger as extremely valuable in the discovery of the epistemics of nursing knowledge and in the advancement of other dimensions of nursing. Leininger presents ethnomethods as a means of explicating transcultural nursing knowledge. She explains how this knowledge can provide meaningful and congruent care to people of diverse and similar cultures.

Morse, J. M., & English, J. (1986). The incorporation of cultural concepts into basic nursing texts. *Nursing Papers, 18*(2), 69–76.

Morse and English describe the findings of their study of the incorporation of cultural aspects of care in seven basic nursing texts used by first-year nursing students. A content analysis revealed that cultural concepts are inadequately integrated in the nursing texts. Implications of these findings on faculty members' and authors' responsibilities are discussed.

Rosenbaum, J. N. (1990). Cultural care of older Greek Canadian widows. *Journal of Transcultural Nursing, 2*(1), 37–47.

Rosenbaum reports the cultural care themes extracted from the data collected for her study of older Greek Canadian widows. The study was conceptualized within Leininger's theory.

Spangler, Z. (1992). Transcultural care values and nursing practices of Philippine-American nurses. *Journal of Transcultural Nursing, 4*(2), 28–37.

Spangler reports the findings of her study, which was derived from Leininger's theory, of the nursing care values and caregiving practices of Philippine nurses working in an American hospital.

Vallarruel, A. M., & Ortiz de Montellano, B. (1992). Culture and pain: A Mesoamerican perspective. *Advances in Nursing Science, 15*(1), 21–32.

Vallarruel and Ortiz de Montellano explain that culture influences a person's reaction to and expression of pain. The findings of their ethnohistoric study of the beliefs related to the experience of pain within ancient Mesoamerica revealed six themes: pain was an accepted, an anticipated, and a necessary part of human life; humans had an obligation to the gods and to the community of man to endure pain in relation to the performance of duties; the ability to endure pain and suffering stoically was valued; the type and amount of pain a person experienced was in part predetermined by the gods; pain and suffering were viewed as a consequence of immoral behavior; and specific methods of pain alleviation were directed toward maintaining balance within the person and the surrounding environment. They commented that the findings facilitate understanding of Mexican-American meanings, expressions, and care associated with pain.

Doctoral Dissertations

Cameron, C. F. (1991). An ethnonursing study of the influence of extended caregiving on the health status of elderly Anglo-Canadian wives caring for physically disabled husbands. *Dissertation Abstracts International, 52,* 746B.

Campinha, J. A. (1988). Consideration of the cultural belief systems of individuals experiencing conjure illness by public health nurses and emergency room nurses: An exploratory study. *Dissertation Abstracts International, 48,* 2923B.

Cunningham-Warburton, P. A. (1989). A study of the relationship between cross-cultural training, the scale to assess world views, and the quality of care given by nurses in a psychiatric setting. *Dissertation Abstracts International, 49,* 3102B.

Gates, M. F. G. (1989). Care and cure meanings, experiences and orientations of persons who are dying in hospital and hospice settings. *Dissertation Abstracts International, 50,* 493B.

Hansen, M. M. (1986). The southern Appalachian mountain families: Cultural determinants of health related characteristics. *Dissertation Abstracts International, 46,* 2259B.

Ingle, J. R. (1989). The business of caring: The perspective of men in nursing. *Dissertation Abstracts International, 50,* 495B.

Johnson, R. W. (1988). The impact of training in transcultural nursing on health care practices. *Dissertation Abstracts International, 49,* 1620B.

Jones, J. A. (1984). Social distance and the baccalaureate transcultural nursing program. *Dissertation Abstracts International, 45,* 1023A.

Lee, M. C. (1991). Cross-cultural comparison of patients' perceptions of pain. *Dissertation Abstracts International, 51,* 3325B.

Luna, L. J. (1990). Care and cultural context of Lebanese Muslims in an urban U.S. community: An ethnographic and ethnonursing study conceptualized within Leininger's theory. *Dissertation Abstracts International, 51,* 2818B.

McDonald, V. E. (1986). Associate degree nurse educators' perception of need for transcultural concepts in nursing education. *Dissertation Abstracts International, 46,* 3393B.

Parnicza, D. R. (1991). Analysis of rural Appalachian caregivers' use of social support. *Dissertation Abstracts International, 51,* 4781B.

Pokorny, M. E. (1990). The effect of nursing care on human dignity in the critically ill adult. *Dissertation Abstracts International, 50,* 3924B.

Ray, M. A. (1981). A study of caring within an institutional culture. *Dissertation Abstracts International, 42,* 2310B.

Rosenbaum, J. N. (1991). Cultural care, cultural health, and grief phenomena related to older Greek Canadian widows within Leininger's theory of culture care. *Dissertation Abstracts International, 52,* 1959B.

Spangler, Z. (1991). Nursing care values and caregiving practices of Anglo-American and Philippine-American nurses conceptualized within Leininger's theory. *Dissertation Abstracts International, 52,* 1960B.

Thompson, T. L. C. (1991). A qualitative investigation of rehabilitation nursing care in an inpatient rehabilitation unit using Leininger's theory. *Dissertation Abstracts International, 52,* 752B.

Tom-Orme, L. (1988). Diabetes in a Navajo community: A qualitative study of health/illness beliefs and practice. *Dissertation Abstracts International, 49,* 1622B.

Wenger, A. F. Z. (1989). The phenomenon of care in a high context culture: The old order Amish. *Dissertation Abstracts International, 50,* 500B.

Master's Theses

Dory, V. B. (1987). Nursing behaviors perceived as caring by gerontological patients. *Master's Abstracts International, 27,* 93.

Dowe, D. S. (1990). African-American diversity in nursing inservice programs. *Master's Abstracts International, 29,* 261.

Eggleston, E. D. (1988). Nurses' attitudes toward geriatric patients and the relationship to the supportive nursing care provided: Implications for nursing administration. *Master's Abstracts International, 27,* 375.

Evans, R. (1987). Labor patterns of Oglala Sioux indians compared to caucasian labor patterns. *Master's Abstracts International, 26,* 236.

Moore, S. J. (1989). The relationship between expressive touch and patients' perceptions of nurses' caring. *Master's Abstracts International, 28,* 579.

Weaver, R. A. (1990). A phenomenological study of caring in the nurse-patient relationship: The patient's perspective. *Master's Abstracts International, 29,* 269.

4

Newman's Theory of Health as Expanding Consciousness_____

Margaret Newman's ideas about health were greatly influenced by her mother's struggle with amyotrophic lateral sclerosis and her experiences as a graduate student (Newman, 1986), as well as her concern "for those for whom health as the absence of disease is not a reality" (Newman, 1992, p. 650). She began to formalize her ideas in preparation for a paper delivered at the Nurse Educator Conference held in New York City in 1978, and she published the first version of the theory in her 1979 book, *Theory Development in Nursing*. The theory continued to evolve and became known as the Theory of Health as Expanding Consciousness with the publication of Newman's 1986 book *Health as Expanding Consciousness*. This chapter presents an analysis and evaluation of that theory.

The concepts of the Theory of Health as Expanding Consciousness are listed below. Each concept is defined and described later in this chapter.

KEY CONCEPTS_____

Time	Consciousness
Space	Pattern
Movement	

ANALYSIS OF THE THEORY OF HEALTH AS EXPANDING CONSCIOUSNESS

This section presents an analysis of Newman's theory. The analysis is based on Newman's publications about her theory, drawing heavily from her 1986 book as well as from a recent journal article entitled "Newman's Theory of Health as Praxis" (Newman, 1990a) and a book chapter titled "Shifting to a Higher Consciousness" (Newman, 1990b).

Scope of the Theory

The central thesis of the Theory of Health as Expanding Consciousness is that health is the expansion of consciousness. The meaning of life and health are, according to Newman (1986), found in the evolving process of expanding consciousness. More specifically, the theory "asserts that *every* person in *every* situation, no matter how disordered and hopeless it may seem, is part of the universal process of expanding consciousness" (Newman, 1992, p. 650). The description of health, the definitions of the concepts of the theory, and the propositions all are at a relatively abstract level, which resulted in the classification of the theory as a grand theory.

Context of the Theory

Metaparadigm Concepts and Propositions

Newman alluded to the metaparadigm of nursing when she made the following comments:

> What we are concerned with is the health of persons in interaction with the environment. (Newman, 1986, p. 33)

> Sometimes I think of my theory strictly in terms of health (as expanding consciousness), but students point out to me that I have not been talking solely about health: I have been talking about the relationship that exists between nurse and client and the mutuality that occurs in the process of assisting clients in making and implementing their choices. (Newman, 1990b, p. 130)

Those comments indicate that the Theory of Health as Expanding Consciousness focuses primarily on the metaparadigm concept *health* and the proposition *the patterning of human behavior in interaction with the environment in normal life events and critical life situations.* The secondary foci are the metaparadigm concepts *person* and *nursing* and the proposition *the [nursing] processes by which positive changes in [the client's] health status are affected.*

Philosophical Claims

Newman has not yet identified the philosophical claims undergirding the Theory of Health as Expanding Consciousness. Sarter (1988) maintained that Newman's theory is based on philosophical claims rooted in "relativity and quantum theory, mysticism, and early Greek and Eastern philosophy" (p. 55). The analysis of Newman's published works resulted in the identification of several statements that could be considered philosophical claims:

1. A universe of undivided wholeness (Newman, 1986, p. 68).
2. The assumption is made that consciousness is coextensive in the universe and resides in all matter (Newman, 1986, p. 33).
3. Persons as individuals, and human beings as a species, are identified by their patterns of consciousness. The person does not *possess* consciousness—the person *is* consciousness. (Newman, 1986, p. 33).
4. The highest form of knowing is loving (Newman, 1986, p. 68).
5. Health encompasses disease as a meaningful aspect of health, as a manifestation of the underlying pattern of person-environment interaction (Newman, 1990b, p. 133).
6. Health encompasses conditions heretofore described as disease (Newman, 1983, p. 163).
7. These disease conditions can be considered a manifestation of the unitary pattern of the person (Newman, 1983, p. 163).
8. The physical manifestations of disease may be considered evidence of how one is interacting with environment (Newman, 1986, p. 43).
9. If developing a disease is the only way an individual['s pattern] can manifest itself, then that is health for that person (Newman, 1983, p. 164).
10. The pattern of the person that eventually manifests itself as disease is part of a larger ongoing pattern (Newman, 1983, p. 164).
11. Elimination of the disease condition in itself will not change the pattern of the person (Newman, 1983, p. 164).
12. Health and illness [are viewed] as a single process and, like rhythmic phenomena, becoming manifest in ups and downs, or peaks and troughs, moving through varying degrees of organization and disorganization, but all as one unitary process (Newman, 1986, p. 4).
13. "Ill" or "illness" refers to a subjective sense of diminished health (Newman, 1983, p. 163).
14. Health . . . is not a utopian state to be achieved, but the totality of the life process to be experienced (Newman, 1983, p. 168).
15. There is no basis for rejecting any experience as irrelevant. The important factor is to get in touch with one's own pattern of interaction and recognize that whatever it is, the process is in progress and the experience is one of expanding consciousness (Newman, 1986, p. 67).

Newman's implicit philosophical claims are consistent with holism (Sarter, 1988) and the *simultaneous action* worldview. Indeed, Newman (1990a) maintained that her view of health "requires a nonfragmentary worldview" (p. 39). More specifically, she noted that her theory of health reflects a "patterned, unpredictable unitary, intuitive, and innovative" view of the world (Newman, personal communication, November 30, 1992).

Conceptual Model

The conceptual base for the Theory of Health as Expanding Consciousness is, according to Newman (1990a), "a paradigm of evolving pattern of the whole" (p. 40). That paradigm, as Newman (1986, 1990a, 1990b) has repeatedly pointed out, is Rogers's (1970) Life Process Model, which is now known as the Science of Unitary Human Beings (Rogers, 1990). Newman (1990a) explained, "Rogers' assumptions regarding the patterning of persons in interaction with the environment are basic to my view that consciousness is a manifestation of an evolving pattern of person-environment interaction" (p. 38). She went on to say, "Rogers' insistence that health and illness are simply manifestations of the rhythmic fluctuations of the life process led me to view health and illness as a unitary process moving through variations in order-disorder" (p. 38).

Newman (1990b) identified two assumptions from Rogers's conceptual model regarding pattern that are basic to the Theory of Health as Expanding Consciousness: (1) pattern identifies the wholeness of the person, (2) pattern evolves unidirectionally. She then explained:

> If you can accept these two assumptions, then you can begin to think of disease as a manifestation of expanding consciousness. If you accept that pattern is a manifestation of the person, and that the process of life moves in the direction of increasing complexity, diversity, and higher consciousness, then when something appears or becomes manifest, it follows that it is a manifestation of the evolving pattern; it is not something separate to be gotten rid of or squelched, but something to be regarded as a clue to the underlying pattern. (p. 132)

The goal of nursing for Newman (1979) "is not to make people well, or to prevent their getting sick, but to assist people to utilize the power that is within them as they evolve toward higher levels of consciousness" (p. 67).

Antecedent Knowledge

Newman (1986) has acknowledged the contributions of several scholars to the development and refinement of her ideas about health.

She noted that de Chardin's (1959) belief "that a person's consciousness continues to develop beyond the physical life and becomes a part of a universal consciousness . . . made sense to me" (p. 5). In addition, she cited Bohm's (1980) theory of the implicate order as a significant contribution to her notions about pattern manifestation and "the interconnectedness and omnipresence of all that there is" (p. 5). Newman (1987) also acknowledged Bateson's (1979) contributions to her understanding of pattern.

Moreover, Newman stated that Young's (1976a, 1976b) theory of human evolution "was the impetus for my efforts to integrate the basic concepts of my theory . . . into a dynamic portrayal of life and health" (p. 6). She also noted that Moss's (1981) idea of "love as the highest level of consciousness provided affirmation and elaboration of my intuition regarding the nature of health" (p. 6). Furthermore, Newman commented that Bentov's (1978) work "provided logical explanations for many things I had taken on faith" (p. 5). Newman also commented that Prigogine's (1980) theory of change contributed to her understanding of the evolution of consciousness.

Content of the Theory

An analysis of Newman's 1986 book and other publications revealed that the concepts of the Theory of Health as Expanding Consciousness are *time, space, movement, consciousness,* and *pattern.*

Time and Space

The analysis of Newman's publications dealing with the Theory of Health as Expanding Consciousness did not yield specific definitions for **time** and **space.** Newman (1979) did, however, note that the world contains time aspects and space aspects.

With regard to time, Newman (1983) mentioned subjective time, which she defined as "the amount of time perceived to be passing" (p. 166), and objective time, which she equated with clock time. Moreover, she identified subjective time, objective time, and use of time as dimensions of time relevant for the individual and private time, coordinated time, and shared time as dimensions relevant for the family.

With regard to space, Newman (1979) mentioned three-dimensional space, life space, personal space, and inner space. In a later publication, Newman (1983) identified personal space, inner space, and life space as dimensions of space relevant to the individual, and territoriality, shared space, and distancing as dimensions relevant to the family. None of these terms were, however, defined.

Newman (1979) views "the concept of space [as] inextricably linked to the concept of time" (p. 61). She has expressed that link with the terms *space-time* and *time-space* in various publications (1986, 1990a).

Movement

Newman (1979) described **movement** as "an essential property of matter" (p. 61) and "a means of communicating" (p. 62). She views movement as "the means whereby one perceives reality and, therefore, [the] means of becoming aware of self" (Newman, 1983, p. 165). Furthermore, movement "is the natural condition of life. When movement ceases, one fears that life has gone out of the organism" (Newman, 1986, p. 58).

Consciousness

Consciousness is defined as "the informational capacity of the . . . human being, that is, the ability of the [person] to interact with the environment" (Newman, 1990a, p. 38). Consciousness encompasses interconnected cognitive and affective awareness, physiochemical maintenance including the nervous and endocrine systems, growth processes, the immune system, and the genetic code (Newman, 1986, 1990a).

Newman (1986) maintained that consciousness can be seen in the quantity and quality of the interaction between the human being and the environment. She explained that "the process of life is toward higher levels of consciousness. Sometimes this process is smooth, pleasant, harmonious; other times it is difficult and disharmonious, as in disease" (p. 31).

Newman (1992) defined the process of expanding consciousness as "a process of becoming more of oneself, of finding greater meaning in life, and of reaching new heights of connectedness with other people and the world in which one lives" (p. 650). She proposed that consciousness expands in a series of stages that are parallel to Young's (1976a, 1976b) stages of human evolution. The corresponding stages are listed in Table 4–1.

Newman (1986) explained that Young proposed that human beings evolve from a loss of potential freedom to real freedom through a process of interactions with each other and the social state. Freedom is lost as the person binds in with the larger network. Subsequently, identity, self-consciousness, and self-determination emerge through centering. When things that worked in the past no longer work, choice operates and the person evolves by decentering and unbinding, finally achieving real freedom. The states of unbinding and real freedom are not physical but may manifest in such superhuman powers as healings and appearances in different forms.

TABLE 4-1.   Comparison of Young's Stages of Evolution and Newman's Stages of Expanding Consciousness

Stage	*Young* *Evolution of Human Beings*	*Newman* *Expanding Consciousness*
1	Potential freedom	Potential consciousness
2	Binding	Time
3	Centering	Space
4	Choice	Movement
5	Decentering	Infinite space or boundarylessness
6	Unbinding	Timelessness
7	Real freedom	Absolute consciousness

Source: Adapted from "Newman's Theory of Health as Praxis" by M. A. Newman, 1990, *Nursing Science Quarterly, 3*, pp. 37–41. Copyright 1990 by Chestnut House Publications. Re-Adapted by permission.

Newman (1986) described the progression of expanding consciousness as follows:

> We come into being from a state of potential consciousness, are bound in time, find our identity in space, and through movement learn the "law" of the way things work and make choices that ultimately take us beyond space and time to a state of absolute consciousness. (p. 46)

The integration of Young's and Newman's theories is evident in the following quotation:

> A person comes into being from the ground of *consciousness* and loses freedom as one is bound in *time* and finds one's identity in *space*. Matters of time-space are very much involved in one's struggles for self-determination and status. *Movement* represents the choice point. It is central to understanding the nature of reality. Through movement one discovers the world of time-space and establishes personal territory. It is also when movement is restricted that one becomes aware of personal limitations and the fact that the old rules don't work anymore. When one no longer has the power of movement (either physical or social), it is necessary to go beyond oneself. As one is able to recognize the *boundarylessness* and *timelessness* of human existence, one gains the freedom of returning to the ground of *consciousness*. (Newman, 1990a, pp. 39–40)

Newman (1986) equated the process of expanding consciousness with the process of health. She also equated absolute consciousness, the last stage of the process, with love. More specifically:

> In [the last stage] all opposites are reconciled. This kind of love embraces all experience equally and unconditionally: pain as well as pleasure, failure as well as success, ugliness as well as beauty, disease as well as non-disease. (p. 47)

Pattern

Drawing from Rogers (1970), Newman (1986) defined **pattern** as "a fundamental attribute of all there is and gives unity in diversity" and as "information that depicts the whole, understanding of the meaning of all the relationships at once" (p. 13). She went on to say that pattern "is relatedness" (p. 14). Furthermore, "a person is identified by her or his pattern" (Newman, 1990a, p. 39). Stated in a slightly different manner, "Pattern [is] an identification of the wholeness of the person" (Newman, 1990b, p. 132). It follows, then, that Newman (1987) regards pattern as "the essence of a holistic view of health" (p. 36).

Newman (1986) identified the characteristics or dimensions of pattern as *movement, diversity,* and *rhythm.* She explained, "The pattern is in constant movement or change, the parts are diverse and are changing in relation to each other, and rhythm identifies the pattern" (p. 14). Furthermore, "the pattern of movement reflects the overall organization of the thought and feeling processes of a person" (p. 59).

Propositions

The definitions and descriptions of the concepts of the Theory of Health as Expanding Consciousness are nonrelational propositions. The theory also contains several relational propositions. *Time* and *space* are linked in a relational proposition that asserts "Time and space have a complementary relationship" (Newman, 1979, p. 60).

Time is linked with *movement* in a relational proposition asserting "Time is a function of movement" (Newman, 1979, p. 60).

Time and *space* are linked with *movement* in the following two relational propositions:

> Movement is a means whereby space and time become a reality (Newman, 1979, p. 60).

> Through movement one discovers the world of time-space and establishes personal territory (Newman, 1990a, p. 39).

Newman (1979) viewed *time, space,* and *movement* as "correlates of developing consciousness" (p. 66). The following relational propositions specify the linkages:

> Time is a measure of consciousness. (Newman, 1979, p. 60)

> A person comes into being from the ground of consciousness and loses freedom as one is bound in time and finds one's identity in space. (Newman, 1990a, p. 39).

> Movement is a reflection of consciousness (Newman, 1979, p. 60).

> The consciousness that characterizes any form of life is expressed in its movement (Newman, 1986, p. 58).

Another relational proposition links *consciousness* with *pattern:* "Consciousness is a manifestation of an evolving pattern of person-environment interaction" (Newman, 1990a, p. 38).

Still another relational proposition links the *rhythm* dimension of pattern to *movement:* "Rhythm is basic to movement . . . [and] the rhythm of movement is an integrating experience" (Newman, 1986, pp. 59–60).

EVALUATION OF THE THEORY OF HEALTH AS EXPANDING CONSCIOUSNESS

This section presents an evaluation of Newman's Theory of Health as Expanding Consciousness. The evaluation is based on the results of the analysis of the theory as well as on publications by others who have used or commented on this nursing theory.

Significance

The metaparadigmatic origins of the Theory of Health as Expanding Consciousness are evident in Newman's publications. In fact, although she did not label it as a concept of the nursing metaparadigm, she explicitly stated that her primary focus was the concept of health. In contrast, Newman did not identify any specific philosophical claims. Such claims were, however, extracted from her publications.

Newman explicitly identified the conceptual model from which the Theory of Health as Expanding Consciousness was derived. Rogers's (1970) model, especially the idea of pattern, clearly served as a starting point for development of the theory. Newman also explicitly acknowledged and cited the scholars from other disciplines whose works provided support for her ideas and contributed to their refinement.

The significance of the Theory of Health as Expanding Consciousness lies in the theory's contributions to our understanding of wellness and illness as different forms of pattern manifestation, as well as the dimensions of pattern manifestation. A special feature of the theory is the focus on the evolution of expanded consciousness.

Internal Consistency

Sarter's (1988) philosophical analysis of the Theory of Health as Expanding Consciousness indicates congruence in philosophical viewpoints among the scholars on whose works the theory is based. For example, she noted that the writings of Moss (1981), Young (1976a, 1976b), and de Chardin (1959) all reflect process philosophy and mysticism. In contrast, Mitchell and Cody (1992) pointed out that Newman's view of human beings as unitary seems to be inconsistent with her discussion of physiological structures and functions. In an attempt to reconcile the inconsistency, they offered the following interpretation of Newman's views:

> The unity of the human "system," for Newman, is predicated on the idea that "mind and matter are made of the same basic stuff" (1986, p. 37). It is apparently quite appropriate within Newman's model to discuss the physiological, psychological, and emotional processes of the "human system" in conventional terms, so long as one remembers that everything, from the atom to the human being and beyond, is a manifestation of the implicate order, or "absolute consciousness" (Newman, 1986, pp. 36–37). (p. 57)

Semantic clarity is evident in the definitions and descriptions Newman gave for the concepts of the theory and their dimensions. Although precise definitions were not given for time and space, those definitions are self-evident. Furthermore, Newman's identification of various dimensions of time and space provided some clarification of the meaning she ascribes to those concepts. Semantic consistency is evident in the consistent use of terms and the consistent meaning attached to each term across various publications.

The analysis of the Theory of Health as Expanding Consciousness revealed one possible concept redundancy: Movement is regarded as both a concept and a dimension of the concept pattern. It is unclear from Newman's (1986) statement that "the pattern is in constant movement or change" (p. 14) whether the dimension of pattern is movement in the sense of a person moving through space or movement as change.

A concept redundancy was avoided by the decision *not* to include health as a separate concept. That decision was supported by Newman's (1990a) statement that "Health and the evolving pattern of consciousness are the same" (p. 38). Inasmuch as health and consciousness are equivalent, the inclusion of both would have created a redundancy.

The analysis of Newman's theory revealed structural consistency, but only when relational propositions were extracted from different published versions of the theory. No one publication contains all of the propositions required to support Newman's (1979) assertion that movement, space, and time are correlates of consciousness. In fact, some of the required propositions are not included in the most recent publications about the theory (Newman, 1990a, 1990b).

Parsimony

The Theory of Health as Expanding Consciousness is parsimonious. The analysis of the theory yielded five concepts and several relational propositions. Although several readings of Newman's publications about the theory were required to extract all concepts and propositions, no extraneous terms or statements were identified. The decision to include pattern as a separate concept was based on Newman's frequent reference to the concept and the central role it plays in the theory. In fact, she stated that "Pattern . . . is basic to the theory" (1990b, p. 132). Thus, although Newman (1979, 1986) explicitly identified just four concepts (movement, space, time, and consciousness), the addition of pattern as the fifth concept avoided oversimplification of the theory.

Testability

The propositions of the Theory of Health as Expanding Consciousness cannot be directly tested because they were written at the grand theory level of abstraction. The theory can, however, be indirectly tested by means of a research methodology that can lead to the development of middle-range theories (Newman, 1990a).

The purpose of research is to develop descriptions of phenomena that represent pattern recognition. The phenomena of interest are patterns of relations and parameters of wholeness as expressed in sequential configurations of the evolving pattern that is the expanding consciousness of the person. The primary data collection method is the interview.

The components of the research methodology that facilitates elaboration of the pattern of expanding consciousness are:

1. Establishing the mutuality of the process of inquiry.
2. Focusing on the most meaningful persons and events in the interviewee's life.
3. Organizing the data in narrative form and displaying it as sequential patterns over time.
4. Sharing the interviewer's perception of the pattern with the interviewee and seeking revision or confirmation. (Newman, 1990a, pp. 40–41).

Newman (1990a) pointed out that the use of the research methodology "embodies negotiation, reciprocity, and empowerment" (p. 41). The methodology, then, precludes viewing the person as an object and requires the nurse to participate in the evolving pattern of consciousness. Indeed, "the nurse-researcher cannot stand outside the person being researched in a subject-object fashion" (p. 40). Rather, clients serve as partners or coresearchers in the search for health patterns (Newman, 1986).

No specific instruments associated with the research methodology have been published, although the interview schedule Moch (1990) used for her study of women's experiences with breast cancer could be used as a prototype for other studies guided by Newman's theory. That interview schedule included the following questions:

1. Tell me what it has been like living with cancer.
2. What is meaningful to you?
3. What do you think about what we have been talking about? (Moch, 1990, p. 1429)

Thus more attention needs to be directed toward formulation of precise definitions and empirical indicators for the concepts of the Theory of Health as Expanding Consciousness at the middle-range theory level. Speaking to that need, Ray (1990) noted:

Abstract categories of wholeness, such as health as expanded consciousness, are timeless and have no real perceptual attributes, but are among the most significant categories for understanding the human relational realm. Knowledge-based praxis, however, requires clear articulation and levels of precision in the cycles of perception-action in the organization of the structures of human experience. . . . Thus, phenomenological clarification is still required at the level of referential meaning. (p. 45)

Furthermore, Boyd (1990) urged refinement of the interview method as well as development of other data collection strategies that would be consistent with the Theory of Health as Expanding Consciousness. She stated:

Explicit incorporation of nursing practice modalities of care in research methods need not be limited to interview, as . . . Newman . . . impl[ies], nor does data need to be limited to participants' verbal descriptions. Further development of these and other methods for nursing research will profit from the search for and admittance of a variety of data forms that include a fuller range of human expression. (p. 42)

Empirical Adequacy

As noted in the preceding section on testability, the Theory of Health as Expanding Consciousness cannot be empirically tested directly because it is a grand theory. Consequently, the research associated with the theory provides only indirect evidence of the theory's empirical adequacy.

Newman (1986) noted that when viewed from the perspective of Bentov's (1978) conceptualization of a relation between subjective and objective time, the findings from her early studies of perceived duration of time (Newman, 1976, 1982) provided support for her notion of expanding consciousness across the life span. In a later publication, however, she stated that "some of the early research purported to test

[her] theory stemmed from a mechanistic view of movement-space-time-consciousness and failed to honor the basic assumptions of the [theory]" (Newman, 1990a, p. 41).

A review of recent research dealing with the Theory of Health as Expanding Consciousness revealed some indirect empirical support for the theory. Moch (1989, 1990) found that women with breast cancer described health according to the pattern dimensions of relating, moving, perceiving, and knowing. She maintained that her study results are consistent with Newman's (1986) notion that "tension in illness may have allowed patterns of expanding consciousness to emerge and facilitated desired change for the person" (Moch, 1990, p. 1430).

Fryback (1991) reported that her study sample of persons with cancer or AIDS/HIV disease described health within physical, health promotion, and spiritual domains. She concluded that her findings were similar to the concepts of Newman's theory. She explained:

> Although the main concepts in [Newman's theory] are different [from the study findings], many of the philosophical underpinnings are the same. One of the areas of agreement is that the informants felt that their disease was a part of their health. . . . In accord with Newman, many informants believed that they had become healthier as a result of having their diagnosis. (p. 1951B)

Pragmatic Adequacy

Nursing Education

Within the context of the Theory of Health as Expanding Consciousness, research is regarded as praxis, or practice. Hence, teaching the research methodology associated with the theory also teaches the student a practice methodology that is congruent with the theory. Indeed, Newman (1990b) commented, "It seems to me that my theory is an *explication* of the experience of many nurses"(p. 131). She went on to say, "I now see the theory, the research, and the practice as one process—not separate entities" (p. 131).

Education for use of the theory of Health as Expanding Consciousness requires a curriculum that reflects a shift in thinking from the traditional view of health as a dichotomy of wellness and illness, or even a continuum from high-level wellness through disease to death, to a new, synthesized view of disease as a meaningful aspect of health. Furthermore, the nurse has to learn to let go of wanting to control the situation. The client's choices have to be respected and supported, even when those choices conflict with the nurse's personal values (Newman, 1990b; Newman, Lamb, & Michaels, 1991).

Students and practicing nurses who plan to use the Theory of Health as Expanding Consciousness have to be prepared for personal transformation. In fact, "personal growth of the student/practitioner [is] paramount" (Newman, 1986, p. 89). Sensitive to this issue, Newman (1986) commented:

> The pathway is uncertain and the feeling is unsure. Those who have gone before us assure us that in letting go and experiencing the moment fully the transformation will take place, and through us others will find a new level of integration and growth. (p. 78)

Despite the potential difficulties of personal transformation, Newman (1992) claimed that nurses who practice within the context of the Theory of Health as Expanding Consciousness will "experience the joy of participating in the expanding process of others and find that their own lives are enhanced and expanded by the process" (p. 650).

Moreover, use of the theory requires the ability to recognize patterns in such observable phenomena as body temperature, blood pressure, heart rate, neoplasms, biochemical variations, diet, exercise, and communication. Pattern, then, is substance, process, and method. Newman (1986) suggested that recognition of patterns occurs when the nurse gets in touch with his or her own pattern and, through that, gets in touch with the client's pattern. She recommended use of Gendlin's (1978) process of focusing as a starting point. That process involves directed concentration on and naming of one's bodily feelings, which results in a feeling of relaxation that, in turn, releases energy for growth.

Nursing Practice

"Pattern recognition," Newman (1986) maintained, "is the essence of practice" (p. 18) and, therefore, "the task in intervention is pattern recognition" (p. 72). Pattern recognition, which is equated with insight and intuition, "illuminates the possibilities for action" (Newman, 1990a, p. 40). In fact, the objective of nursing practice, according to Newman (1986), is "an authentic involvement of [the nurse] with the patient in a mutual relationship of pattern recognition and augmentation" (p. 88).

Newman (1987) pointed out that "pattern recognition comes from within the observer" (p. 38). She went on to explain that nurses help clients to recognize patterns in their interactions with the environment. Consequently, nurses can assist people in their search for understanding the evolving patterns of their lives through application of the Theory of Health as Expanding Consciousness (Newman, 1990a). The nurse facilitates the recognition of pattern by connecting with the person in an authentic way and assisting the person to discover new rules for a higher level of organization or consciousness. The nurse and the person come together when old rules do not work and the person must make a choice. The choice involves learning how things work, discovering new rules, and moving on—evolving—to a new level of being and understanding, that is, to a higher level of consciousness. The rules deal with how to engage in meaningful relationships with other people, and recognition of patterns leads to higher levels of consciousness.

Nurses and patients become partners in pattern recognition and give up the traditional roles of "nurse" and "patient." Instead, they are "participants in a greater whole . . . [and] are not separate persons. They are persons experiencing the pattern of consciousness formed by their interaction. Their relationship is based not only on problems and solutions . . . but is a manifestation of the evolving consciousness of the whole" (Newman, 1986, p. 89). Nurses are also partners with other nurses and other health care professionals and thereby form an integrated team (Newman, 1986; 1990b).

Newman (1986) noted that an assessment framework identified by the nurse theorist group of the North American Nursing Diagnosis Association (NANDA) (Roy et al., 1982) "may be useful in initial efforts to identify pattern" (p. 73). The framework is made up of nine dimensions—exchanging, communicating, relating, valuing, choosing, moving, perceiving, feeling, and knowing. Newman (1986) modified the NANDA group's definitions of the dimensions so that they would be consistent with her theory. The dimensions and modified definitions are given in Table 4–2. In addition, Newman (1987) stated that the way a person talks and moves, as well as genetic patterns, are enduring patterns or characteristics that identify the whole person across the life span. She indicated that the data obtained from the assessment format can be viewed from "the standpoint of movement-space-time patterns of consciousness" (1986, p. 75).

Publications dealing with the application of the theory provide some evidence of pragmatic adequacy. The Theory of Health as Expanding Consciousness may be used with individuals, families, and

TABLE 4–2. **Dimensions and Definitions of Pattern**

Dimension	Definition
Exchanging	Interchanging matter and energy between person and environment and transforming energy from one form to another
Communicating	Interchanging information from one system to another
Relating	Connecting with other persons and the environment
Valuing	Assigning worth
Choosing	Selecting one or more alternatives
Moving	Rhythmic alternating between activity and rest
Perceiving	Receiving and interpreting information
Feeling	Sensing physical and intuitive awareness
Knowing	Personal recognizing of self and world

Source: From Newman, 1986, p. 74; with permission.

communities (Marchione, 1986; Newman, 1986). Situations for which the theory is appropriate include childbirth, parenting, caring for a loved one with long-term illness, and one's own health concerns (Newman, 1986). The feasibility of implementing clinical protocols that reflect the theory is becoming evident (Newman, Lamb, & Michaels, 1991), and clinicians have the legal ability to implement assessment formats and interventions dealing with pattern recognition. The extent to which use of those formats and interventions is compatible with expectations for nursing practice and the actual effects of their use on health care professionals and patients has begun to be explored. Ethridge (1991) reported that nursing case management that reflects the Theory of Health as Expanding Consciousness has resulted in increased job satisfaction and decreased job stress for nurses, increased patient satisfaction with nursing services, and considerable savings of health care dollars due to decreased incidence of hospitalization and decreased length of hospital stay. Controlled experimental studies are necessary, however, to determine the relative contributions of case management and the use of the theory.

CONCLUSION

Newman has made a meaningful contribution to nursing by explicating a theory of health that expands Rogers's (1970, 1990) concept of pattern in person-environment interactions. Evidence of the empirical and pragmatic adequacy of the theory is beginning to accumulate. Evidence from one practice setting, in which nurses have established a health maintenance organization (Ethridge, 1991; Newman, Lamb, & Michaels, 1991), is especially impressive. Continued documentation of outcomes of the use of the Theory of Health as Expanding Consciousness is needed, with attention given to the design and conduct of carefully controlled experimental studies.

REFERENCES

Bateson, G. (1979). *Mind and nature: A necessary unity.* Toronto: Bantam.
Bentov, I. (1978). *Stalking the wild pendulum.* New York: E. P. Dutton.
Bohm, D. (1980). *Wholeness and the implicate order.* London: Routledge and Kegan Paul.
Boyd, C. O. (1990). Critical appraisal of developing nursing research methods. *Nursing Science Quarterly, 3,* 42–43.
de Chardin, T. (1959). *The phenomenon of man.* New York: Harper and Brothers.
Ethridge, P. (1991). A nursing HMO: Carondelet St. Mary's experience. *Nursing Management, 22*(7), 22–27.
Fryback, P. B. (1991). Perceptions of health by persons with a terminal disease: Implications for nursing. *Dissertation Abstracts International, 52,* 1951B.
Gendlin, E. T. (1978). *Focusing.* New York: Everest.

Marchione, J. M. (1986). Application of the new paradigm of health to individuals, families, and communities. In M. A. Newman, *Health as expanding consciousness* (pp. 107–134). St. Louis: C. V. Mosby.

Mitchell, G. J., & Cody, W. K. (1992). Nursing knowledge and human science: Ontological and epistemological considerations. *Nursing Science Quarterly, 5*, 54–61.

Moch, S. D. (1989). Health in illness: Experiences with breast cancer. *Dissertation Abstracts International, 50*, 497B.

Moch, S. D. (1990). Health within the experience of breast cancer. *Journal of Advanced Nursing, 15*, 1426–1435.

Moss, R. (1981). *The I that is we.* Millbrae, CA: Celestial Arts.

Newman, M. A. (1978, December). *Toward a theory of health.* Paper presented at the Second Annual Nurse Educator Conference, New York. (Cassette recording)

Newman, M. A. (1979). *Theory development in nursing.* Philadelphia: F.A. Davis.

Newman, M. A. (1983). Newman's health theory. In I. Clements & F. Roberts (Eds.), *Family health: A theoretical approach to nursing care* (pp. 333–336). New York: John Wiley & Sons.

Newman, M. A. (1986). *Health as expanding consciousness.* St. Louis: C. V. Mosby.

Newman, M. A. (1987). Patterning. In M. E. Duffy and N. J. Pender (Eds.), *Conceptual issues in health promotion: A report of proceedings of a Wingspread conference* (pp. 36–50). Indianapolis: Sigma Theta Tau.

Newman, M. A. (1990a). Newman's theory of health as praxis. *Nursing Science Quarterly, 3*, 37–41.

Newman, M. A. (1990b). Shifting to higher consciousness. In M. E. Parker (Ed.), *Nursing theories in practice* (pp. 129–139). New York: National League for Nursing.

Newman, M. A. (1992). Window on health as expanding consciousness. In M. O'Toole (Ed.), *Miller-Keane encyclopedia & dictionary of medicine, nursing, & allied health* (5th ed., p. 650). Philadelphia: W. B. Saunders.

Newman, M. A., Lamb, G. S., & Michaels, C. (1991). Nurse case management. The coming together of theory and practice. *Nursing and Heatlh Care, 12*, 404–408.

Prigogine, I. (1980). *From being to becoming.* San Francisco: W.H. Freeman.

Ray, M. A. (1990). Critical reflective analysis of Parse's and Newman's research methodologies. *Nursing Science Quarterly, 3*, 44–46.

Rogers, M. E. (1970). *An introduction to the theoretical basis of nursing.* Philadelphia: F. A. Davis.

Rogers, M. E. (1990). Space-age paradigm for new frontiers in nursing. In M. E. Parker (Ed.), *Nursing theories in practice* (pp. 105–113). New York: National League for Nursing.

Roy, C., Rogers, M. E., Fitzpatrick, J. J., Newman, M. A., Orem, D., Field, L., Stafford, M. J., Weber, S., Rossi, L., & Krekeler, K. (1982). Nursing diagnosis and nursing theory. In M. J. Kim & D. A. Moritz (Eds.), *Classification of nursing diagnosis* (pp. 214–278). New York: McGraw-Hill.

Sarter, B. (1988). Philosophical sources of nursing theory. *Nursing Science Quarterly, 1*, 52–59.

Young, A. M. (1976a) *The geometry of meaning.* San Francisco: Robert Briggs.

Young, A. M. (1976b). *The reflexive universe: Evolution of consciousness.* San Francisco: Robert Briggs.

ANNOTATED BIBLIOGRAPHY

Primary Sources

Newman, M. A. (1979). *Theory development in nursing.* Philadelphia: F. A. Davis.
Newman describes the process of theory analysis and presents the first published version of her theory of health.

Newman, M. A. (1981). The meaning of health. In G. E. Lasker (Ed.). *Applied systems and cybernetics: Proceedings of the International Congress on Applied Systems Research and Cybernetics: Vol. 4. Systems research in health care, biocybernetics and ecology* (pp. 1739–1743). New York: Pergamon.
Newman discusses her ideas about health.

Newman, M. A. (1983). Newman's health theory. In I. Clements & F. Roberts (Eds.), *Family health: A theoretical approach to nursing care* (pp. 333–336). New York: Wiley.
In this chapter, Newman outlines the basic assumptions and major concepts of her theory of health. The broad generalizations linking the major concepts are discussed. Finally, the author illustrates the application of the theory of health to families.

Newman, M. A. (1986). *Health as expanding consciousness.* St. Louis: C. V. Mosby.
Newman describes her theory of health as expanding consciousness. The book includes a chapter by Joanne Marchione that presents an application of Newman's theory to individuals, families, and the community.

Newman, M. A. (1987). Patterning. In M. Duffy & N. J. Pender (Eds.), *Conceptual issues in health promotion: Report of Proceedings of a Wingspread Conference* (pp. 36–50). Indianapolis: Sigma Theta Tau.
Newman discusses her approach to pattern recognition and illustrates the approach with case studies of individuals at various developmental stages.

Newman, M. A. (1990). Newman's theory of health as praxis. *Nursing Science Quarterly, 3,* 37–41.
Newman presents an overview of her theory of health as expanding consciousness and an emerging research methodology. As an expansion of Rogers's theory of unitary human beings, the author identifies the theories of Bohm, Prigogine, and Young as supportive of her theory of health. Newman advocates research as praxis and emphasizes process as content. She describes the elements of the research methodology used to elaborate the pattern of expanding consciousness as: establishing the mutuality of the inquiry process, focusing on the most meaningful persons and events in the interviewee's life, organizing data in narrative form and displaying sequential patterns over time, and sharing the interviewer's perception of the pattern with the interviewee for revision or confirmation.

Newman, M. A. (1990). Shifting to higher consciousness. In M. E. Parker (Ed.), *Nursing theories in practice* (pp. 129–139). New York: National League for Nursing.
Newman presents elements of her theory of health as expanding consciousness.

Newman, M. A. (1992). Window on health as expanding consciousness. In M. O'Toole (Ed.), *Miller-Keane encyclopedia & dictionary of medicine, nursing, & allied health* (5th ed., p. 650). Philadelphia: W. B. Saunders.
Newman provides a very brief overview of her theory.

Commentary by Newman and Others

Adams, T. (1991). The idea of revolution in the development of nursing theory. *Journal of Advanced Nursing, 16,* 1487–1491.
Adams examines Newman's assertion, following from Kuhn's work on scientific revolutions, that theory development in nursing proceeds by means of revolution (c.f. annotation in this section for Newman, M. A. (1983). The continuing revolution: A history of nursing science. In N. L. Chaska (Ed.), *The nursing profession: A time to speak* (pp. 385–393). St. Louis: C. V. Mosby). He concludes that the idea of theory development through revolution is useful, but that the cumulative approach is also useful in nursing.

Engle, V. (1983). Newman's model of health. In J. J. Fitzpatrick & A. L. Whall, *Conceptual models of nursing: Analysis and application* (pp. 263–273). Bowie, MD: Brady.

Engle, V. (1989). Newman's model of health. In J. J. Fitzpatrick & A. L. Whall, *Conceptual models of nursing: Analysis and application* (2nd ed., pp. 301–312). Norwalk, CT: Appleton and Lange.
Engle describes Newman's theory, presents an analysis of the theory, and briefly discusses its relation to nursing research, education, and practice.

George, J. B. (1990). Other extant theories. In J. B. George (Ed.), *Nursing theories: The base for professional nursing practice* (3rd ed., pp. 373–379). Norwalk, CT: Appleton and Lange.
George presents a very brief description of Newman's theory.

Hensley, D. M., Kilgore, K. A., Langfitt, J. V., & Peterson, L. (1986). Margaret A. Newman:

Model of health. In A. Marriner, *Nursing theorists and their work* (pp. 369–377). St. Louis: C. V. Mosby.

Hensley, D. M., Keffer, M. J., Kilgore-Keever, K. A., Langfitt, J. V., & Peterson, L. (1989). Margaret A. Newman: Model of health. In A. Marriner-Tomey, *Nursing theorists and their work* (2nd ed. pp. 432–447). St. Louis: C. V. Mosby.
The authors describe Newman's academic and experiential credentials and present a rudimentary analysis of her theory. They also include a cursory critique of the theory.

Marchione, J. (1993). *Margaret Newman: Health as expanding consciousness.* Newbury Park, CA: Sage.
Marchione presents an interpretation and analysis of Newman's theory of health as expanding consciousness. Two case studies focusing on identifying patterns of the whole are included. A very brief discussion of Newman's theory and family health also is included, as well as a brief review of research methods and studies derived from the theory.

McCarthy, M. P., Craig, C., Bergstrom, L., Whitley, E. M., Stoner, M. H., & Magilvy, J. K. (1991). Caring conceptualized for community nursing practice: Beyond caring for individuals. In P. L. Chinn (Ed.), *Anthology on caring* (pp. 85–93). New York: National League for Nursing.
The authors describe their idea regarding caring at the community level and use a definition of community health based on Newman's theory of health as the underpinning for their notion of community competence.

Mitchell, G. J., & Cody, W. K. (1992). Nursing knowledge and human science: Ontological and epistemological considerations. *Nursing Science Quarterly, 5,* 54–61.
Mitchell and Cody define and describe human science from Dilthey's perspective. They conclude that Newman's view represents an objectivist reality that is not completely consistent with the human science view of reality as a complex multidimensional whole.

Newman, M. A. (1972). Nursing's theoretical evolution. *Nursing Outlook, 20,* 449–453.
Newman describes the evolution of nursing science and discusses three approaches to nursing theory development: borrowing theory from other disciplines, analyzing nursing practice situations for theoretical underpinnings, and creating conceptual models from which theories can be derived.

Newman, M. A. (1983). The continuing revolution: A history of nursing science. In N. L. Chaska (Ed.), *The nursing profession: A time to speak* (pp. 385–393). St. Louis: C. V. Mosby.
Newman discusses the development of nursing science and nursing theory, as well as the continuing emphasis, since the time of Nightingale, on the nurse, the patient, the nurse-patient situation, and the health of the patient.

Newman, M. A. (1990). Nursing paradigms and realities. In N. L. Chaska (Ed.), *The nursing profession: Turning points* (pp. 230–235). St. Louis: C. V. Mosby.
The author presents the major paradigms of health and illustrates how they guide the conceptualization and interpretation of research as well as nursing practice. Inasmuch as any one paradigm captures just one level of reality, Newman proposes that nurses be able to practice from a paradigm broad enough to incorporate different perspectives and methods.

Newman, M. A. (1990). Professionalism: Myth or reality. In N. L. Chaska (Ed.), *The nursing profession. Turning points* (pp. 49–52). St. Louis: C. V. Mosby.
Newman maintains that the fulfillment of a professional role in nursing is primarily a myth. She claims that increased emphasis on a nursing paradigm that incorporates feminist principles of caring, cooperation, collaboration, and mutuality would advance the reality of professionalism in nursing practice.

Newman, M. A. (1991). Health conceptualizations. In J. J. Fitzpatrick, R. L. Taunton, & A. K. Jacox (Eds.), *Annual review of nursing research* (Vol. 9, pp. 221–243). New York: Springer.
Newman presents an overview of various conceptualizations of health found in the nursing literature. She discusses conceptualizations that reflect the wellness-illness

continuum, including well-being, quality of life, adaptation, and functional ability, as well as conceptualizations reflecting health as a developmental phenomenon, including self-actualization, expanding consciousness, and personal transformation.

Newman, M. A. (1992). Nightingale's vision of nursing theory and health. In F. Nightingale, *Notes on nursing: What it is, and what it is not* (Commemorative edition, pp. 44–47). Philadelphia: J. B. Lippincott. (Original work published in 1859).
Newman explains the influence of Nightingale's work on her own theory of health and patterning.

Sarter, B. (1988). Philosophical sources of nursing theory. *Nursing Science Quarterly, 1,* 52–59.
Sarter identifies the philosophical roots of Newman's theory as relativity and quantum theory, mysticism, and early Greek and Eastern philosophy.

Schroeder, C., & Smith, M. C. (1991). Nursing conceptual frameworks arising from field theory: A critique of the body as manifestation of underlying field. Commentary: Disembodiment or "Where's the body in field theory?" [Schroeder]. Response: Affirming the unitary perspective [Smith]. *Nursing Science Quarterly, 4,* 146–152.
Schroeder notes that Newman builds on Martha Rogers's concept of energy field and discusses Newman's idea of expansion of consciousness, pointing out that the body, for Newman, is manifest only in patterns of energy exchange with the environment. Smith focuses on the unitary perspective and agrees with Schroeder that Newman discounts the body as the source of all experience. She notes that a unitary perspective does not treat body, mind, and spirit as separate entities.

Watts, R. J. (1990). Democratization of health care: Challenge for nursing. *Advances in Nursing Science, 12*(2), 37–46.
In her discussion of the need for democratic institutions and processes within the health care system, Watts notes that Newman's definition of health as the expansion of consciousness and Dewey's view of the purpose of democracy as the creation of a new human potential are consistent.

Practice

Bramlett, M. H., Gueldner, S. H., & Sowell, R. L. (1990). Consumer-centric advocacy: Its connection to nursing frameworks. *Nursing Science Quarterly, 3,* 156–161.
The authors include a discussion of consumer-centric advocacy, as it is operationalized in Newman's theory. They explain that for Newman, advocacy is accomplished through interpersonal encounters involving the nurse and the client, with emphasis on the client's freedom to implement decisions.

Gustafson, W. (1990). Application of Newman's theory of health: Pattern recognition as nursing practice. In M. E. Parker (Ed.), *Nursing theories in practice* (pp. 141–161). New York: National League for Nursing.
Gustafson describes the application of Newman's theory of health, with emphasis on the who, when and where, and doing of pattern recognition, in her practice as a parish nurse at Gloria Dei Lutheran Church in Duluth, Minnesota.

Kalb, K. A. (1990). The gift: Applying Newman's theory of health in nursing practice. In M. E. Parker (Ed.), *Nursing theories in practice* (pp. 163–186). New York: National League for Nursing.
Kalb describes pattern recognition as it is applied in a comprehensive program of care for high-risk pregnant women.

Keene, L. (1985). Nursing as a partnership. *New Zealand Nursing Journal, 78*(12), 10–11.
Keene, an editorial assistant for the journal, presents her interview with Margaret Newman. Keene describes Newman's views about health and an alternative approach to nursing. Newman explains how the assessment of the person's total pattern of health should be the focus of the nurse's diagnosis. In discussing the limitations of the medical model, Newman emphasizes the importance of primary nursing as an essential element in the holographic model of intervention.

Magan, S. J., Gibbon, E. J., & Mrozek, R. (1990). Nursing theory applications: A practice model. *Issues in Mental Health Nursing, 11,* 297–312.
Based on the open system nursing principles of Parse, Newman, and Rogers, the

authors describe the implementation of nursing theory-based assessment and interventions for hospitalized, chronically mentally ill patients. They also discuss the empirical testing of the practice model.

Nelson, J. I. (1991). A crab or a dolphin: A new paradigm for nursing practice. *Nursing Outlook, 39,* 136–137.

Nelson discusses the application of Newman's theory to a case study of professional nursing practice, with emphasis on the nurse's struggle to practice in a professional manner. She maintains that nurses need to improve their vision to see what is happening in the practice setting and to change the nursing paradigm from a crab (a metaphor referring to others pulling one who is rising back down to their level) to a dolphin (a metaphor referring to warning others of impending danger, supporting one another, and using intelligence to promote harmony in the environment).

Newman, M. A. (1984). Nursing diagnosis: Looking at the whole. *American Journal of Nursing, 84,* 1496–1999.

Newman discusses the development of the taxonomy for nursing diagnosis as proposed by the North American Nursing Diagnosis Association (NANDA). The use of an organizing framework with an unifying focus on the person is proposed.

Newman, M. A. (1987). Nursing's emerging paradigm: The diagnosis of pattern. In A. M. McLane (Ed.), *Classification of nursing diagnoses: Proceedings of the Seventh Conference, North American Nursing Diagnosis Association* (pp. 53–60). St. Louis: C. V. Mosby.

In this chapter, Newman presents nursing's new paradigm, which is based on pattern recognition of the person-environment interaction. Drawing from Rogers's theory of the unitary nature of human beings, Newman explains how the identification of sequential patterns is crucial for nursing practice. A description of the nurse's role within a paradigm of pattern is presented. Newman proposes the use of the holographic model of intervention to guide nursing diagnosis.

Newman, M. A. (1989). The spirit of nursing. *Holistic Nursing Practice, 3*(3), 1–6.

According to Newman, human interaction encompasses a spiritual dimension. Inasmuch as nursing is concerned with human interaction in regard to health matters, Newman describes how nurses can assist clients to experience the reality of the patterns of their lives. The author illustrates the activities of the nurse, which include the processes of pattern recognition and sensing into one's own being. Newman believes that the essence of nursing is being open to whatever arises in the interaction with the client.

Newman, M. A. (1990). Toward an integrative model of professional practice. *Journal of Professional Nursing, 6,* 167–173.

Newman notes that a review of nursing practice demonstrates repeated attempts to focus on direct professional responsibilities to clients but failure to do so consistently in an effective professional model. The cycles of growth of the profession depict the long-standing subordination of nursing to hospital administration and medicine and suggest that nursing is ready to move into an integrative, collaborative stage of development. Newman proposes a trilevel model of professional practice, based on differentiated roles for graduate, baccalaureate, and associate degree levels of education.

Smith, M. C. (1990). Pattern in nursing practice. *Nursing Science Quarterly, 3,* 57–59.

Smith traces the discussion of the concept of pattern in the nursing literature, starting with Martha Rogers and continuing with Parse's and Newman's notions of pattern. She notes that for Newman, pattern recognition is the essence of nursing practice.

Administration

Ethridge, P. (1991). A nursing HMO: Carondelet St. Mary's experience. *Nursing Management, 22*(7), 22–27.

Ethridge explains the organizational structure of the nursing services at Carondelet St. Mary's Hospital and Health Center in Tucson, Arizona and identifies several favorable fiscal, nurse, and client outcomes. She also explains that the quality and cost outcomes of professional nurse case management reflect Newman's theory of health as expanding consciousness.

Michaels, C. (1992). Carondelet St. Mary's nursing enterprise. *Nursing Clinics of North America, 27,* 77–85.
Michaels explains the development and current organizational structure of nursing services at Carondelet St. Mary's Hospital and Health Center in Tuscon, Arizona. As noted in another article, the nurse case management delivery system uses Newman's theory of health to facilitate clients' pattern recognition (c.f. annotation in this section for Newman, M. A., Lamb, G. S., & Michaels, C. (1991). Nurse case management. The coming together of theory and practice. *Nursing and Health Care, 12,* 404–408).

Newman, M. A., Lamb, G. S., & Michaels, C. (1991). Nurse case management. The coming together of theory and practice. *Nursing and Health Care, 12,* 404–408.
The authors discuss the application of Newman's theory of health at Carondelet St. Mary's Hospital and Health Center in Tucson, Arizona. They explain that nurse case managers use pattern recognition to engage clients in viewing and managing their health in creative ways.

Education

Bunkers, S. S., Brendtro, M., Holmes, P. K., Howell, J., Johnson, S., Koerner, J., Larson, J., Nelson, J., & Weaver, R. (1992). The healing web: A transformative model for nursing. *Nursing and Health Care, 13,* 68–73.
The Healing Web is a model designed to integrate nursing education and nursing service, and to bring together private and public educational programs for baccalaureate and associate degree nursing. The project involved the Augustana College Department of Nursing, Sioux Valley Hospital Department of Nursing, and the University of South Dakota Department of Nursing and School of Medicine. Newman's theory of health as expanding consciousness provided some of the content for the project philosophy, conceptual framework, and outline of the nurse's caring capabilities.

Research

Boyd, C. O. (1990). Critical appraisal of developing nursing research methods. *Nursing Science Quarterly, 3,* 42–43.
Boyd discusses Newman's and Parse's orientations to research and notes that both have contributed to the needed clarification of processes of analysis in qualitative research.

Butrin, J., & Newman, M. A. (1986). Health promotion in Zaire: Time perspective and cerebral hemispheric dominance as relevant factors. *Public Health Nursing, 3,* 183–191.
Butrin and Newman report the results of a study that examined the relationship between time perspective and cerebral hemispheric dominance, and the variables of education and setting (rural and urban) in 100 Zairians. Educated Zairians were found to place a greater emphasis on the future than the noneducated group who was more oriented in the present. The concept of time, which is an integral factor in Newman's work, was found to be important in Zairians' health behaviors. Implications of such knowledge in developing health-promotion activities is addressed.

Engle, V. F. (1984). Newman's conceptual framework and the measurement of older adults' health. *Advances in Nursing Science, 7*(1), 24–36.
Engle reports that her study findings supported the postulated relationship between personal tempo and time perception. Contrary to hypothesized expectations, self-assessment of health was not related to personal tempo or time perception.

Engle, V. F. (1986). The relationship of movement and time to older adults' functional health. *Research in Nursing and Health, 9,* 123–129.
Engle reports that the study results revealed significant relationships between functional health and walking cadence, and between walking cadence and perceived duration of time. She contends that the findings support Newman's conceptualization of movement as a dimension of health and her proposition that movement and time are interrelated.

Engle, V. F., & Graney, M. J. (1985–1986). Self-assessed and functional health of older women. *International Journal of Aging and Human Development, 22,* 301–313.

This study examined the relationships of self-assessment of health to functional health, age self-concept, attitudes, and demographic variables. Results demonstrated that body care and movement, emotional behavior activities, age self-concept, self-assessment of speed, and identity as a homemaker explained almost 40 percent of the variance in self-assessment of health.

Gulick, E. E., & Bugg, A. (1992). Holistic health patterning in multiple sclerosis. *Research in Nursing and Health, 15*, 175–185.

The investigators report the findings of a study of changes in health patterning in persons with multiple sclerosis. Although the study is not directly derived from Newman's theory, Gulick and Bugg note that Newman identifies the task of the nurse as facilitating the patient's insight into health patterns and patterning.

Marchione, J. M. (1986). Pattern as methodology for assessing family health: Newman's theory of health. In P. Winstead-Fry (Ed.), *Case studies in nursing theory* (pp. 215–240). New York: National League for Nursing.

Marchione presents a brief overview of Newman's theory of health and describes the use of pattern assessment in a study of family health. The pattern assessment format was based on Newman's theory of health and Kantor and Lehr's family process theory.

Mentzer, C. A., & Schorr, J. A. (1986). Perceived situational control and perceived duration of time: Expressions of life patterns. *Advances in Nursing Science, 9*(1), 12–20.

Newman's notion of perceived duration of time as an index to consciousness provided the theoretical framework for the study. Contrary to hypothesized expectations, the investigators found that perceived duration of time was not related to age or perceived control in a sample of 40 aged women living in an extended care facility. Additional data analysis revealed that length of institutionalization was positively related to perceived control.

Moch, S. D. (1990). Health within the experience of breast cancer. *Journal of Advanced Nursing, 15*, 1426–1435.

Moch reports the results of her study of women's experiences of breast cancer, which was based on Newman's perspective of illness as a meaningful aspect of health as expanding consciousness. Themes of the experience included: getting information and making choices, coping with the physical aspects, dealing with lack of control or possible recurrence, being hopeful about the prognosis and optimistic about life, changing relatedness, and identifying meaning and adding new perspectives of life. Health within the experience of breast cancer emerged as changing patterns of relating, moving, perceiving, and knowing.

Newman, M. A. (1966). Identifying and meeting patients' needs in short-span nurse-patient relationships. *Nursing Forum, 5*(1), 76–86.

Newman reports the findings of her descriptive study on the needs of hospitalized patients. She points out that the identification and meeting of patients' needs is a function of nurse-patient communication. Effective communication is necessary for the achievement of quality in nursing. This study was conducted several years before Newman's formulation of her theory of health.

Newman, M. A. (1972). Time estimation in relation to gait tempo. *Perceptual and Motor Skills, 34*, 359–366.

Newman reports the results of her initial study of the effect of accelerated and decelerated rates of walking on judgment of a 40-second interval in 52 healthy males. No difference was found in time estimation in response to the imposed gait tempos. Newman concluded that accurate time estimation is a characteristic of healthy young men even when they are placed in a situation that imposes an external rhythm in the form of movement.

Newman, M. A. (1976). Movement tempo and the experience of time. *Nursing Research, 25*, 273–279.

Newman reports that the hypothesized relationship between preferred rate of movement and time estimation was not supported in a sample of 90 healthy subjects. In contrast, the hypothesis that time estimation would be greater under the condition of 50 percent decelerated rate of walking than under 30 percent decelerated rate, and that time estimation would be greater under 30 percent decelerated rate than the preferred rate, was supported.

Newman, M. A. (1982). Time as an index of expanding consciousness with age. *Nursing Research, 31*, 290–293.
Newman reports the results of her study of subjective time, which was viewed as a developmental phenomenon of man's expanding consciousness. No evidence was found of relationships between age or preferred walking rate and perceived duration of a 40-second interval of time.

Newman, M. A. (1982). What differentiates clinical research? *Image, 14*, 86–88.
Newman examines the meaning of clinical nursing research within the context of the relationship between research design and level of theory development. She notes that the purpose of a study is the crucial factor in determining its clinical relevance. In addition, she recommends that investigators identify their assumptions regarding health and incorporate health goals in the research process.

Newman, M. A. (1983). [Editorial]. *Advances in Nursing Science, 5*(2), x–xi.
Newman introduces the articles in this issue of the journal, which is devoted to research methods. She notes that although the prevailing methodology of nursing research is the context stripping scientific method, the human experience—the focus of nursing inquiry—requires methods that are context dependent.

Newman, M. A. (1987). Aging as increasing complexity. *Journal of Gerontological Nursing, 13*, 16–18.
Drawing from research on the relationship between age and subjective time, Newman identifies the multiple factors that often accompany aging that may influence one's subjective time. The factors include: emotional state attention, external events, body movements, metabolism, and depressive mood. The use of subjective time as an indicator of quality of life for older adults is discussed.

Newman, M. A. (1987). Commentary: Perception of time among Japanese inpatients. *Western Journal of Nursing Research, 9*, 299–300.
Newman interprets the findings of a study by Yoshiko Nojima et al. of time as an index of consciousness within the context of her theory of health and explains the difference between her theory and the study framework, which dichotomizes wholeness (wellness) and obstructed wholeness (illness).

Newman, M. A., & Batey, M. (1991). The research-practice relationship. Commentary [Newman]. Response [Batey]. *Nursing Science Quarterly, 4*, 100–103.
Newman reviews her idea of research as practice and explains that, for her, the most meaningful research reflects on or creates the practice relationship in a fully authentic manner and is immediately applicable to nursing practice. She also explains that the form that nursing research takes is the form of practice, that is, a real relationship between nurse (researcher-practitioner) and client focusing on a real concern of nursing practice. She emphasizes that practice, however, is not research. Batey responds that the primary goals of research are to search for, develop, and use research methods that will provide credible insights into relevant phenomena, whereas the goals of professional practice focus on client needs. She claims that Newman's approach blurs the goals of research and practice.

Newman, M. A., & Guadiano, J. K. (1984). Depression as an explanation for decreased subjective time in the elderly. *Nursing Research, 33*, 137–139.
The investigators report that their study findings revealed evidence of the hypothesized relationship between depression and decreased subjective time in a sample of women over 65 years of age. They comment that the result provides a tentative explanation for deviations from the documented trend toward increased subjective time with aging.

Newman, M. A., & Moch, S. D. (1991). Life patterns of persons with coronary heart disease. *Nursing Science Quarterly, 4*, 161–167.
Newman and Moch report the findings of a study using the method of cooperative inquiry that involved 11 clients in a cardiac rehabilitation center, a cardiovascular nursing specialist, and the investigators. Patterns that emerged from the inquiry are similar to some previously reported behaviors associated with coronary heart disease: the need to excel and a tendency to be repressed and externally controlled.

Phillips, J. R. (1990). New methods of research: Beyond the shadows of nursing science [Guest editorial]. *Nursing Science Quarterly, 3*, 1–2.

Phillips notes that Newman's research method (c.f. annotation in the Primary Sources section for Newman, M. A. (1990). Newman's theory of health as praxis. *Nursing Science Quarterly, 3,* 27–41) addresses Bohm's notion of the implicate order and facilitates understanding of individuals' experiences rather than gathering data from them as objects.

Ray, M. A. (1990). Critical reflective analysis of Parse's and Newman's research methodologies. *Nursing Science Quarterly, 3,* 44–46.
Ray presents an analysis of Newman's research methodology. She points out that the method addresses assertoric knowledge, that is, knowledge claims that use practical reasoning and argumentation (negotiation, reciprocity, and empowerment) as a means to improve the character of relationships.

Schorr, J. A., Farnham, R. C., & Ervin, S. M. (1991). Health patterns in aging women as expanding consciousness. *Advances in Nursing Science, 13*(4), 52–63.
The authors report the findings of their study of powerlessness in aging women, which was based on Newman's theory of health. Findings indicated that the subjects manifested high levels of perceived situational control or powerfulness, with little variance in powerlessness scores. They maintain that those findings are consistent with Newman's theory.

Schorr, J. A., & Schroeder, C. A. (1989). Consciousness as a dissipative structure: An extension of the Newman model. *Nursing Science Quarterly, 2,* 183–193.
The authors describe their model of consciousness as a dissipative structure, which they derived from Newman's theory of health and Prigogine's theory of dissipative structures. They examine relationships among Type A behavior, temporal orientation, and death anxiety from the perspective of their model and report preliminary research findings. They claim that Type A behavior, future time orientation, and death anxiety are manifestations of consciousness with the potential to evolve to higher levels.

Schorr, J. A., & Schroeder, C. A. (1991). Movement and time: Exertion and perceived duration. *Nursing Science Quarterly, 4,* 104–112.
Using Newman's theory of health and Prigogine's theory of dissipative structures, the investigators examined differences in consciousness indexes, operationalized as perceived duration of time, at different levels of physical exertion. Significant differences were found between the resting consciousness index and those at preferred, increased, and decreased exertion levels.

Silva, M. C. (1986). Research testing nursing theory: State of the art. *Advances in Nursing Science, 9*(1), 1–11.
Silva includes a review of Engle's study of older adult's health, which was derived from Newman's theory (c.f. annotation in this section for Engle, V. F. (1984). Newman's conceptual framework and the measurement of older adults' health. *Advances in Nursing Science, 7*(1), 24–36).

Doctoral Dissertations

Brenner, P. S. (1987). Temporal perspective, professional identity, and perceived well-being. *Dissertation Abstracts International, 47,* 4821B.

Butrin, J. E. (1990). The experience of culturally diverse nurse-client encounters. *Dissertation Abstracts International, 51,* 2815B.

DeBrun, K. T. (1989). An investigation of the relationships among standing, sitting, recumbent postures, judgment of time duration and preferred personal space in adult females. *Dissertation Abstracts International, 50,* 122B.

Engle, V. F. (1981). A study of the relationship between self-assessment of health, function, personal tempo, and time perception in elderly women. *Dissertation Abstracts International, 42,* 967B.

Fryback, P. B. (1991). Perceptions of health by persons with a terminal disease: Implications for nursing. *Dissertation Abstracts International, 52,* 1951B.

Kelley, F. J. (1990). Spatial temporal experiences and self-assessed health in the older adult. *Dissertation Abstracts International, 51,* 1194B.

Leners, D. W. (1990). The deep connection: An echo of transpersonal caring. *Dissertation Abstracts International, 51,* 2818B.

Moch, S. D. (1989). Health in illness: Experiences with breast cancer. *Dissertation Abstracts International, 50,* 497B.

Newman, M. A. (1971). An investigation of the relationship between gait tempo and time perception. *Dissertation Abstracts International, 32,* 2821B.

Page, G. (1989). An exploration of the relationship between daily patterning and weight loss maintenance. *Dissertation Abstracts International, 50,* 497B.

Schmitt, N. A. (1992). Caregiving couples: The experience of giving and receiving social support. *Dissertation Abstracts International, 52,* 5761B.

Smith, C. T. (1990). The lived experience of staying healthy in rural black families. *Dissertation Abstracts International, 50,* 3925B.

Master's Theses

Burress, Y. (1988). An investigation of the relationships among systolic blood pressure, rate of speech, and perceived duration of time. *Masters Abstracts International, 27,* 373.

Kuhn, M. E. (1989). Comparison of health beliefs of adolescents with diabetes and those of their mothers. *Masters Abstracts International, 28,* 412.

Terhaar, N. C. (1989). Blood sugar and cognition patterns in the elderly. *Masters Abstracts International, 28,* 116.

Orlando's Theory of the Deliberative Nursing Process_____

Ida Jean Orlando Pelletier discovered the Theory of the Deliberative Nursing Process in the data collected for a study of experiences in
nursing and teaching that was funded by the National Institute of Mental Health, United States Public Health Service, and conducted under
the auspices of the Yale University School of Nursing. Orlando (1989)
explained that as she sorted the data into the categories of good and bad
outcomes, she realized that the good outcomes were the result of effective nursing practice in the form of the nurse's nonobservable reaction
and observable actions in response to the patient's behavior. She
pointed out that the fundamental idea of her work

> is directed toward the organization, development and implementa-
> tion of a system of understanding which makes it possible for nurses
> to develop and maintain professional responsibility for the patient's
> care and mutual job responsibility with others who may affect the
> nurse's care of patients. (Orlando, 1972, p. 3)

Orlando (1961) originally labeled her work a theory of effective
nursing practice but later—in the preface to the 1990 reprint of her
book—referred to it as the nursing process theory. Explaining the
change in label, she stated:

> If I had been more courageous in 1961, when this book was first writ-
> ten, I would have proposed it as "nursing process theory" instead of

as a "theory of effective nursing practice." A "deliberative" process was presented as a guide for nurses to practice "effectively." Conversely, an "automatic" process was shown to be "ineffective." "Effectiveness" was conceptualized and illustrated as "improvement" in the patient's behavior. The "improvement" stemmed from the fact that the deliberative process made it possible for the nurse to identify and meet the patient's *need for help*. (Orlando Pelletier, 1990, p. vii)

The concepts of the Theory of the Deliberative Nursing Process and their dimensions are listed below. Each concept and dimension is defined and described later in this chapter.

KEY CONCEPTS

Patient's Behavior	Thought
Need for Help	Feeling
Improvement	Nurse's Activity
Nurse's Reaction	Automatic Nursing Process
Perception	Deliberative Nursing Process

ANALYSIS OF THE THEORY OF THE DELIBERATIVE NURSING PROCESS

This section presents an analysis of Orlando's Theory of the Deliberative Nursing Process. The analysis is based on the content of Orlando's 1961 book, *The Dynamic Nurse-Patient Relationship: Function, Process and Principles*, and her 1972 book, *The Discipline and Teaching of Nursing Process (An Evaluation Study)*.

Scope of the Theory

The Theory of the Deliberative Nursing Process focuses exclusively on the interpersonal process between people and is directed toward facilitating identification of "the nature of the patient's distress and his need for help" (Orlando, 1961, p. viii). The central thesis of the theory is that "(often marvelous) [outcomes are] a result of finding out and meeting the patient's immediate needs for help" (Orlando Pelletier, 1990, p. viii). Orlando's work is appropriately classified as a middle-range predictive theory that specifies the effects of a particular nursing process on the patient's behavior.

Context of the Theory

Metaparadigm Concepts and Proposition

Even a cursory review of Orlando's books indicates that the Theory of the Deliberative Nursing Process is based on the metaparadigm concepts *person* and *nursing*. In fact, Orlando (1961) maintained that "Learning how to understand what is happening between herself and the patient is the central core of the nurse's practice and comprises the basic framework for the help she gives to patients" (p. 4).

Orlando focused on a particular nursing process that leads to improvement in the patient's behavior. She stated, "What a nurse says or does is the exclusive mode through which she serves the patient" (1961, p. 6). Hence the metaparadigm proposition that is most relevant is the *[nursing] processes by which positive changes in [the patient's] health status are affected.*

Philosophical Claims

Orlando (1961, 1972) made many statements that represent the philosophical basis for the Theory of the Deliberative Nursing Process. Some of those statements reflect Orlando's claims about patients:

1. A patient *may* react with distress to any aspect of an environment which was designed for therapeutic and helpful purposes. (1961, p. 17)
2. The patient's reactions in the setting which may cause him distress are generally based on an inadequate or incorrect understanding of an experience in the setting. (1961, p. 17)
3. It is safe to assume that patients become distressed when, without help, they cannot cope with their needs. (1961, p. 11)

Other statements represent philosophical claims about nursing:

1. Nursing is historically rooted in an immediate responsiveness to individuals assumed to be suffering helplessness in immediate situations. Traditionally, the responsiveness has been specific to the individual's cry for help and has provided direct assistance for the purpose of avoiding, relieving or diminishing the helplessness suffered or anticipated. (1972, p. 8)
2. It may be assumed that [the nurse's] intention is to be of help. (1961, p. 70)
3. Any nursing, whether one is caring for the self or is being cared for by another, should result in some measure of curative value which is specific to the helplessness suffered or anticipated by individuals in immediate experiences. (1972, p. 9)
4. The nurse is responsible for helping the patient avoid or alleviate the distress of unmet needs. (1961, p. 6)

5. It is important for the nurse to concern herself with the patient's distress because the treatment and prevention of disease proceeds best when conditions extraneous to the disease itself and its management do not cause the patient additional suffering. (1961, pp. 22–23)
6. Nursing in its professional character does not add to the distress of the patient. Instead the nurse assumes the professional responsibility of seeking out and obviating impediments to the patient's mental and physical comfort. (1961, p. 9)
7. It is the nurse's direct responsibility to see to it that the patient's needs for help are met either by her own activity or by calling in the help of others. (1961, p. 22)
8. The focus and stimulus of the professional nurse's service is therefore the patient and his needs. (1961, p. 8)
9. All nursing activities are designed for the benefit of the patient, but sometimes they do not suit the patient because at the same moment he may require something entirely different. (1961, p. 8)
10. It is reasonable to assume that any activity performed with or for the patient is designed, at least ultimately, for the patient's benefit. But, it sometimes happens that professional and non-professional personnel alike carry out activities which not only do not help the patient but may even hinder his progress. (1961, p. 19)

Still other statements reflect Orlando's philosophical position with regard to interactions between nurses and patients. Those statements are:

1. Since the nurse and patient are both people, they interact, and a process goes on between them. (1961, p. 8)
2. The nurse-patient situation [is] a dynamic whole—how the patient behaves affects the nurse and the nurse in turn affects the patient. (1961, p. 36)
3. In order for the nurse to develop and maintain the professional character of her work she must know and be able to validate how her actions and reactions help or do not help the patient or know and be able to validate that the patient does not require her help at a given time. (1961, p. 9)
4. The nurse . . . must first realize that the patient cannot clearly state the nature and meaning of his distress or his need without her help or without her first having established a helpful relationship with him. (1961, p. 23)

Two additional statements represent the philosophical basis for Orlando's (1972) research methodology:

1. The process discipline [the deliberative nursing process] was most effective when an explicit verbal form was used. (p. 51)
2. The use of the process discipline [the deliberative nursing process] would enable the nurse to fulfill her professional and job functions. (p. 54)

Forchuk (1991) and Sellers (1991) both noted that some of the philo-sophical claims on which Orlando's theory is based reflect the totality worldview. Sellers also noted that the theory

> illustrates a mechanistic, deterministic, persistence worldview. Orlando proposes a reductionistic view of person, in which human behavior is perceived from within a stimulus-response framework and a closed system notion of tension reduction and comfort mainte-nance. All behavioral activities are considered as purposeful and directed toward the reduction of discomfort from unmet needs. (p. 144)

At the same time, however, the theory "focuses on the reciprocal interaction between the [patient] and the nurse. Both the [patient] and the nurse are affected by the other's behavior" (Sellers, 1991, p. 144). Furthermore, although Orlando's separation of behaviors, perceptions, thoughts, and feelings reflects the totality worldview, "she sees each person as unique and as providing her or his own meaning to the situ-ation, as in the simultaneity [worldview]" (Forchuk, 1991, p. 41). Thus it can be concluded that Orlando's philosophical claims most closely reflect the *reciprocal interaction* worldview.

Conceptual Model

Although Orlando did not explicitly identify the conceptual under-pinnings of her theory, she did describe the person and nursing in some detail. The person is described as a patient. People become patients when they submit to medical procedures. Orlando (1972) explained:

> Once an individual undergoes medical diagnosis, treatment or super-vision, he automatically assumes the status of patient and is vulnerable to the predicament of being a patient. That is, the patient may not be in a position to control all that happens to him and may suffer help-lessness as a result. (1972, p. 10)

Patients in need of nursing are those who "require help when their distresses stem from (1) physical limitations, (2) adverse reactions to the setting and (3) experiences which prevent the patient from communi-cating his needs" (Orlando, 1961, p. 11). Conversely, "When the patient is able to meet his own needs and is able to carry out prescribed mea-sures unaided, he is not dependent [on] the nurse for help" (pp. 5–6).

Orlando (1961) regarded nursing as distinct from medicine. She explained:

> There is a clear distinction between the medical management of a patient and the way the patient would manage his own affairs and his own comforts if he were able to do so. . . . The doctor places the patient under the care of the nurse for either or both of the following

> reasons: (1) the patient cannot deal with what he needs, or (2) he cannot carry out the prescribed treatment or diagnostic plan alone. . . .
> The responsibility of the nurse is necessarily different [from that of the physician]; it offers whatever help the patient may require for his needs to be met, i.e., for his physical and mental comfort to be assured as far as possible while he is undergoing some form of medical treatment or supervision. (p. 5)

Hence the purpose of nursing "is to supply the help a patient requires in order for his needs to be met" (Orlando, 1961, p. 8). Stated in other words, the nurse's function, which is dictated by patients' predicaments, is "to find out and meet patients' immediate needs for help while undergoing treatment in prescribed settings" (Pelletier, 1967, p. 27).

In a further comparison of nursing and medicine, Orlando (1972) commented:

> Nursing (not necessarily the nurse) is responsive to individuals who suffer or anticipate a sense of helplessness; it is focused on the process of care in an immediate experience; it is concerned with providing direct assistance to individuals in whatever setting they are found for the purpose of avoiding, relieving, diminishing or curing the individual's sense of helplessness. Nursing by another person may take place when an individual is unable to nurse himself and may function independently of whether or not the individual is under medical care. In contrast, medicine is responsive to individuals who suffer or are apt to suffer ill health and commits itself to those who are willing to undergo medical diagnosis, treatment or supervision; it is thus focused on the process of disease; it is concerned with diagnosis and treatment, carried out by advising or directing patients to follow or undergo specific diagnostic, medical, surgical or psychiatric procedures in settings where patients are found or in whatever setting individuals are placed for the purpose of curing, alleviating or preventing disease. Medical practice functions independently of whether or not the patient is able to nurse himself. (p. 12)

The distinction between nursing and medicine is also evident in Orlando's (1961) comment about medically prescribed activities. She stated, "It is important to recognize that the nurse is using a doctor's order for the patient and is not carrying out orders for the doctor" (p. 72). She went on to point out that her position was logical, since "if the patient were able to carry out the diagnostic or treatment plan alone, in all probability the nurse would not become involved in the first place" (p. 72).

Orlando (1961) provided only a brief description of health, referring to mental health and physical health and to a person's sense of well-being and adequacy. She did not describe environment, although she implied that the immediate situation is the environment of interest.

Antecedent Knowledge

Orlando did not identify sources of antecedent knowledge. In fact, as Forchuk (1991) noted, "neither book [Orlando, 1961, 1972] contains even a reference list for a hint of other influences" (p. 40). Rather, the Theory of the Deliberative Nursing Process was induced from clinical observations of nurses and patients made as part of a research project. It represents Orlando's (1961) "synthesis of experience in working and learning with teachers, students, nurses, patients, friends and colleagues" (p. ix).

Orlando (1989) recalled that she rejected preexisting frameworks from psychology, social work, and other disciplines for the analysis of the research project data. She explained, "I found what was there [in the data describing nursing outcomes]—I didn't make it up." Elaborating, Schmieding (1990b) explained:

> Orlando was one of the first to use field methodology to develop her theoretical perspectives long before it was accepted as appropriate. From participant-observer notes, she devised an ingenious conception of the elements and relationships involved as the nurse determines the meaning of the patient's immediate behavior. (p. xviii)

Content of the Theory

Analysis of Orlando's publications revealed that the concepts of the Theory of the Deliberative Nursing Process are *patient's behavior, nurse's reaction,* and *nurse's activity.* "The interaction of these [concepts] with each other is," according to Orlando (1961), "nursing process" (p. 36).

Patient's Behavior

The concept **patient's behavior** is defined as "behavior which is observed by the nurse in an immediate nurse-patient situation" (Orlando, 1961, p. 36). The concept has two dimensions: *need for help* and *improvement.*

The label for the dimension *need for help* is a modification of Orlando's original label, need. In the preface to the 1990 reprint of her book, she explained, "Throughout this text, only the phrase *need for help* should have been used and not the word *need* (Orlando Pelletier, 1990, p. vii). The patient's need for help is defined as follows: "Need [for help] is situationally defined as a requirement of the patient which, if supplied, relieves or diminishes his immediate distress or improves his immediate sense of adequacy or well-being" (Orlando, 1961, p. 5).

Improvement is formally defined as "to grow better, to turn to profit, to use to advantage" (Orlando, 1961, p. 6). When used with regard to patient behavior, improvement refers to an increase in patients' mental and physical health, their well-being, and their sense of adequacy (Orlando, 1961). In her 1972 book, Orlando used the term helpful outcome as an apparent synonym for improvement. She defined that term as "a change in the behavior of the [person] indicating either relief from distress or symptoms or that a solution to a living or work problem had been found" (p. 61).

Improvement (or helpful outcome) is, as Orlando (1961) pointed out,

> always relative to "what was" when the [nursing process] started, and is concerned with the patient's increased sense of well-being or a change for the better in his condition. The help received by the patient may also have cumulative value as it affects or contributes toward the individual's adequacy in taking better care of himself. (p. 9)

The two dimensions of the patient's behavior—need for help and improvement—can be expressed in both nonverbal and verbal forms. Visual manifestations of nonverbal behavior include such motor activities as eating, walking, twitching, and trembling, as well as such physiological forms as urinating, defecating, temperature and blood pressure readings, respiratory rate, and skin color. Vocal forms of nonverbal behavior—nonverbal behavior that is heard—include crying, moaning, laughing, coughing, sneezing, sighing, yelling, screaming, groaning, and singing. Verbal behavior refers to what a patient says, including complaints, requests, questions, refusals, demands, and comments or statements. Orlando (1961) pointed out that "verbal and nonverbal behavior can of course be observed simultaneously" (p. 37).

Orlando (1961) also pointed out that some patient behaviors, such as refusals or demands, may be regarded as ineffective, that is, "behavior which prevents the nurse from carrying out her concerns for the patient's care or from maintaining a satisfactory relationship to the patient" (p. 78). She urged nurses not to dismiss or ignore such behavior, however, because it is "a possible signal of distress or a manifestation of an unmet need" (p. 79).

Nurse's Reaction

The concept **nurse's reaction** is defined as the nurse's nonobservable response to the patient's behavior. The three dimensions of the concept are *perceptions, thoughts,* and *feelings.*

Perception is defined as "a physical stimulation of any one of a person's five senses" (Orlando, 1972, p. 59). In the nursing situation, perceptions are of the patient's behavior. Orlando (1961) claimed that "the perception of the nurse is more often than not correct. It is unlikely that the patient would deny the statement of it if he is aware of the stimulus at the moment the event transpires" (p. 43).

Thought is defined as "an idea which occurs in the mind of a person" (Orlando, 1972, p. 59). Orlando (1961) focused on thoughts stimulated by the nurse's perceptions of the patient's behavior. She maintained that "the individual and automatic thought the nurse has about her perception is likely to be inadequate or not completely correct unless it is first investigated with the patient. Indeed, thoughts are sometimes completely incorrect" (p. 43).

Feeling is defined as "a state of mind inclining a person toward or against a perception, thought or action" (Orlando, 1972, p. 59). In the nursing situation, feelings are in response to the nurse's perceptions and thoughts. Orlando (1961) pointed out that the nurse's feelings must be expressed if they are to benefit the patient. She explained:

> Even if feelings are positive but derived from thoughts which are not first checked with the patient, they do not benefit him. . . . The patient can make use of the nurse's feeling when she expresses it, provided she explains the basis for it and allows the patient to correct or validate what her feeling is about. (p. 49)

Orlando (1961) acknowledged the difficulty of separating perceptions from thoughts and feelings. She maintained, however, that "it is worth trying to do so in order to focus attention on how one aspect of the nurse's reaction may affect the other aspects" (p. 40).

Nurse's Activity

The concept **nurse's activity** refers to the observable action taken by the nurse in response to her reaction. More specifically, Orlando (1972) defined action as "observable behavior, i.e., what the individual says verbally and/or manifests nonverbally" (p. 60). The nurse's action "includes only what she says or does with or for the benefit of the patient" (Orlando, 1961, p. 60). Examples of nursing actions are instructions, suggestions, directions, explanations, information, requests, and questions directed toward the patient; making decisions for the patient; handling the patient's body; administering medications or treatments; and changing the patient's immediate environment (Orlando, 1961).

The two dimensions of nurse's activity are *automatic nursing process* and *deliberative nursing process*. The *automatic nursing process* dimension of the nurse's activity, which Orlando later referred to as "the nursing process 'without discipline'" (Orlando Pelletier, 1990, p. vii), refers to actions decided on by the nurse "for reasons other than the patient's immediate need" (Orlando, 1961, p. 60). Orlando explained:

> Some automatic activities are ordered by the doctor; others are concerned with routines of caring for patients, and still others are based on principles pertinent to protecting and fostering the health of people in general. (p. 60)

Orlando called the other dimension of the nurse's activity the *deliberative nursing process* in her 1961 book and the *process discipline* in her 1972 book. She explained, "the deliberative nursing process was renamed nursing process 'with discipline'" (Orlando Pelletier, 1990, p. vii). Both terms refer to a specific set of nurse behaviors or actions directed toward the patient's behavior. Deliberatively decided actions are "those which ascertain or meet the patient's immediate need" (Orlando, 1961, p. 60). The *deliberative nursing process* is specifically described as follows:

> In order to meet the patient's needs [for help], the nurse (1) initiates a process of helping the patient express the specific meaning of his behavior in order to ascertain his distress and (2) helps the patient explore the distress in order to ascertain the help he requires so that his distress may be relieved. (Orlando, 1961, p. 29)

Orlando (1961) explained that the deliberative nursing process follows a definite sequence:

> First, [the nurse] shares with the patient aspects of her perceptions, thoughts and feelings by expressing in words or nonverbal gestures or tones her wondering, thinking, or questioning in order to learn how accurate or adequate her reaction is. The response of the patient gives rise to fresh reactions which she continues to express and explore. She must do this so that both can find out what each is thinking, and why, so that an understanding of the patient's need can be arrived at. When the patient's need is clearly discerned, the nurse can decide on an appropriate course of action. The nurse then does or says something with or for the patient, or together they decide that the help of another person is required. Whatever the action, the nurse asks the patient about it in order to find out how her action affects him. (pp. 67–68)

In her 1972 book, Orlando identified three specific requirements for the process discipline, that is, the deliberative nursing process:

1. What the nurse says to the individual in the contact must match *(be consistent with)* any or all of the items contained in the immediate reaction and what the nurse does nonverbally must be verbally expressed, and the expression must match one or all of the items contained in the immediate reaction.
2. The nurse must clearly communicate to the individual that the item being expressed belongs to herself.
3. The nurse must ask the individual about the item expressed in order to obtain correction or verification from that same individual. (pp. 29–30)

Elaborating on the third requirement, Orlando (1972) stated:

> The use of the process discipline is "effective" when a specific verbal form is used . . . in a given person-to-person contact. Specifically, the

item expressed is explicitly self-designated (with the use of a personal pronoun) and a question is asked about the same item. (p. 30)

Examples of the third requirement are:

> I am afraid you will hit me if I ask you a question. Should I be afraid? (p. 30)
>
> I don't think you trust anyone. Do you think you do? (p. 60)

Clearly, then, the deliberative nursing process "has elements of continuous reflection as the nurse tries to understand the meaning to the patient of the behavior she observes and what he needs from her in order to be helped" (Orlando, 1961, p. 67).

Orlando (1961) pointed out that deliberative nursing activities are effective—that is, they meet the patient's need for help. In contrast, automatic nursing activities may be "correct" (p. 87), but they are ineffective in meeting the patient's need for help. Thus, although automatic activities may be designed to help the patient, "deliberation is needed to determine whether the activity actually achieves its intended purpose and whether the patient is helped by it" (p. 60). Table 5–1 lists the reasons Orlando gave for the opposing outcomes of the two dimensions of the nurse's activity.

TABLE 5–1.   Reasons for Ineffective and Effective Nursing Activities

Automatic Nursing Activities Are Ineffective Because	*Deliberative Nursing Activities Are Effective Because*
The activity is decided on for reasons other than the meaning of the patient's behavior and the unmet need giving rise to it.	The activity comes about after the nurse knows the meaning of the patient's behavior and the specific activity that is required to meet his need.
The activity does not enable the patient to let the nurse know how the activity affects him.	The activity is carried out in such a way that the patient is helped to inform the nurse as to how her activity affects him.
The activity is unrelated to the patient's immediate need for help.	The specific required activity meets the patient's need for help and achieves the nurse's purpose of having helped the patient.
The activity may occur because the nurse is not free to explore her reaction to the patient's behavior.	The nurse is available to respond to the patient's need for help.
The nurse is unaware of how her activity affects the patient.	The nurse knows how her activity affects the patient.

Source: Adapted from Orlando, 1961, p. 65, with permission.

Nonrelational Propositions

The definitions and descriptions of the concepts of the Theory of the Deliberative Nursing Process are nonrelational propositions. Other nonrelational propositions enhance understanding of the theory concepts and their dimensions.

The following proposition elaborates the concept *patient's behavior:* "The presenting behavior of the patient, regardless of the form in which it appears, may represent a plea for help" (Orlando, 1961, p. 40).

Other propositions further delineate the concept *nurse's reaction:*

> The nurse does not assume that any aspect of her reaction to the patient is correct, helpful or appropriate until she checks the validity of it in exploration with the patient. (Orlando, 1961, p. 56)

> Reactions which the nurse does not resolve may interfere with the interaction between herself and a patient. These reactions may stem from her personal or professional frame of reference, i.e., her personal codes of behavior, her personal value system or her own ideas as to what a nurse should or should not do and say. (Orlando, 1961, p. 56)

Still another proposition, which provides a general guide for the nurse's activity dimension of *deliberative nursing process,* asserts: "The nurse initiates a process of exploration to ascertain how the patient is affected by what she says or does." (Orlando, 1961, p. 67)

Relational Propositions

Relational propositions link the concepts of the Theory of the Deliberative Nursing Process and their dimensions. The patient behavior dimension of *Need for help* and the nurse's reaction dimension of *Perception* are linked in this proposition: "The behavior which the nurse perceives must be viewed as a possible manifestation of an unmet need [for help] or a signal of distress . . . unless she has evidence to the contrary" (Orlando, 1961, p. 39).

The *perception* and *thought* dimensions of the nurse's reaction are linked in this proposition: "When the nurse perceives a patient, the thoughts which automatically occur to her reflect the meaning or interpretation she attaches to her perception" (Orlando, 1961, p. 40).

The concepts *nurse's reaction* and *nurse's activity* are linked in the following general proposition: "What a nurse says or does is necessarily an outcome of her reaction to something in the situation (Orlando, 1961, p. 61).

More specifically, the dimensions of the *nurse's reaction* are linked to the *nurse's activity* in the following sequential proposition that describes what Orlando (1972) called the action process:

> The process of a nurse's activity is based on a specific formulation of the process by which any individual acts. . . . The process . . . is com-

prised of four distinct items. These separate items reside within an individual and at any given moment occur in the following automatic, sometimes instantaneous, sequence: (1) The person perceives with any one of his five sense organs an object or objects; (2) the perceptions stimulate automatic thought; (3) each thought stimulates an automatic feeling; and (4) then the person acts. (pp. 24–25)

The concept's *nurse's activity* and *patient behavior* are linked in the following propositions:

> Any observation shared and explored with the nurse is immediately useful in ascertaining and meeting his need [for help] or finding out that he is not in need at that time. (Orlando, 1961, p. 36)

> If the nurse automatically decides on the "right" activity but holds in abeyance what she wants to achieve until she ascertains and meets the patient's need, she helps the patient and achieves her primary objective. If the nurse is not able to carry out what she thinks is indicated, she helps the patient tell her why her judgment is inappropriate or incorrect. She then makes a new decision or continues to explore what is going on so that the patient will understand and accept what the nurse believes is indicated. In either case the purpose is to help the patient. Another way to think of this is that either the patient is willing to go along with the nurse, or the nurse is willing to go along with the patient. They have to move together to achieve a common goal. (Orlando, 1961, p. 89)

The concept *nurse's activity* is linked with the patient behavior dimension of *improvement* (outcome) in the following proposition: "There are . . . three possible ways for the patient to be affected by nursing activities—the activity may help, may not help, or the result may be unknown." (Orlando, 1961, p. 67)

The concept *nurse's activity* is linked more precisely with the patient behavior dimension *improvement* in the following propositions:

> The nurse recognizes if she has met the patient's need for help by noting the presence or absence of improvement in his presenting behavior. In the absence of improvement, the nurse knows the patient's need has not yet been met, and, if she remains available, she starts the process all over again with whatever presenting behavior is then observed. (Orlando, 1961, p. 68)

> The product of meeting the patient's immediate need for help is . . . "improvement" in the immediate verbal and nonverbal behavior of the patient. This observable change allows the nurse to believe or disbelieve that her activity relieved, prevented or diminished the patient's sense of helplessness. In subjective but at least conceptual terms the "improvement" has a measure of curative value to the helplessness suffered by patients in immediate experiences. In this conceptual sense the professional function of nursing is fulfilled and its product is achieved. (Orlando, 1972, pp. 21–22)

The nurse, in achieving her purpose contributes simultaneously to the mental and physical health of her patient. This is so because in helping him she affects for the better his sense of adequacy or well-being. (Orlando, 1961, p. 9)

EVALUATION OF THE THEORY OF THE DELIBERATIVE NURSING PROCESS

This section presents an evaluation of Orlando's Theory of the Deliberative Nursing Process. The evaluation is based on the results of the analysis of the theory as well as on publications by others who have used or commented on this nursing theory.

Significance

Orlando did not explicitly identify the metaparadigmatic or paradigmatic origins of the Theory of the Deliberative Nursing Process. The relevant metaparadigm concepts and proposition were, however, readily extracted from the contents of her books, and a rudimentary conceptual model that describes the person, health, and nursing was extracted from Orlando's publications. Moreover, although Orlando did not label all of her assumptions as such, the statements that represent the philosophical claims undergirding the Theory of the Deliberative Nursing Process were easily identified in her writings.

Orlando claimed no influences from antecedent knowledge on development of the Theory of the Deliberative Nursing Process. In fact, systematic examination of her publications about the theory revealed no evidence of its derivation from other nursing theories or theories from other disciplines.

The Theory of the Deliberative Nursing Process is, then, a distinctive nursing theory. Indeed, as Forchuk (1991) stated, "Orlando's most significant contribution may have been her move away from any existing nursing or nonnursing theory to build her theory entirely on grounded research of actual nursing practice" (p. 43).

The Theory of the Deliberative Nursing Process has definitely enhanced understanding of the nurse-patient relationship as well as understanding of the nurse's professional role and identity. A special feature of the theory is the precise specification of the requirements making up the deliberative nursing process.

Speaking to the special significance of the theory in a foreword to the 1990 reprint of Orlando's 1961 book, Schmieding (1990b) stated:

Orlando's work was a major force in shifting the nurse's focus from the medical diagnosis to the patient's immediate experience. In her book, Orlando clearly articulates the uniqueness of each patient's immediate need for help as well as the uniqueness of the nurse's deliberative process in determining with the patient his or her specific need. The use of Orlando's theory thus prevents the nurse from acting on invalidated assumptions. . . . Orlando's theory [emphasizes] the necessity of involving patients in all aspects of their care. Nursing care has become more individualized as a result of this involvement. (p. hr xvii)

Internal Consistency

The Theory of the Deliberative Nursing Process is congruent with Orlando's philosophical claims. In addition, it is clearly based on her conceptualization of the person and nursing.

Semantic clarity is evident in the definitions given for the concepts of the Theory of the Deliberative Nursing Process and their dimensions. As Schmieding (1990b) pointed out, Orlando provided

succinct descriptions of the nursing process [which] express elegantly what nurses perceive as the essence of nursing, namely, determining and meeting, directly or indirectly, the patient's need for help in the immediate nurse-patient contact. (p. xvii)

Semantic inconsistency is, however, evident in the progressive change in certain terms, but that appears to be the result of Orlando's (1961, 1972; Orlando Pelletier, 1990) attempt to find terms that would more effectively convey her ideas. Inconsistencies were noted in the following terms: help (1961) and need for help (1990), improvement (1961) and helpful outcome (1972), automatic nursing process (1961) and nursing process without discipline (1972), and deliberative nursing process (1961) and process discipline or nursing process with discipline (1972).

The analysis of the Theory of the Deliberative Nursing Process presented earlier in this chapter yielded no concept redundancies. The potential for a redundancy in the concept of patient behavior was introduced by Schmieding (1990a) and Forchuk (1991), who regarded improvement as a separate concept in the theory. Repeated readings of Orlando's books, however, led to the conclusion that improvement is more accurately regarded as a dimension of patient behavior.

The analysis of the Theory of the Deliberative Nursing Process revealed structural consistency. The concepts are adequately linked by means of relational propositions, and the progression from patient's behavior (need for help) to nurse reaction to nurse's activity and back to patient's behavior (improvement) is clearly specified.

Parsimony

The Theory of the Deliberative Nursing Process is parsimonious. Indeed, it is elegant in the paucity of words used to convey complex ideas. The theory may, however, be oversimplified. Schmieding (1987) explained:

> A criticism of Orlando's work, despite its elegant specificity, is the lack of repetition and full explanation to accompany important concepts and formulations. The thought may occur to the reader, 'if a feature is mentioned, isn't that sufficient?' When learning complex formulations, even if they are clear and precise, and in grasping the meaning and use of abstract concepts, . . . repetition and more detailed explanations are necessary strategies. (p. 440)

Schmieding went on to say, "This criticism does not detract from the soundness of Orlando's theory; rather it highlights the fact that practical theories are noted for their simplicity and precision" (p. 440).

In a later commentary, Schmieding (1990b) pointed out that

> the simplicity of [Orlando's] formulations . . . disguises the complexity of the nurse-patient interaction. The importance of using perceptions, thoughts, or feelings to understand the meaning of the patient's immediate behavior is not something a person does naturally. It must be developed. (p. xviii)

Testability

The Theory of the Deliberative Nursing Process is testable by means of a specific research methodology developed by Orlando (1972). The primary purpose of research designed to test the theory is to determine the effects of the use of the process discipline (that is, the deliberative nursing process) on behavior of patients and other persons (staff and supervisees) in the nursing system. Another purpose is to test the effects of training in the use of the process discipline on its actual use in practice. The phenomena of interest are the person's behavior, the nurse's reactions, and the nurse's activity.

The purposes of research and the phenomena of interest are reflected in several of Orlando's (1961, 1972) statements. Although she labeled some of the statements assumptions, they are more appropriately labeled testable propositions or hypotheses. Some statements refer to the effects of using or not using the process discipline:

> Once the patient has been helped, he feels safer to communicate the distress of which he is aware. . . . Once he trusts the nurse, his communications are more explicit and he is more likely to spontaneously discuss the experiences which distress him. (1961, p. 26)

> When the reaction of the nurse, in any of its aspects, is not explored with the patient, his condition remains unchanged or becomes worse. (1961, p. 45)

> If a nurse automatically acts on any perception, thought, or feeling without exploring it further with the patient, the activity may very well

be ineffective in achieving its purpose or in helping the patient. On the other hand, if the nurse checks her thoughts and explores her reactions with the patient before deciding on which action to follow, what she does is more likely to achieve its purpose and help the patient. (1961, p. 61)

Other statements refer to the effects of training nurses to use the process discipline:

Training would increase the nurse's use of the process discipline. (1972, p. 66)

Trained nurses would use the process discipline more than untrained ones. (1972, p. 66)

TABLE 5–2.   Operational Definitions for Orlando's Research Methodology

Characteristics of Verbal Expressions

X	An item is verbally expressed.
Y	An item is asked about.
Z	An item which is verbally expressed is designated to the self with a personal pronoun.
XY	An item is first expressed and the same item is asked about.
XZ	An item expressed is designated to the self.
XYZ	An item first expressed is designated to the self and the same item is asked about.

Outcome

High	Verbal and vocal nonverbal indications of helpful outcome.
Medium	Verbal or nonverbal indications of helpful outcome.
Low	No indication of helpful outcome but understanding increased.
Zero	No indications of high, medium or low outcome; or no indication of distress, symptom, or problem or indication of increased distress or symptom or manifestation of a problem.

Consistency between Reactions and Verbal Expressions

Consistency	Whether or not verbal behavior matched the reaction.
Self-designated consistency	Whether self-designated verbal expressions were or were not consistent with the reaction.
No self-designated consistency	Whether verbal expressions that were not self-designated were or were not consistent with the reaction.
Codes	Consistent and self-designated. Consistent and not self-designated. Inconsistent and self-designated. Inconsistent and not self-designated.

Source: Adapted from Orlando, 1972, pp. 60–61, 63, with permission.

Orlando (1972) used the definitions of the three aspects of the nurse's reaction (perception, thought, feeling); the nurse's activity, in the form of action; and helpful outcome given in the analysis section of this chapter for research purposes. She also developed precise operational definitions to code the characteristics of verbally expressed items, the outcome, and the consistency of the nurse's verbal expression with the nurse's reaction. Those definitions are given in Table 5–2.

The primary data collection methods are nonparticipant observation, tape-recorded person-to-person contacts, and process recordings. Other methods of data collection could include questionnaires and devices designed to measure particular manifestations of patient distress and specific symptoms. For example, Dumas and Leonard (1963) measured the incidence of postoperative vomiting, and Anderson and her colleagues (1965) measured blood pressure, pulse rate, and such observable behaviors as sobbing and movements of limbs.

Empirical Adequacy

A review of the research designed to test the Theory of the Deliberative Nursing Process revealed considerable empirical support. In fact, several studies conducted in the early 1960s by faculty and students at the Yale University School of Nursing provided impressive evidence of the beneficial effects of using the deliberative nursing process (see especially Anderson, Mertz, & Leonard, 1965; Barron, 1966; Bochnak, 1963; Cameron, 1963; Dumas, 1963; Dumas & Leonard, 1963; Dye, 1963; Elms & Leonard, 1966, Faulkner, 1963; Fischelis, 1963; Mertz, 1963; Rhymes, 1964; Tryon, 1963, 1966; Tryon & Leonard, 1964). The specific findings of relevant studies are summarized in the annotated bibliography at the end of this chapter.

Although the Yale studies "came to an abrupt halt," Orlando explained that she "continued to develop and refine" her original formulations (Orlando Pelletier, 1990, p. vii). The result of her effort was the publication of the findings of a major quasi-experimental study, funded by the National Institute of Mental Health, which Orlando conducted at McLean Hospital, a psychiatric facility located in Belmont, Massachusetts (Orlando, 1972). The purpose of the research was to test the effectiveness of the use of the process discipline (the deliberative nursing process) and the value of its use in patient, staff, and supervisee contacts. The study participants were staff nurses and supervisors, whose contacts with patients, other staff, and supervisees were observed and tape-recorded. Data included 144 transcribed tape recordings of contacts made by six staff nurses and six supervisors who had been trained in the process discipline, as well as 280 written records of verbal exchanges submitted by 28 trainees. Use of the process discipline was found to have a significant positive effect on patient and staff behavior, as indicated by a relief from distress or symptoms or the identification of a solution to a living or work problem. Summarizing the results of her research, Orlando (1972) stated:

> The research findings amply document that a verbal form of a process discipline can be isolated, tested and then evaluated in relation to an operational concept of effectiveness in patient, staff and supervisee contacts. Further, the same verbal form is sufficient to measure the use of the process discipline and, therefore, sufficient to measure training results. Still further, findings show that the process discipline and training in its use is effective in achieving helpful outcomes in patient and/or staff and/or supervisee contacts. . . . These findings, specific to this research, strongly suggest that the process discipline and training in its use is directly relevant to solving the more general problem of inadequate patient care. (p. viii)

Pragmatic Adequacy

Nursing Education

Special training is required to learn how to apply the Theory of the Deliberative Nursing Process. Training in the nursing process discipline (the deliberative nursing process) is predicated on Orlando's (1961) claim that:

> What the individual nurse happens to perceive or think (relevant or otherwise) is not so important as what she does with it. What the nurse automatically perceives or thinks cannot ordinarily be controlled, but she can learn a responsive discipline, the discipline which phrases or formulates her perceptions or thoughts by questioning and wondering about the meaning of them to the patient. (p. 41)

Orlando (1972) used the term "training" to refer to "the process of preparing nurses to impose a specific discipline on the nursing process to fulfill a specific function and achieve a specific product" (p. 2). The purpose of training "is to change the responsiveness of the nurse from the one described as *personal* and *automatic* to one which is *disciplined* and *professional*" (p. 33).

Emphasis in training is, therefore, placed on the nurse's response or activity rather than on the components of the reaction (perception, thought, feeling). Consequently, the two major tasks for the training instructor and their outcomes are:

> 1. To help the trainee express in full detail (in retrospect) all of the items contained in the immediate reaction in the particular nurse-patient contact being examined. In effect, this helps the trainee experience freedom to acknowledge what the reaction was.

2. To find out what formerly acquired expectation and of what origin explains whatever the activity of the trainee was in the same contact being examined; and further, to authoritatively release the trainee from the relevance of the expectation to the same contact being examined. In effect, this helps the trainee not only to experience freedom from expectations of what the trainee "should" perceive, think, feel, say and do, but to further acknowledge that what she "actually" perceived, thought and felt [and] what she "actually" said and did in the contact being examined. (p. 34)

Orlando (1972) found that the process discipline can be successfully taught to staff nurses in 6 weeks and to supervisors in 3 months. Training is facilitated by use of process recordings of the trainee's reaction and activity. The process recordings are then discussed in individual and group conferences between the trainees and training instructor. The following is an outline of the steps of training nurses to use the process discipline.

1. Initially, the training instructor focuses exclusively on eliciting all of the items contained in the trainee's immediate reaction and activity and identifying each item— perception, thought, feeling, and action.
2. The trainee records his or her own reaction and activity on a process record that contains parallel columns for "perception of or about the patient," "thought and/or feeling about the perception," and "said and/or did to, with, or for the patient."
3. The instructor helps the trainee to correct any items of the reaction and/or activity that were misplaced on the process record form and to add any items that were not included.
4. The instructor helps the trainee analyze how the particular reaction and activity affected finding out and meeting the patient's immediate need for help.
5. The instructor "literally, but lovingly, coerces the trainee to be herself with the specified discipline" (p. 42) when there are inconsistencies between the trainee's verbal action and the reaction. In that case, the trainee returns to the patient, expresses and explores his or her immediate reaction, and thereby acquires the additional data needed to find out the patient's perception, thought, and/or feeling and to explain the patient's reaction.

The need for training is supported by the results of Schmieding's (1988) study of the action process used by nurse administrators in response to hypothetical problematic staff situations. She found that the administrators either did not regard the situations as problematic or responded in an automatic manner. Schmieding indicated that her findings supported Orlando's (1972) contention that special training is required for use of the deliberative nursing process.

The effort expended in training leads to rewards when the Theory of the Deliberative Nursing Process is applied. Orlando (1989) commented, "Nurses who practice their process with discipline will enjoy their practice and can control their practice." Furthermore, nurses who use the process discipline express "greater comfort and satisfaction in work situations" (Orlando, 1972, p. 36). Finally, "the trainee's understanding of the process by which she can help a patient in an immediate situation enables her to find her own identity as a professional nurse" (1972, p. 43).

Nursing Practice

The purpose of nursing practice is, according to Orlando (1961), "to supply the help a patient requires in order for his needs to be met" (p. 8). More specifically, the function of professional nursing "is conceptualized as finding out and meeting the patient's immediate needs for help" (Orlando, 1972, p. 20). Consequently, emphasis in practice is placed on the immediate experience of the patient, and a nurse's activity is regarded as professional "only when it deliberatively achieves the purpose of helping the patient" (1961, p. 70).

Orlando (1961, 1972) maintained that the purpose of nursing is achieved when the nurse initiates "a process which ascertains the patient's immediate need and helps to meet the need directly or indirectly" (1961, p. 8). The nurse meets the patient's needs directly when the patient is unable to meet his or her own need and when the nurse's activity is confined to the nurse-patient contact. The nurse meets the patient's need indirectly when the activity extends to arranging the services of a person, agency, or resource that the patient cannot contact by himself or herself.

Nursing practice, for Orlando (1961), encompasses "1) observation, 2) reporting, 3) recording, and 4) actions carried out with or for the patient" (p. 31). Observations, which are defined as "any [and] all information pertaining to a patient which the nurse acquires while she is on duty" (p. 6), are "the raw material with which she makes and implements her plans for the patient's care" (p. 6). Observations may be direct or indirect. Direct observations are "any perception, thought, or feeling the nurse has from her own experience of the patient's behavior at any or several moments in time" (p. 32). Direct observations, therefore, constitute the nurse's reaction to the patient's behavior. Indirect observations consist of "any information which is derived from a source other than the patient. This information pertains to, but is not directly derived from, the patient" (p. 31).

Orlando (1961) pointed out that although "the natural consequence of observation is a decision to act or not act in relation to what is observed" (p. 7), the direct and indirect observations of the patient "are not adequate for the individual nurse to carry out her responsibility of helping the patient with his needs" (p. 32). Rather, observations must be shared with and validated by the patient. Indeed, "any observation shared and explored with the patient is immediately useful in ascertaining and meeting his need or finding out that he is not in need at that time" (pp. 35–36). The process used to share and validate the nurse's observations is the deliberative nursing process, which Orlando (1972) considers a disciplined professional response.

Application of the Theory of the Deliberative Nursing Process requires that a relationship be established between the nurse and the patient. Orlando (1961) explained:

> Before the nurse establishes her relationship to the patient he does not clearly tell her about his distress or needs; he cannot do so without her help and he does not do so until he is sure she will meet them. Once the relationship is established, his communications to the nurse become clearer and more explicit. When he spontaneously informs the nurse about the specific nature of his distress or what he needs, the nurse can be fairly certain that her professional relationship is established. (p. 28)

The Theory of the Deliberative Nursing Process is applicable in virtually all person-to-person encounters in the nursing system and, therefore, in all clinical areas. As Orlando (1961) pointed out, "it has been successfully applied in the nursing of patients with medical, surgical, obstetric and psychiatric conditions and is applicable to the nursing of adults and children whether in the home, hospital or clinic" (p. viii). Later, Orlando (1972) noted that the theory can be applied not only to nurse-patient relationships but also to "contacts with other nurses (line-and-staff relationships among nursing personnel) and contacts with other professional and nonprofessional people (other staff relationships)" (p. vii). When the theory is extended beyond patients, all references to the patient and the patient's behavior are modified to focus on the person of interest, such as a staff nurse or a supervisee.

The pragmatic adequacy of the Theory of the Deliberative Nursing Process has been firmly established. Application of the theory yields improvements or helpful outcomes because when one individual in a person-to-person contact expresses and explores his or her own immediate reaction, the other individual in the contact is more able to do the same. Consequently, a more reliable data base is available for professional action and decision making (Orlando, 1972).

Clinicians have the legal ability to use Orlando's theory in practice, and the feasibility of implementing clinical protocols that reflect the theory is almost self-evident—the expression and exploration of perceptions, thoughts, and feelings can, with proper training, occur in any professional nursing situation without sanctions from others. Clinical protocols contain the specific requirements for the deliberative nursing process that were identified in the analysis section of this chapter. In addition, protocols might contain the various techniques that Orlando (1961) suggested to facilitate identification of the patient's immediate need for help. She stated that the nurse may express and explore any aspect of his or her reaction to the patient's behavior—perception, thought, or feeling. She went on to indicate that if exploration of one aspect of the reaction does not result in identification of the patient's need for help, then another aspect of the reaction can be explored. She noted that if exploration of all aspects of the reaction does not yield a verbal response from the patient, then the nurse could use negative expressions to demonstrate continued interest in the patient behavior. Some examples of negative expressions are:

> Is it that you don't think I'll understand?
> Am I wrong?
> It looked like that procedure was very painful, and you didn't say a
>   word about it. (p. 42)

Orlando commented that "when the nurse raises possibilities with negative connotations, the patient experiences the permission and responds with his own 'negative' reaction" (p. 42).

The Theory of the Deliberative Nursing Process seems to be compatible with patients' expectations of nursing practice; there are no reports to date of patients' discomfort or dissatisfaction when the theory has been used. The actual beneficial effects of its use have been documented extensively by Orlando (1972) and other investigators, as discussed in the section of this chapter dealing with empirical adequacy.

Continuing interest in the Theory of the Deliberative Nursing Process is attested to by the reprinting of Orlando's 1961 book in 1990. International interest in the theory is documented by translations of the 1961 book into Japanese, Hebrew, French, Portuguese, and Dutch (Orlando Pelletier, 1990).

CONCLUSION

Orlando has made a substantial and significant contribution to nursing knowledge development by explicating a theory that specifies a nursing process that will meet a person's immediate need for help. "There is no doubt," as Schmieding (1990b) pointed out, "that Orlando's formulations . . . have had substantial influence on the nursing education, practice, research, and literature that followed [the publication of her theory in 1961]" (p. xviii). Despite the already impressive evidence of the empirical adequacy and pragmatic adequacy of the Theory of the Deliberative Nursing Process, continued study is needed to determine if, as Orlando (1972) predicted, "training in the process discipline is directly relevant to the effectiveness of a nursing system designed to improve the care of patients on a massive scale" (p. 126).

REFERENCES

Anderson, B., Mertz, H., & Leonard, R. (1965). Two experimental tests of a patient-centered admission process. *Nursing Research, 14*, 151–156.

Barron, M. A. (1966). The effects varied nursing approaches have on patients' complaints of pain. *Nursing Research, 15*, 90–91. (Abstract)

Bochnak, M. A. (1963). The effect of an automatic and deliberative process of nursing activity on the relief of patients' pain: A clinical experiment. *Nursing Research, 12*, 191–192. (Abstract)

Cameron, J. (1963). An exploratory study of the verbal responses of the nurses in 20 nurse-patient interactions. *Nursing Research, 12*, 192. (Abstract)

Dumas, R. G. (1963). Psychological preparation for surgery. *American Journal of Nursing, 63*(8), 52–55.

Dumas, R., & Leonard, R. C. (1963). The effect of nursing on the incidence of postoperative vomiting. *Nursing Research, 12*, 12–15.

Dye, M. (1963). A descriptive study of conditions conductive to an effective process of nursing activity. *Nursing Research, 12*, 194. (Abstract)

Elms, R. R., & Leonard, R. C. (1966). Effects of nursing approaches during admission. *Nursing Research, 15*, 39–48.

Faulkner, S. (1963). A descriptive study of needs communicated to the nurse by some mothers on a postpartum service. *Nursing Research, 12*, 26. (Abstract)

Fischelis, M. (1963). An exploratory study of labels nurses attach to patient behavior and their effect on nursing activities. *Nursing Research, 12*, 195. (Abstract)

Forchuk, C. (1991). A comparison of the works of Peplau and Orlando. *Archives of Psychiatric Nursing, 5*, 38–45.

Mertz, H. (1963). A study of the process of the nurse's activity as it affects the blood pressure readings and pulse ratings of patients admitted to the emergency room. *Nursing Research, 12*, 197–198. (Abstract)

Orlando, I. J. (1961). *The dynamic nurse-patient relationship: Function, process and principles.* New York: G.P. Putnam's Sons. Reprinted 1990. New York: National League for Nursing.

Orlando, I. J. (1972). *The discipline and teaching of nursing process (An evaluation study).* New York: G.P. Putnam's Sons.

Orlando, I. J. (1989). The nurse theorists: Portraits of excellence. Athens, OH: Fuld Institute for Technology in Nursing Education. (Videocassette recording)

Orlando Pelletier, I. J. (1990). Preface to the NLN edition. In I. J. Orlando, *The dynamic nurse-patient relationship: Function, process, and principles* (pp. vii–viii). New York: National League for Nursing.

Pelletier, I. O. (1967). The patient's predicament and nursing function. *Psychiatric Opinion, 4*(1), 25–30.

Rhymes, J. (1964). A description of nurse-patient interaction in effective nursing activity. *Nursing Research, 13*, 365. (Abstract)

Schmieding, N. J. (1987). Problematic situations in nursing: Analysis of Orlando's theory based on Dewey's theory of inquiry. *Journal of Advanced Nursing, 12*, 431–440.

Schmieding, N. J. (1988). Action process of nurse administrators to problematic situations based on Orlando's theory. *Journal of Advanced Nursing, 13*, 99–107.

Schmieding, N. J. (1990a). The analysis of the patient's immediate experience through the use of Orlando's theory. In *Proceedings of the First and Second Rosemary Ellis Scholars' Retreat* (pp. 155–158). Cleveland, OH: Frances Payne Bolton School of Nursing, Case Western Reserve University. (Abstract)

Schmieding, N. J. (1990b). Foreword. In I. J. Orlando, *The dynamic nurse-patient relationship: Function, process, and principles* (pp. xvii–xix). New York: National League for Nursing.

Sellers, S. C. (1991). A philosophical analysis of conceptual models of nursing. *Dissertation Abstracts International, 52*, 1937B. (University Microfilms No. AAC9126248)

Tryon, P. A. (1963). An experiment of the effect of patients' participation in planning the administration of a nursing procedure. *Nursing Research, 12*, 262. (Abstract)

Tryon, P. A. (1966). Use of comfort measures as support during labor. *Nursing Research, 15*, 109–118.

Tryon, P. A., & Leonard, R. C. (1964). The effect of patients' participation on the outcome of a nursing procedure. *Nursing Forum, 3*, 79–89.

ANNOTATED BIBLIOGRAPHY

Primary Sources

Orlando, I. J. (1961). *The dynamic nurse-patient relationship: Function, process and principles.* New York: G. P. Putnam's Sons. [Reprinted 1990. New York: National League for Nursing]

Orlando presents the elements of her theory of nursing as a deliberative process that can identify and meet the patient's immediate need for help. In the Preface to the 1990 edition, she explains the background of her work. In the Foreword of the 1990 edition, Schmieding points out that Orlando's work was a major force in shifting nurses' focus from medical diagnosis to the patient's immediate need for help.

Orlando, I. J. (1962). Function, process and principle of professional nursing practice. In *Integration of mental health concepts in the human relations professions.* New York: Bank Street College of Education.

Orlando discusses her approach to identifying the patient's immediate needs for help. This chapter is an overview of the content of Orlando's book, *The Dynamic Nurse-Patient Relationship.*

Orlando, I. J. (1972). *The discipline and teaching of nursing process.* New York: G. P. Putnam's Sons.

Orlando reports the findings of her study of the application of her theory in a psychiatric hospital. She elaborates on the theory and fully explains the elements of the deliberative nursing process/nursing process discipline.

Commentary by Orlando and Others

Andrews, C. M. (1983). Ida Orlando's model of nursing. In J. J. Fitzpatrick & A. L. Whall, *Conceptual models of nursing: Analysis and application* (pp. 47–65). Bowie, MD: Brady.

Andrews, C. M. (1989). Ida Orlando's model of nursing practice. In J. J. Fitzpatrick & A. L. Whall, *Conceptual models of nursing: Analysis and application* (2nd ed., pp. 69–87). Norwalk, CT: Appleton and Lange.

Andrews describes Orlando's theory, which she mistakenly refers to as a model, presents an analysis of the theory, and briefly discusses its relation to nursing research, education, and practice.

Beckstrand, J. (1980). A critique of several conceptions of practice model in nursing. *Research in Nursing and Health, 3*, 69–79.

Beckstrand contends that the Dickoff, James, and Wiedenbach conception of a practice theory is essentially equivalent to a plan of action. She contrasts their idea of practice theory with other conceptions of a prescriptive practice theory, especially the set-of-rules conception explicated by Jacox. She points out that the set-of-rules conception is untenable and that other conceptions of practice theory are nothing more than established forms of knowledge. She regards Orlando's theory as a beginning metatheory of nursing practice.

Crane, M. D. (1980). Ida Jean Orlando. In Nursing Theories Conference Group, J. B. George (Chairperson), Nursing theories: The base for professional nursing practice (pp. 123–137). Englewood Cliffs, NJ: Prentice-Hall.

Crane, M. D. (1985). Ida Jean Orlando. In J. B. George (Ed.), Nursing theories: The base for professional nursing practice (2nd ed., pp. 158–179). Englewood Cliffs, NJ: Prentice-Hall.

Leonard, M. K., & Crane, M. D. (1990). Ida Jean Orlando. In J. B. George (Ed.), Nursing theories: The base for professional nursing practice (3rd ed., pp. 145–164). Norwalk, CT: Appleton and Lange.
The chapter in each edition of the book contains a description of Orlando's academic and experiential credentials and a description and analysis of her theory.

de la Cuesta, C. (1983). The nursing process: From development to implementation. Journal of Advanced Nursing, 8, 365–371.
In this study, the author analyzes in sociological terms the nursing process development and describes its implementation through a review of the literature, interviews of American and British nurses, and observations in US and United Kingdom hospitals. Analysis of the data revealed that the nursing process, originally developed in the United States is not congruent with the nursing context in the United Kingdom. The usefulness of the nursing process in nursing education, practice, and research is questioned. The author notes that Orlando introduced the concept of nursing process in her 1961 book.

Flynn, J-B. M., & Heffron P. B. (1984). Nursing: From concept to practice. Bowie, MD: Brady.
The authors include a brief overview of Orlando's theory.

Forchuk, C. (1991). A comparison of the works of Peplau and Orlando. Archives of Psychiatric Nursing, 5, 38–45.
Forchuk comments that Peplau and Orlando have had a great impact on past and current mental health nursing practice. She compares and critiques their works, pointing out that Peplau places a greater emphasis on the development of the individual, whereas Orlando focuses on the immediate needs of the client.

Henderson, V. (1978). The concept of nursing. Journal of Advanced Nursing, 3, 113–130.
Henderson presents her views on the different definitions of nursing, the functions of nurses, and legal barriers to these functions. Drawing from the works of several nursing theorists, the author outlines nursing activities and the educational preparation required for nurses to be effective. Proposals for a basic nursing program are suggested. She credits Orlando with coining the term "nursing process."

Lego, S. (1980). The one-to-one nurse-patient relationship. Perspectives in Psychiatric Care, 18, 67–89.
Lego presents a review of the theory and practice of psychiatric nursing from 1946 to 1974. The issue of nurses doing psychotherapy is examined. The author discusses the history and trends of psychiatric nursing and critically assesses the theory, practice, and published research reported by psychiatric nurses. A summary of patterns from the literature, which have provided a direction for the one-to-one relationship in psychiatric nursing is presented. An overview of Orlando's theory is included.

McBride, A. B. (1986). Present issues and future perspectives of psychosocial nursing. Theory and research. Journal of Psychosocial Nursing and Mental Health Services, 24(9), 27–32.
In this article, McBride examines the developments in nursing and, in particular, in psychosocial nursing. An overview of nursing theorists' contributions to nursing and the increasing need for nurses to engage in research activities are presented. Theoretical and research influences on the development of psychosocial nursing are described. She notes that both Orlando and Peplau were prime movers in the development of psychosocial nursing practice. She goes on to address the importance of research as a means for theory development.

McGilloway, F. (1980). The nursing process: A problem solving approach to patient care. *International Journal of Nursing Studies, 17,* 79–80.

McGilloway notes that Peplau and Orlando made early attempts to analyze nursing actions and recognized that nursing intervention is an interpersonal process.

Orlando, I. J. (1987). Nursing in the 21st century: Alternate paths. *Journal of Advanced Nursing, 12,* 405–412.

Orlando presents her views about the distinct nature of nursing and the need for nursing to establish its independence from other professions. Factors that have influenced nursing's choice of a dependent path stem from the collective failure of nursing to articulate and implement a distinct function and product from medicine. The author shares her concerns about the dependent and independent paths nursing will face in the future.

Orlando, I. J., & Dugan, A. B. (1989). Independent and dependent paths: The fundamental issue for the nursing profession. *Nursing and Health Care, 10,* 76–80.

Concerned with the unclear definition of nursing's function and product, Orlando and Dugan reexamine the tension between independent and dependent paths. They maintain that the articulation of a product for nursing's distinct function is important for the viability of the profession.

Pelletier, I. O. (1963). Behind the theory of nursing practice. [Interview with Ida Orlando Pelletier by the staff of the *American Journal of Nursing.*] *American Journal of Nursing, 63*(8), 54.

In this interview, Orlando Pelletier discusses her nursing career and the development of her theory.

Schmieding, N. J. (1983). An analysis of Orlando's theory based on Kuhn's theory of science. In P. L. Chinn (Ed.), *Advances in nursing theory development,* (pp. 63–87). Rockville, MD: Aspen.

Schmieding presents an analysis and evaluation of Orlando's theory.

Schmieding, N. J. (1987). Problematic situations in nursing: Analysis of Orlando's theory based on Dewey's theory of inquiry. *Journal of Advanced Nursing, 12,* 431–440.

Schmieding presents an analysis of Orlando's theory using Dewey's theory of inquiry. This analysis revealed that Orlando's concepts are remarkably similar to those of Dewey. Each used an organizing principle that was derived from the meaning of experience and both view investigation as a serial process using facts and ideas to determine the problem and its solution. Several areas in Orlando's work could be enhanced and extended through Dewey's formulations. The analysis supports the use of Orlando's theory in problematic situations.

Schmieding, N. J. (1989). Time spent on MDs work is astronomical [Letter to the editor]. *Nursing Management, 20*(5), 18–19.

In her letter addressing an editorial in the December 1988 issue of the journal, Schmieding suggests using Orlando's theory to delineate the nurse's professional responsibility. She explains that focusing on activities that help the nurse find out and meet the patient's immediate need for help clarifies nursing's professional role responsibilities and relieves nurses of nonnursing activities.

Torres, G. (1986). *Theoretical foundations of nursing.* Norwalk, CT: Appleton-Century-Crofts.

Torres presents a brief description and an evaluation of Orlando's theory. She also describes the application of the theory within the context of the nursing process framework of assessment, diagnosis, planning, implementation, and evaluation.

Winder, A. (1984). A mental health professional looks at nursing care. *Nursing Forum, 21,* 184–188.

Winder presents her views about the process of caring as nursing's distinct professional function. An analysis of the concept of care and nursing care is provided. Drawing from Orlando's conceptualization of the nursing process, the author addresses the need for teaching the caring process to nursing students.

Practice

Harrison, C. (1966). Deliberative nursing process versus automatic nurse action. The care of a chronically ill man. *Nursing Clinics of North America, 1,* 387–397.

Harrison presents a case study of a patient regarded as "uncooperative." She cites the benefits of using Orlando's deliberative nursing process in the care of such patients.

Hughes, M. M. (1983). Nursing theories and emergency nursing. *Journal of Emergency Nursing, 9*, 95–97.
Hughes briefly discusses the works of Henderson, King, Orem, Orlando, and Roy as frameworks for the practice of emergency nursing.

Pelletier, I. O. (1967). The patient's predicament and nursing function. *Psychiatric Opinion, 4*(1), 25–30.
Orlando Pelletier describes nursing function as a distinct entity in the life of patients. She maintains that the nursing function of identifying and meeting patient's needs provides a basis for the analysis and direction of nurses' activities in relation to other nurses and health professionals.

Schmidt, J. (1972). Availability: A concept of nursing practice. *American Journal of Nursing, 72*, 1986–1989.
Drawing from Orlando's concept of deliberative nursing, the author discusses how the effectiveness of a nurse-patient interaction varies with the nurse's availability. This article presents the various tools nurses use to increase their receptive availability and the various stages of problem solving in the nursing process. Through several excerpts of a nurse-patient interaction, the author illustrates the concept of availability.

Schmieding, N. J. (1970). Relationship of nursing to the process of chronicity. *Nursing Outlook, 18*, 58–62.
Schmieding maintains that nurses must focus their attention on patients and their immediate needs for help. That focus, she claims, prevents the development of undesired outcomes of hospitalization.

Schmieding, N. J. (1986). Orlando's theory. In P. Winstead-Fry (Ed.), *Case studies in nursing theory* (pp. 1–36). New York: National League for Nursing.
Schmieding describes Orlando's theory and presents several case studies that illustrate the use of the theory in practice.

Administration

Schmieding, N. J. (1984). Putting Orlando's theory into practice. *American Journal of Nursing, 84*, 759–761.
Schmieding describes the implementation of Orlando's theory in a hospital nursing department. The author discusses how Orlando's theory can be helpful in defining nursing's function, in analyzing nursing practice, in facilitating patient care, and in management decisions.

Schmieding, N. J. (1987). Face-to-face contacts: Exploring their meaning. *Nursing Management, 18*(11), 82–86.
Schmieding explains how Orlando's theory can help nurse managers to interact effectively with their staffs. (c.f. annotations in the Research section for Schmieding, N. J. (1987). Analyzing managerial responses in face-to-face contacts. *Journal of Advanced Nursing, 12*, 357–365; Schmieding, N. J. (1988). Action process of nurse administrators to problematic situations based on Orlando's theory. *Journal of Advanced Nursing, 13*, 99–107; Schmieding, N. J. (1990). Do head nurses include staff nurses in problem solving? *Nursing Management, 21*(3), 58–60; Schmieding, N. J. (1990). A model of assessing nursing administrators' actions. *Western Journal of Nursing Research, 12*, 293–306; and Schmieding, N. J (1991). Relationship between head nurse responses to staff nurses and staff nurse responses to patients. *Western Journal of Nursing Research, 13*, 746–760).

Schmieding, N. J. (1990). An integrative nursing theoretical framework. *Journal of Advanced Nursing, 15*, 463–467.
The use of an integrative nursing theoretical framework for both clinical and administrative practice has recently been suggested. Schmieding describes a theoretical framework that incorporates key concepts from the writings of Orlando and Henderson and proposes its use as an integrative framework. The rationale for using the framework is discussed along with clinical and administrative examples of how to

integrate concepts from the proposed framework. The premise of the article is that benefits are derived from the use of a nursing theoretical framework because it provides a specific vision of nursing.

Sheafor, M. (1991). Productive work groups in complex hospital units: Proposed contributions of the nurse executive. *Journal of Nursing Administration, 21*(5), 25–30.
  Sheafor explains Schmieding's application of Orlando's theory to nursing administration and describes ways to achieve a stress-free environment on hospital units.

Research

Anderson, B., Mertz, H., & Leonard, R. (1965). Two experimental tests of a patient-centered admission process. *Nursing Research, 14,* 151–156.
  This article describes two experiments that were conducted in the emergency room of an urban hospital and a state mental hospital. The effects on patient welfare of a patient-centered nursing approach, consistent with Orlando's work, and a task-centered approach were tested. Findings indicated that patients who received the patient-centered nursing approach exhibited less distress and decreased blood pressure than the patients in the task-oriented group.

Bochnak, M. A., Rhymes, J. P., & Leonard, R. C. (1962). The comparison of two types of nursing activity on the relief of pain. In *Innovations in nurse-patient relationships: Automatic or reasoned nurse action* (Clinical papers no. 6, pp. 5–11). New York: American Nurses' Association.
  The authors report the findings of Bochnak's master's thesis, which examined the effect of deliberative and automatic nursing processes on patients' pain relief. Observations of the giving of pain-relieving medications and patients' verbal and nonverbal behaviors were used as dependent variables. Consistent with Orlando's work, the findings indicated that patients who received deliberative nursing care were more effectively relieved than those in the automatic nursing process group.

Diers, D. (1970). Faculty research development at Yale. *Nursing Research, 19,* 64–71.
  Diers describes the outcomes of the Faculty Research Development Grant program, funded by the United States Public Health Service, at Yale University School of Nursing. She notes that Orlando's work was an early and major contribution to the theoretical base for many of the studies, which focused on the effectiveness of nursing care.

Dracup, K., & Breu, C. (1978). Using nursing research findings to meet the needs of grieving spouses. *Nursing Research, 27,* 212–216.
  The authors describe the utilization of nursing research findings in a coronary care setting. They used Orlando's definition of need when investigating the effects of research-based nursing interventions on spouses' needs.

Dumas, R. G. (1963). Psychological preparation for surgery. *American Journal of Nursing, 63*(8), 52–55.
  Dumas demonstrates that through the deliberative nursing process, the nurse can be effective in relieving the emotional distress of patients during the preoperative period. Using two case histories, the author illustrates the effectiveness of the nursing process.

Dumas, R. G., Anderson, B. J., & Leonard, R. C. (1965). The importance of the expressive function in preoperative preparation. In J. K. Skipper & R. C. Leonard (Eds.), *Social interaction and patient care* (pp. 16–29). Philadelphia: J. B. Lippincott.
  The authors describe the beneficial results of psychological preparation of surgical patients by a nurse on the incidence of postoperative vomiting, as documented by the findings from three studies. The intervention of psychological preparation was based on Orlando's theory.

Dumas, R. G., & Leonard, R. C. (1963). The effect of nursing on the incidence of postoperative vomiting. *Nursing Research, 12,* 12–15.
  The authors describe three experiments that tested the effect of two nursing approaches on the incidence of postoperative vomiting in surgical patients. The findings indicated that in all three experiments, patients who received the experimental nursing approach, which was based on Orlando's theory and was directed toward

reducing patients' emotional distress, had a lower incidence of postoperative vomiting than control patients who received routine preoperative nursing care. Implications for nursing practice are discussed.

Dye, M. C. (1963). Clarifying patients' communications. *American Journal of Nursing,* 63(8), 56–59.

Dye reports the findings of her study, which explored the effectiveness of the nursing process as described by Orlando, on helping patients express their needs and in reducing their distress. Observations of 16 nurse-patient situations revealed that most patients experienced distress related to misunderstandings about their illnesses and treatments. Through several examples, the author illustrates the use of the nursing process to improve communication between patients and nurses.

Eisler, J., Wolfer, J., & Diers, D. (1972). Relationship between need for social approval and postoperative recovery and welfare. *Nursing Research, 21,* 520–525.

The investigators describe their study of factors influencing postoperative recovery. In the discussion of the findings, they note that although Orlando advocates validating nursing observations with patients, patients may respond as they think they are expected to, rather than on the basis of their inner experiences.

Elms, R. R. (1964). Effects of varied nursing approaches during hospital admission: An exploratory study. *Nursing Research, 13,* 266–268.

This exploratory study demonstrated the feasibility and usefulness of assessing patients' responses to varied nursing approaches during the hospital admission. Specifically, the effect of experimental, control, and hospital nursing approaches on patients' responses to stress was examined. The findings revealed that the experimental nursing approach, which was based on Orlando's theory, was more effective in relieving patients' distress than were the control and hospital nursing approaches.

Elms, R. R., & Leonard, R. C. (1966). Effects of nursing approaches during admission. *Nursing Research, 15,* 39–48.

This study examined the effectiveness of an experimental approach, congruent with Orlando's and Peplau's works, in relieving distress experienced by patients during an elective admission to a general hospital. Although the somatic and subjective indicators of distress failed to show consistent differences between the experimental and control groups, they indicate that a patient-centered nursing approach is more apt to alleviate distress than approaches that emphasize technical tasks. The authors discuss the need for instrument development and for testing theories.

Gillis, L. (1976). Sleeplessness: Can you help? *Canadian Nurse, 72*(7), 32–34.

Gillis reports the results of a study that examined the influence of automatic and deliberative nursing approaches on patients' inability to sleep. Patients unable to sleep were randomly assigned to control and experimental groups. The investigator recorded patients' behaviors and the activities of the nurses in responses to patients' complaints of sleeplessness as well as their effectiveness. Consistent with Orlando's work, the study supports the use of deliberative nursing as an effective approach to patient welfare.

Gowan, N., & Morris, M. (1964). Nurses' responses to expressed patient needs. *Nursing Research, 13,* 68–71.

This study explored 52 surgical patients' needs for nursing care as well as their satisfaction with nurses' responses to their requests. Data on patients' needs and length of time elapsed between the request and nurses' actions revealed that 52 percent of the nurses' responses were delayed from 15 minutes to 2.5 hours. The investiators discuss patients' reports related to their satisfaction with the quality of nursing care.

Haggerty, L. (1987). An analysis of senior nursing students' immediate response to distressed patients. *Journal of Advanced Nursing, 12,* 451–461.

Based on Orlando's theory, this study examined whether the effectiveness of senior nursing students' immediate responses to distressed patients is related to type of student educational preparation (ADN/BSN) or to type of patient's distress (physical/emotional). After viewing videotaped simulations of patients displaying complaints of pain and emotional distress, ADN and BSN students were interviewed. Findings revealed that type of distress was related to response effectiveness, but the type of education was not. The author addresses the need for improving the communication and psychosocial skills of nursing students.

Hampe, S. (1975). Needs of the grieving spouse in a hospital setting. Nursing Research, 24, 113–120.

Hampe reports that spouses were able to identify their own needs but perceived nurses and physicians as being too busy to be concerned with them. Orlando's definition of need was used.

Houfek, J. F. (1992). Nurses' perceptions of the dimensions of nursing care episodes. Nursing Research, 41, 280–285.

Houfek claims that Orlando incorporates the principles of symbolic interactionism into her conceptualization of nursing practice. She reports that nurses regarded care episodes that required activity participation by patients as having the most potential to promote independence.

Larson, P. (1977). Nurse perceptions of patient characteristics. Nursing Research, 26, 416–421.

Larson notes that the nurse utilizes a form of systematic problem solving to plan care that is individualized on the basis of data obtained from each patient. She cites Orlando's approach as one way to elicit relevant data from the patient.

Madden, B. P. (1990). The hybrid model for concept development: Its value for the study of therapeutic alliance. Advances in Nursing Science, 12(3), 75–87.

The investigator noted that the definition of therapeutic alliance as "a process that emerges within a provider-client interaction in which both the client and the provider are (1) actively working toward the goal of developing client health behaviors chosen for consistency with the client's current health status and life style, (2) focusing on mutual negotiation to determine activities to be carried out toward that goal, and (3) using a supportive and equitable therapeutic relationship to facilitate that goal" (p. 85) is consistent with Peplau's and Travelbee's perspectives, as well as with Orlando's notion of the primacy of the nurse-client relationship.

Mertz, H. (1962). Nurse actions that reduce stress in patients. In Emergency intervention by the nurse (Clinical papers no. 1, pp. 10–14). New York: American Nurses' Association.

Mertz reports the results of a study that tested the effects of deliberative and automatic processes of nursing on the condition of the patients treated in the emergency room. The findings indicated that the patients who received the deliberative process tended to have their immediate needs met and, consequently, showed improvements in pulse rates and blood pressure readings. Consistent with Orlando's work, this study supports the need for nurses to use a deliberative approach.

Nelson, B. (1978). A practice application of nursing theory. Nursing Clinics of North America, 13, 157–169.

Nelson reports the results of her study of the concerns of renal transplant patients, which was based on Orlando's theory. The categories of identified concerns were: depersonalization, communication difficulties, family distress, psychologic decompensation, limitation intolerance, unsatisfactory self-image, and physiologic disorders.

Peitchinis, L. (1972). Therapeutic effectiveness of counseling by nursing personnel: Review of the literature. Nursing Research, 21, 138–147.

Peitchinis presents a review of the literature on nurses' use of the elements of therapeutic effectiveness, including empathy, nonpossessive warmth, and genuineness. She points out that the studies conducted at Yale University School of Nursing provided support for Orlando's theory. She maintains that some of the studies have been replicated, but others require replication.

Pienschke, D. (1973). Guardedness or openness on the cancer unit. Nursing Research, 22, 484–490.

Pienschke reports that although patients are generally satisfied with nursing care regardless of the approach used to reveal cancer diagnosis and prognosis, nursing interventions are more effective when an open approach is used. She cites Orlando as one author who claims that learning whether patients need help, what help is needed, and how assistance might be best provided is a direct nursing responsibility.

Powers, M., & Wooldridge, P. (1982). Factors influencing knowledge, research, and compliance of hypertensive patients. Research in Nursing and Health, 5, 171–182.

The investigators report that an experimental educational program had no significant effects on blood pressure reduction in a sample of 160 hypertensive patients. The educational program was based in part on Orlando's theory of the deliberative nursing process.

Pride, L. F. (1968). An adrenal stress index as a criterion measure of nursing. *Nursing Research, 17*, 292–303.

Pride reports that her study findings revealed that an experimental interpersonal nursing approach had a beneficial effect on patients' hospital-related stress. One aspect of the nursing approach was based on Orlando's theory.

Princeton, J. C. (1986). Incorporating a deliberative nursing approach with breastfeeding mothers. *Health Care for Women International, 7*, 277–293. (See also Clausen, J. C. (1983). Clinical nursing research on the science and art of breastfeeding using a deliberative nursing care approach (Abstract). *Communicating Nursing Research, 16*, 29. Reprinted in *Western Journal of Nursing Research, 5*(3), 29.)

The purpose of this research was to compare deliberative and automatized nursing care approaches for reducing distress among breastfeeding mothers on an obstetrical unit. Distress variables such as the milk ejection reflex and the length of time mothers breastfeed after hospital discharge were measured in a sample of 36 mothers. Results revealed that the deliberative nursing approach significantly reduced maternal distress.

Ramos, M. C. (1992). The nurse-patient relationship: Theme and variations. *Journal of Advanced Nursing, 17*, 496–506.

Ramos reports the findings of her analysis of critical incidents describing nurses' perceptions of their relationships with patients. The study addresses characteristics of relationships in the tradition developed by Orlando and Peplau. The analysis revealed that close relationships, described as modified social relationships, were common.

Schmieding, N. J. (1987). Analyzing managerial responses in face-to-face contacts. *Journal of Advanced Nursing, 12*, 357–365.

Schmieding proposes that Orlando's theory can serve as a framework to analyze managerial actions. The author presents data from previous and current research on the effectiveness of managerial actions in identifying the meaning of the staff's behaviors. The analysis of nurse managers' actions revealed that staff nurses prefer that their managers use exploratory actions. A discussion on how specific types of actions facilitate or hinder problem identification follows.

Schmieding, N. J. (1988). Action process of nurse administrators to problematic situations based on Orlando's theory. *Journal of Advanced Nursing, 13*, 99–107.

Schmieding reports the results of her study, which used Orlando's theory to investigate the action process of nurse administrators to realistic hypothetical situations presented to them by their staff. Ninety subjects recorded their thoughts, feelings, and actions in response to six problematic situations. Findings indicated that over 50 percent of nurse administrators' actions were automatic rather than deliberative. The author discusses the need for nurse administrators to use a specific concept of nursing and an organizing principle to guide their actions to the immediate situation of nursing staff.

Schmieding, N. J. (1990). Do head nurses include staff nurses in problem-solving? *Nursing Management, 21*(3), 58–60.

Schmieding used Orlando's theory as a basis for the development of a model aimed at assessing managerial actions in face-to-face contacts. Using questionnaires containing vignettes of situations about patients, physicians, and nurses, the author examined head nurses' and staff nurses' responses. Findings revealed that a large majority of head nurses' actions did not involve the staff nurses in any way. The relationship between administrative and subordinate behavior and its implications on nursing care are discussed.

Schmieding, N. J. (1990). A model of assessing nursing administrators' actions. *Western Journal of Nursing Research, 12*, 293–306.

Schmieding uses Orlando's theory as a basis for her study of actions taken by nurse administrators. She found that the majority of subjects (staff nurses, head nurses, and supervisors) regard actions that are consistent with Orlando's theory to be most helpful.

Schmieding, N. J. (1991). Relationship between head nurse responses to staff nurses and staff nurse responses to patients. *Western Journal of Nursing Research, 13*, 746–760.
Schmieding reports that her study findings revealed that both head nurses and staff nurses use automatic responses in interactions (head nurses with staff nurses, staff nurses with patients), which Orlando contends block or hinder communication.

Silva, M. C. (1979). Effects of orientation information on spouses' anxieties and attitudes toward hospitalization and surgery. *Research in Nursing and Health, 2*, 127–136.
Silva based her experimental intervention of information-giving and psychological support in part on Orlando's theory. She found that spouses of patients who received the experimental intervention had more positive attitudes toward hospitalization and surgery and reported fewer anxieties than did spouses who received no special information or support.

Stevens, B. (1971). Analysis of structured forms used in nursing curricula. *Nursing Research, 20*, 388–397.
Stevens presents the results of her analysis of the philosophic concepts underlying common curriculum structures, including the logistic, dialectical, operational, and problematic methods. She classifies Orlando's theory as an example of the operational method and notes that Orlando does not define nursing per se, but she does define the elements of the nursing process.

Tarasuk, M. B., Rhymes, J., & Leonard, R. C. (1965). An experimental test of the importance of communication skills for effective nursing. In J. K. Skipper & R. C. Leonard (Eds.), *Social interaction and patient care* (pp. 110–120). Philadelphia: J. B. Lippincott.
The authors report the findings of a study that tested an experimental nursing intervention, based on Orlando's theory, on the administration of pain medication. The use of the experimental intervention permitted accurate assessment of the patients' problems, which they initially expressed as pain.

Thibaudeau, M., & Reidy, M. (1977). Nursing makes a difference: A comparative study of the health behavior of mothers in three primary care agencies. *International Journal of Nursing Studies, 14*, 97–107.
Based on Wiedenbach's and Orlando's works, this study examined the effect of an experimental nursing intervention on improving mothers' knowledge and compliance with their children's medical regimen. Subjects were recruited from three different types of health services and formed two experimental groups and three control groups (routine care). Findings indicated that mothers in the experimental group had significantly more knowledge of child's diagnosis, causes, and complications than mothers in the control groups. Moreover, experimental groups included a higher proportion of compliant mothers than the other group.

Tryon, P. A. (1962). The effect of patient participation in decision making on the outcome of a nursing procedure. In *Nursing and the patients' motivation* (Clinical papers no. 19, pp. 14–18). New York: American Nurses' Association.
Tryon reports the results of a study that tested the effect of patient participation in planning for the administration of the predelivery enema on the results of the treatment. Fifty women in labor were assigned to control and experimental groups. Based on Orlando's theory of nursing care, subjects in the experimental group received a deliberative nursing approach whereas those in the control group received routine care. Findings indicated that experimental subjects participated in planning for the administration of the enema and had more effective outcomes than subjects in the control group. The author discusses the benefits of the experimental approach on the progress of labor.

Tyon, P. A. (1966). Use of comfort measures as support during labor. *Nursing Research, 15*, 109–118.
Tryon reports the results of a study that examined the use of comfort measures for 30 women during labor, randomly assigned to a control group receiving routine nursing care, and to an experimental group receiving deliberative nursing care. Consistent with Orlando's work, the findings showed that the use of comfort measures was more effective in the experimental group than in the control group.

Tryon, P. A., & Leonard, R. C. (1964). The effect of patients' participation on the outcome of a nursing procedure. *Nursing Forum, 3,* 79–89.

Tryon and Leonard report the findings of two studies comparing the effects of two types of nursing approaches, experimental and control, on nurse-patient relationships, as well as patient acceptance and participation in the predelivery enema procedure. Findings indicated that the experimental approach patients were encouraged to participate in the predelivery enema and that they experienced more effective results from the procedure than women in the control group. These results are supportive of Orlando's work.

Williamson, J. (1978). Methodological dilemmas in tapping the concept of patient needs. *Nursing Research, 27,* 172–177.

Williamson notes that Orlando emphasizes the importance to the recovery process of recognizing and meeting patients' needs. She studied the reliability of an instrument designed to measure patients' and nurses' awareness of patients' physical and emotional needs. The data failed to support the reliability of the instrument.

Wolfer, J., & Visintainer, M. (1975). Pediatric surgical patients' and parents' stress responses and adjustment as a function of psychological preparation and stress point nursing care. *Nursing Research, 24,* 244–255.

The study reported by Wolfer and Visintainer was based on Orlando's theory of deliberative nursing process. They found that hospitalized children who received an experimental nursing intervention of systematic psychological preparation and continued supportive care were less upset, more cooperative, and had fewer posthospital adjustment problems than those who did not receive the experimental nursing intervention (control group). The parents of the experimental group children had less anxiety and were more satisfied with the information and care than the control group parents.

Doctoral Dissertations

Reid Ponte, P. A. (1990). The relationships among empathy and the use of Orlando's deliberative process by the primary nurse and the distress of the adult cancer patient. *Dissertation Abstracts International, 50,* 2848B.

Schmieding, N. J. (1983). A description and analysis of the directive process used by directors of nursing, supervisors, and head nurses in problematic situations based on Orlando's theory of nursing experience. *Dissertation Abstracts International, 44,* 1414B.

Master's Theses

The following master's theses were conducted at Yale University School of Nursing.

Barron, M. A. (1966). The effects varied nursing approaches have on patients' complaints of pain (Abstract). *Nursing Research, 15,* 90–91.

Bochnak, M. A. (1963). The effect of an automatic and deliberative process of nursing activity on the relief of patients' pain: A clinical experiment (Abstract). *Nursing Research, 12,* 191–192.

Cameron, J. (1963). An exploratory study of the verbal responses of the nurses in 20 nurse-patient interactions (Abstract). *Nursing Research, 12,* 192.

Diers, D. K. (1966). The nurse orientation system: A method for analyzing the nurse-patient interactions (Abstract). *Nursing Research, 15,* 91.

Dye, M. (1963). A descriptive study of conditions conductive to an effective process of nursing activity (Abstract). *Nursing Research, 12,* 194.

Faulkner, S. (1963). A descriptive study of needs communicated to the nurse by some mothers on a postpartum service (Abstract). *Nursing Research, 12,* 26.

Fischelis, M. (1963). An exploratory study of labels nurses attach to patient behavior and their effect on nursing activities (Abstract). *Nursing Research, 12,* 195.

Mertz, H. (1963). A study of the process of the nurse's activity as it affects the blood pressure readings and pulse ratings of patients admitted to the emergency room (Abstract). *Nursing Research, 12,* 197–198.

Rhymes, J. (1964). A description of nurse-patient interaction in effective nursing activity (Abstract). *Nursing Research, 13,* 365.

Taylor, S. K. (1963). A measure of nurse-patient verbal interaction (Abstract). *Nursing Research, 12,* 262.

Tryon, P. A. (1963). An experiment of the effect of patients' participation in planning the administration of a nursing procedure (Abstract). *Nursing Research, 12,* 262.

CHAPTER

6

Parse's Theory of Human Becoming_____

Rosemarie Rizzo Parse set out to create a theory based in the human sciences that would enhance nursing knowledge. She explained:

> The idea to create such a theory began many years ago when I began to wonder and wander and ask why not? The theory itself . . . surfaced in me in Janusian fashion over the years in interrelationship with others primarily through my lived experience with nursing. The creation of it has been long and arduous, but with many moments of joy. (Parse, 1981, p. xiii)

The result of Parse's intellectual effort was the theory of Man-Living-Health, which was first published in her 1981 book. The theory was renamed the Theory of Human Becoming in 1990 because although the term "man" formerly referred to "mankind," it currently connotes the male gender (Parse, 1992).

The concepts and subconcepts of the Theory of Human Becoming are listed below. Each one is defined and described later in this chapter.

KEY CONCEPTS_____

Human Becoming	Enabling-Limiting
Meaning	Connecting-Separating
Imaging	Cotranscendence
Valuing	Powering
Languaging	Originating
Rhythmicity	Transforming
Revealing-Concealing	

ANALYSIS OF THE THEORY OF HUMAN BECOMING

This section presents an analysis of Parse's theory. The analysis is based on Parse's publications about her theory, drawing primarily from her 1981 book, *Man-Living-Health: A Theory of Nursing*, and her 1992 journal article, "Human Becoming: Parse's Theory of Nursing." The 1992 article presented a rephrasing of the philosophical claims and theoretical propositions to reflect the change in the name of the theory.

Scope of the Theory

The central thesis of the Theory of Human Becoming is that "humans participate with the universe in the cocreation of health" (Parse, 1992, p. 37). "Human becoming," according to Parse, "refers to the human being structuring meaning multidimensionally while cocreating rhythmical patterns of relating and cotranscending with possibles" (cited in Takahashi, 1992, p. 86). The concepts and propositions of the theory are written at a relatively abstract level of discourse, which resulted in the theory's classification as a grand theory.

Context of the Theory

Metaparadigm Concepts and Proposition

Parse's (1981) statement that her theory "is a system of interrelated concepts describing unitary man's interrelating with the environment while cocreating health" (p. 13) indicates that the metaparadigm concepts of interest are *person, environment,* and *health.* Furthermore, her statement suggests that the metaparadigm proposition of particular interest is *the wholeness or health of human beings, recognizing that they are in continuous interaction with their environments.*

Philosophical Claims and Conceptual Model

The Theory of Human Becoming is derived from existential-phenomenological philosophy and Rogers's (1980) conceptual model of nursing. Parse has so interwoven the philosophical and conceptual foundations of her theory that they must be discussed together.

The philosophical foundation of the Theory of Human Becoming encompasses the concepts of coconstitution, coexistence, and situated freedom, along with the tenets of intentionality and human subjectivity. The conceptual foundation draws from Rogers's (1980) concepts of energy field, openness, pattern and organization, and four-dimensionality and the principles of helicy, complementarity, and resonancy. Parse (1981) combined those concepts, tenets, and principles in four assumptions about man and five assumptions about health. She later rephrased the assumptions by substituting "the human" for "man," "becoming" for "health," and the "universe" for the "environment" (Parse, 1992). The assumptions about the human are:

1. The human is coexisting while coconstituting rhythmical patterns with the universe.
2. The human is an open being, freely choosing meaning in situations, bearing responsibility for decisions.
3. The human is a living unity continuously coconstituting patterns of relating.
4. The human is transcending multidimensionally with the possibles. (Parse, 1992, p. 38)

The assumptions about becoming are:

1. Becoming is an open process, experienced by the human.
2. Becoming is a rhythmically coconstituting process of the human-universe interrelationship.
3. Becoming is the human's pattern of relating value priorities.
4. Becoming is an intersubjective process of transcending with the possibles.
5. Becoming is human unfolding. (Parse, 1992, p. 38)

Three other assumptions were presented in a 1985 book by Parse, Coyne, and Smith. Those assumptions, which represent a synthesis of the assumptions about man (the human) and health (becoming), were rephrased in Parse's 1992 article by substituting "human becoming" for "man-living-health." They are:

1. Human becoming is freely choosing personal meaning in situations in the intersubjective process of relating value priorities.
2. Human becoming is cocreating rhythmical patterns of relating in open interchange with the universe.
3. Human becoming is cotranscending multidimensionally with the unfolding possibles. (Parse, 1992, p. 38)

Five additional assumptions, some of which are combinations or restatements of the assumptions about humans, becoming, and human becoming, are the basis for Parse's research methodology. Those assumptions are:

1. Humans are open beings in mutual process with the universe. The construct human becoming refers to the human-universe-health process.
2. Human becoming is uniquely lived by individuals. People make reflective and prereflective choices in connection with others and the universe which incarnate their health.

3. Descriptions of lived experiences enhance knowledge of human becoming. Individuals and families can describe their own experiences in ways that shed light on the meaning of health.
4. Researcher-participant dialogical engagement uncovers the meaning of phenomena as humanly lived. The researcher in true presence with the participant can elicit authentic information about lived experiences.
5. The researcher, through inventing, abiding with logic, and adhering to semantic consistency during the extraction-synthesis and heuristic interpretation processes, creates structures of lived experiences and weaves the structure with the theory in ways that enhance the knowledge base of nursing. (Parse, 1992, p. 41)

Coyne (1981) explained that Parse's theory is a synthesis of the phenomenal (known through the senses) and the nuomenal (known only to the mind) worlds. The theory, according to Coyne, captures White's (1938) notion of sciencing, that is, doing science, or science as an action, an activity. Parse (1981) commented that her theory is "rooted in the human sciences" (p. 13).

Parse's philosophical claims reflect the *simultaneous action* worldview. In fact, Parse (1981, 1987, 1992) explicitly categorized her theory as grounded in the human sciences and an example of the simultaneity perspective. Moreover, she noted that "human becoming reflects the unity of the construct man-living-health [and that] there are no references to particular aspects of humans, such as biological, psychological, or spiritual" (1992, p. 37). Even more to the point, Parse commented that her theory "is in contradistinction to a [philosophical perspective] that views man as the sum of parts, acted upon and delimited by such terms as disease and pathology" (1981, p. 7).

In keeping with Rogers's (1980) conceptual system, Parse (1981, 1992) regards the person as a unitary being who simultaneously and mutually cocreates with the rhythmical patterns of the environment (the universe) and who freely chooses in situations. Health is regarded as "ongoing participation with the world" (1981, p. 39), as well as a "process of becoming as experienced and described by the person" (1992, p. 36). The goal of nursing is "quality of life" (1992, p. 36).

Antecedent Knowledge

Parse (1981) stated that her assumptions about man (the human) and health (becoming) emerged from Rogers's (1980) conceptual model and from the existential-phenomenological thinking of Heidegger (1962), Merleau-Ponty (1974), and Sartre (1966). She also cited numerous other scholars as she defined and discussed the concepts of the theory, including Schutz (1967), Greene (1978), Raths, Harmin, and Simon (1978), Bandler and Grinder (1975), Watzlawick (1978), Buber (1965),

Kempler (1974), Dilthey (1961), Tillich (1954), Nietzsche (1968), and van den Berg (1971).

Content of the Theory

The central concept of the Theory of Human Becoming is **Human Becoming.** Becoming is defined as "living health"; human health is defined as "the day-to-day unfolding through human-universe interchanges"; and human becoming is defined as "an ongoing process lived through the changing of value priorities" (Parse, cited in Takahashi, 1992, p. 86).

The other concepts of the Theory of Human Becoming represent themes that emerge from the philosophical claims undergirding the theory. They are *meaning, rhythmicity,* and *cotranscendence.* Analysis of Parse's publications revealed that each of those three concepts is further specified by three subconcepts.

Meaning

No definition is given for the concept **meaning.** A definition is, however, given for each of the subconcepts associated with meaning, which are *imaging, valuing,* and *languaging.* Parse (1981) defined *Imaging* as "symbolizing or picturing" (p. 177) or "making concrete the meaning of multidimensional experiences" (p. 44). Elaborating on that definition, she explained:

> Reality is constructed through man's simultaneous reflective-prereflective imaging. Reflective-prereflective imaging is the shaping of personal knowledge, the creating of reality explicitly and tacitly all at once. (pp. 42–43)

Parse (1981) defined *valuing* as "choosing to confirm a cherished belief" (p. 179) or "the process of confirming cherished beliefs" (p. 45). She commented:

> This confirming of beliefs is choosing from imaged options and owning the choices. The choosings are integrated into one's value system, which is a matrix of principles and ideas that guide one's life. The matrix is the framework through which is screened all that is imaged from one's multidimensional experiences. (p. 45)

Parse defined a value as "a symbol that signifies meaning" (p. 46). Citing Raths, Harmin, and Simon (1978), she identified seven essential elements that, when present, convert an attitude or belief into a value. The essential elements are choosing freely, choosing from alternatives, reflectively choosing, prizing and cherishing, affirming, acting on choices, and repeating.

Parse went on to claim that as new values are appropriated, they are integrated with currently cherished values. Those "ever-changing values reflect a person's move toward greater complexity. A synthesis of values is one's health" (p. 46).

Parse (1981) defined *languaging* as "expressing valued images" (p. 46) or "sharing valued images through symbols of words, gesture, gaze, touch, and posture" (p. 177). She maintained that "through the process of languaging . . . each individual symbolizes unique realities. This symbolizing surfaces in the process of speaking and moving" (p. 47). Elaborating, she stated:

> Languaging is not just the content of what a person says with words but how the whole message is revealed in the context of the situation. It is the rhythmical moments of silence, the choice of words and syntax, the intonation, the facial expressions, the gestures, the posture, and that which is not said that constitute . . . symbolic expression. (p. 48)

Rhythmicity

Although **rhythmicity** is not defined, the adjective form of that term—rhythmical—is defined as "cadent; ordered" (Parse, 1981, p. 178). The subconcepts for rhythmicity are *revealing-concealing, enabling-limiting,* and *connecting-separating.* Each subconcept represents a rhythmical, paradoxical pattern of human becoming. Parse (1992) explained that paradoxical rhythms are only *apparent* opposites. Actually, "these rhythmical patterns are not opposites; they are two sides of the same rhythm that coexist all at once. Both sides of the rhythms are present simultaneously" (p. 38).

Parse (1981) defined *revealing-concealing* as "the simultaneous disclosing of some aspects of self and hiding of others" (p. 52). She later described this subconcept as "a paradoxical rhythm in the pattern of relating with others. One reveals-conceals all at once the who that one is now, which incarnates the who that one was and will be. While revealing, one simultaneously conceals" (Parse, 1992, p. 38).

An explicit definition is not given for *enabling-limiting.* However, Parse (1992) described that subconcept as follows:

> Enabling-limiting is a rhythmical pattern of relating. In choosing, there are an infinite number of opportunities and an infinite number of limitations. Moving in one direction limits movement in another. Within the chosen direction there are inherent opportunities and limitations all at once, thus one is enabled-limited by all choices. (p. 38)

Parse (1992) defined *connecting-separating* as "a rhythmical process of moving together and moving apart" (p. 38). She explained, "In moving together, with one phenomenon, the individual moves away from other phenomena. In moving together, there is both the closeness of togetherness and the distance of moving apart with the same phenomenon" (p. 38). Earlier, Parse (1981) had noted that the rhythm of connecting-separating "can be recognized as man is connecting with one phenomenon and simultaneously separating from others" (pp. 53–54).

Cotranscendence

Cotranscendence is not explicitly defined. However, the participle, cotranscending, is defined as "going beyond the actual in interrelationships with others" (Parse, 1981, p. 177). The subconcepts associated with cotranscendence are *powering, originating,* and *transforming.*

Powering is defined by Parse (1981) as "struggling with the tension of pushing-resisting" (p. 178). It is "a process of man-environment energy interchange, recognized in the continuous affirming of self in light of the possibility of non-being" (p. 57), and "a process in all change and transformation from what one is to what one is not-yet" (p. 58). Elaborating on powering, Parse commented:

> How one lives powering is reflected in one's patterns of relating with the world through the rhythm of pushing-resisting. Pushing-resisting is present in every human encounter, creating tension and sometimes conflict. Possibles unfold through the tension and conflict that create the alternatives from which one can choose in reaching beyond. Tension is the struggling between pushing and resisting while contending with others, issues, ideas, desires, and hopes all at once in the process of striving to reach new possibles. In the struggling an individual emerges in cotranscending toward what is not-yet. (p. 58)

Parse (1992) maintained that powering, "the back and forth experienced by humans in all life situations," is "an energizing force which sparks moving beyond the moment" (p. 38). She went on to explain that although conflict occurs when the pushing-resisting rhythm that is powering is altered, "it is not a negative force, but rather, an opportunity to clarify views" (p. 38).

Parse defined *originating* as "springing from; emerging" (1981, p. 178) or "creating anew, generating unique ways of living which surface through interconnections with people and projects" (1992, p. 38). More specifically, originating "is a continuing process of negentropically unfolding while emerging in mutual energy interchange with the environment. It is choosing a particular way of self-emergence through inventing unique ways of living" (1981, pp. 59–60).

In originating, then, individuals distinguish themselves from each other and become unique. "One is unique," according to Parse (1992), "in that one is irreplaceable in close relationships and in creative projects" (p. 39). Elaborating, Parse (1981) explained:

> To distinguish oneself is to choose a unique way of living the paradoxical unity of conformity-nonconformity and certainty-uncertainty all at once. The paradoxical unity of conformity-nonconformity surfaces in human encounters, as individuals seek to be like others yet, simultaneously, not to be like others. . . . The paradox of living certainty-uncertainty surfaces in human encounter as individuals make concrete or clear their choices in situations yet, simultaneously, live the ambiguity of the unknown outcomes. (p. 60)

Transforming is defined by Parse as "the changing of change, coconstituting anew in a deliberate way" (1981, p. 62) or "the shifting of views of the familiar as different light is shed on what is known" (1992, p. 39). She explained, "Change is an ongoing process; that is, man coparticipates with environment in the simultaneous unfolding called change" (1981, p. 62).

The unfolding that is change, according to Parse (1981), occurs throughout life as the person interacts with the environment (the universe). She explained:

> Innovative discoveries and shifts in worldview are coconstituted through the simultaneous interchange between person and world. The person is open to the discovery, and the phenomenon is open to be discovered. The opportunity for discovery then emerges in the context of the person-world interrelationship. (p. 62)

Furthermore, change

> is recognized by increasing diversity. Increasing diversity is rhythmically lived as experience melts into experience and different priorities arise. . . . One's patterns of relating, then, are both the same and different all at once; threads of what was and is weave with the new and can be recognized in the fabric of one's life. This is transforming. (Parse, 1992, p. 39).

Nonrelational Propositions

The definitions of the concepts and the subconcepts are nonrelational propositions. In addition, Parse (1981, 1992) articulated three principles that can be considered nonrelational propositions. Each principle deals with one of the concepts of the Theory of Human Becoming and its associated subconcepts. The first principle is "Structuring *meaning* multidimensionally is cocreating reality through the *languaging* of *valuing* and *imaging*." Parse (1992) explained that that principle

> means that human beings construct a personal significance by choosing options from the various realms of the universe, as speaking and

moving unveil the cherished beliefs lived explicitly and tacitly all at
once. What is *real* for each individual is structured by that individual.
(p. 37)

In addition, Parse (1981) maintained that meaning changes continuously as the individual grows more diverse and complex and as
diverse images point to the possibilities of new values and original
expression through language.

The second principle is "Cocreating *rhythmical* patterns of relating
is living the paradoxical unity of *revealing-concealing, enabling-limiting* while *connecting-separating*." That principle, Parse (1992)
explained, articulates the rhythmical cocreation of the human-universe process. "The rhythmical patterns of relating are," according to
Parse, "paradoxical in nature. . . . [the] patterns are not opposites; they
are two sides of the same rhythm that coexist all at once. Both sides of
the rhythm are present simultaneously" (p. 38).

The third principle is "*Cotranscending* with the possibles is *powering* unique ways of *originating* in the process of *transforming*." Parse
(1992) noted that that principle "specifies that human beings move
beyond with intended hopes and dreams through pushing-resisting in
creating new ways of viewing the familiar" (p. 38).

Relational Propositions

Parse (1981) linked the concepts of the Theory of Human Becoming
in the following relational proposition:

> Man-Living-Health [*Human Becoming*] is structuring *meaning* multi-
> dimensionally in cocreating *rhythmical* patterns of relating while
> *cotranscending* with the possibles. (p. 67)

Another relational proposition links the concept *human becoming*
with the subconcepts associated with *meaning*. That proposition
asserts:

> Man-Living-Health, man becoming [i.e., *human becoming*], is the
> day-to-day creating of reality through the *languaging* of *valuing* and
> *imaging* (Parse, 1981, p. 67)

Linkages among the subconcepts are evident in the following relational proposition:

> *Languaging* reflects the rhythms of *revealing-concealing, enabling-lim-
> iting,* and *connecting-separating* as people live *powering* as a way of
> *originating transforming*. (Parse, 1981, p. 67)

In addition, Parse has begun to identify other linkages among the
subconcepts across the three principles. Those statements, which she

called theoretical structures, can be classified as relational propositions. As Parse (1992) pointed out, the relational propositions are nondirectional and noncausal. To date, three such relational propositions have been stated:

1. *Powering* is a way of *revealing* and *concealing imaging.*
2. *Originating* is a manifestation of *enabling* and *limiting valuing.*
3. *Transforming* unfolds in the *languaging* of *connecting* and *separating.* (Parse, 1981, p. 72)

EVALUATION OF THE THEORY OF HUMAN BECOMING

This section presents an evaluation of Parse's Theory of Human Becoming. The evaluation is based on the results of the analysis of the theory as well as on publications by others who have used or commented on this nursing theory.

Significance

Parse did not label her focus on the person, the environment, and health and her statement that the Theory of Human Becoming deals with "unitary man's interrelating with the environment while cocreating health" as elements of the nursing metaparadigm. It is obvious, however, that those concepts and that statement represent the metaparadigmatic origin of the theory.

In contrast, Parse clearly and explicitly identified the philosophical assumptions and conceptual model that undergird her theory. The philosophical and conceptual elements are so integrated that, as noted in the analysis section of this chapter, it is not possible to separate them. Parse makes clear that Rogers's conceptual model of nursing was a starting point for her theory. Furthermore, she acknowledged and cited the scholars from other disciplines—especially philosophers—whose works undergird her theory.

The significance of the Theory of Human Becoming lies in its contributions to understanding how people experience health from a human science perspective. As Parse (1992) pointed out, her theory is consistent with human science because its essence "is embedded in meanings, patterns in relationships, and in hopes and dreams" (p. 37).

The significance of the theory also lies in the recognition that values play a part in health. As Parse (1992) noted, "This theory takes into consideration that human beings live their health incarnating personal values which are each individual's unique connectedness with the universe" (p. 37).

A special feature of the theory is its process orientation and the emphasis on paradoxical, rhythmical patterns of interchange between the person and the universe. Another special feature is the focus on the person's participation and connectedness with the universe in cocreating health.

The terminology used by Parse may, however, limit appreciation of the significance of her work. Holmes (1990) commented:

> Unfortunately, [Parse's] efforts have not had the impact on nursing that might have been hoped. Their accessibility is undermined by an obscure style, a penchant for the utterly novel use of familiar words, and a large crop of ill-explained neologisms. These problems are exacerbated if the reader is not familiar with the esoteric language and idiosyncratic conceptual tools of existential phenomenologists. (p. 193)

Internal Consistency

The Theory of Human Becoming is consistent with its philosophical and conceptual origins. In fact, Mitchell and Cody (1992) pointed out that Parse's philosophical claims and the content of the theory are consistent with "human science in Dilthey's traditional sense" (p. 59). Moreover, they claimed that the theory clarifies and expands the human science approach. Furthermore, as Sarter (1988) noted, Parse's synthesis of existentialism and Rogers's conceptual model is creative as well as logically constructed and organized.

Semantic clarity is evident in the explicit definitions or descriptions of all of the concepts and subconcepts of the Theory of Human Becoming except meaning. Parse's discussion of that concept and the associated subconcepts suggests that the definition is the typical one found in any dictionary.

Parse used the participle form—an "ing" ending—for all of the subconcepts. She explained that the terms "were deliberately designed this way to make explicit the process orientation of the theory" (Parse, 1992, p. 37).

Semantic consistency is evident. Parse has been consistent in her use of terms and has attached the same meaning to terms in her various publications. Furthermore, she provided a rationale for the change in the name of the theory and the subsequent rewording of propositions.

There are no concept redundancies. Each concept and subconcept adds something distinctive to the theory.

The analysis of the Theory of Human Becoming revealed structural consistency. Parse (personal communication, April 20, 1990) described the development of her theory as both inductive and deductive. The analysis indicated that the derivation of relational propositions from the concepts and subconcepts contained in the three major nonrelational propositions (Parse's "principles") follows a logical line of deductive reasoning.

Parsimony

The Theory of Human Becoming is relatively parsimonious. The analysis revealed that the major components of the theory encompass four major concepts, nine subconcepts, and three major nonrelational propositions. The decision to divide the elements of the theory into major concepts and subconcepts was based on Parse's (1992) explicit identification of three themes that emerged from her philosophical claims. Inasmuch as those themes (meaning, rhythmicity, cotranscendence) clearly represented major concepts, the concepts that Parse (1981, 1992) associated with each theme were labeled "subconcepts." Furthermore, Parse's recent description of her theory (cited in Takahashi, 1992) led to the identification of human becoming as a distinct concept of the theory. Overall, the arrangement of concepts and subconcepts seen in the analysis section of this chapter provided a parsimonious structure for the theory.

Testability

The relational propositions of the Theory of Human Becoming cannot be directly tested because they were written at the grand theory level of abstraction. Those propositions can, however, be transformed to the more specific and concrete level of the middle-range theory. Parse (1992) offered the three examples given in Table 6–1.

Middle-range theories, which are potentially testable, can be derived from the Theory of Human Becoming by means of a qualitative research methodology developed by Parse (1987, 1990a, 1992). The purpose of research is "to uncover the structure of lived experiences with persons or groups who can articulate the meaning of an experience" (1992, p. 41). The phenomena of interest are "universal human health experiences" (1992, p. 41) or "lived experiences of health" (1990a, p. 10). Examples of relevant lived experiences of health, according to Parse (1981, 1992), include joy, suffering, grieving, struggling with uncovering hidden meaning in a dialogue, struggling in cocreating possibilities for self-disclosure, being different from others, being enabled and limited by choices made, planning for the future, shifting points of view, and critical life decisions.

Research participants can be of any age, but they must be able to give an authentic accounting of the lived experience of interest. Parse (1987) maintained that 2 to 10 participants are sufficient for saturation or redundancy of the data. The criterion for saturation is "a pattern in

TABLE 6-1.   Examples of Propositions Derived from the Theory of Human Becoming

Grand Theory Propositions	Middle-Range Theory Propositions
Powering is a way of revealing-concealing imaging.	Struggling toward goals discloses and hides the significance of situations.
Originating is a manifestation of enabling-limiting valuing.	Creating anew shows one's cherished beliefs and leads in a directional movement.
Transforming unfolds in the languaging of connecting-separating.	Changing views emerge in speaking and moving with others.

Data from Parse, 1987, p. 170 and Parse, 1992, p. 39.

the engagements repeated by a number of participants" (Parse, 1990a, p. 10).

The primary data are symbols that can describe the lived experience of interest, such as pictures, metaphors, or poetry created and interpreted by the research participants. Those data are gathered by means of dialogical engagement and analyzed by using the processes of extraction-synthesis and heuristic interpretation.

Dialogical engagement "is the researcher-participant discussion" (Parse, 1987, p. 176). It is not an interview in the traditional sense; instead, it requires the researcher to be in true presence with the participant. In particular, dialogical engagement is "an intersubjective 'being with' in which researcher and participant live the I-Thou process as they move through an unstructured discussion about the lived experience" (Parse, 1987, p. 176). The researcher prepares for the dialogical engagement by "dwelling with" the meaning of the lived experience, that is, "centering self in a way to be open to a full discussion" (Parse, 1990a, p. 11), and creating some ideas for the direction the dialogue might take. An audio or video tape recording of the discussion is made and later transcribed for analysis.

Parse (1990a) explained that extraction-synthesis "is a process of moving the descriptions from the language of the participants up the levels of abstraction to the language of science" (p. 11). The process requires the researcher to engage in a "multisensory immersion," that is, "a contemplative abiding with" (p. 11) the discussion by reading the typed transcript and listening to the audio tape at the same time. If available, the video tape is viewed after reading the transcript.

Extraction-synthesis represents a creative conceptualization of the discussion through "inventing, which is synthesizing in the researcher's perspective; abstracting, which is moving up the ladder of discourse; and abiding with logic, which is adhering to semantical consistency" (Parse, 1987, p. 176). The researcher's own perspective is, therefore, clearly a part of the data analysis procedure.

Parse (1987) identified five processes that are involved in creative conceptualization:

1. Extracting an essence from the transcribed description to obtain a complete expression of a core idea described by the participant, in the participant's language.
2. Synthesizing the essence to obtain the core idea of the extracted essence as conceptualized by the researcher, in the researcher's language.
3. Formulating a proposition from each participant's description to obtain a nondirectional statement conceptualized by the researcher that joins the core idea of the synthesized essences.
4. Extracting concepts from the formulated propositions of all participants to obtain a term that captures the central meaning of the proposition.
5. Synthesizing a structure of the lived experience from the extracted concepts to obtain a statement conceptualized by the researcher that joins the core concepts.

Heuristic interpretation encompasses structural integration and conceptual interpretation. Parse (1987, 1990a) explained that structural integration involves connecting the synthesized structure to the Theory of Human Becoming, which results in moving the structure of the lived experience up another level of abstraction. "Conceptual interpretation," as viewed by Parse (1990a), "further specifies the structure of the lived experience by using concepts of the theory to create a unique theoretical structure which represents the meaning of the lived experience at the level of the theory" (p. 11). Thus the study finding is the structure of the lived experience. Such structures can be considered middle-range theories and should be empirically testable.

Parse (1981) claimed that her theory "invites empirical verification" (p. 77). She went on to comment, "It is expected that this theory will be verified through descriptive methodologies" (p. 78). Verification through traditional empirical testing, however, does not seem to be a goal for Parse and may not be consistent with the Theory of Human Becoming. In fact, Parse noted that generalizability is not relevant. Instead, "the goal of the Parse methodology is to gain an understanding of the structure of lived experiences thus enhancing the theory and the knowledge base of nursing to guide practice and further research" (Parse, 1990a, p. 11). Similarly, Ray (1990) pointed out that studies actually test Parse's research methodology, which was designed to generate theories.

Empirical Adequacy

Inasmuch as direct empirical testability does not seem to be consistent with the Theory of Human Becoming, the criterion of empirical adequacy must be modified to stipulate that Parse's research methodology does in fact yield descriptions of lived experiences. A review of research associated with the Theory of Human Becoming revealed that the modified criterion of empirical adequacy has been met. More specifically, a review of the results of the studies based on the Theory of Human Becoming revealed that new middle-range descriptive theories of lived experiences of health were indeed generated.

Parse (1992) pointed out that several studies related to the theory were conducted prior to the development of her research methodology. Those studies, which are described in the annotated bibliography at the end of this chapter, were conducted by using such qualitative methods as phenomenology, ethnography, and description rather than the distinctive processes of dialogical engagement, extraction-synthesis, and heuristic interpretation (Banonis, 1989; Jonas, 1992; Nokes & Carver, 1991; Parse, Coyne, & Smith, 1985; Santopinto, 1989; Wondolowski & Davis, 1988, 1991).

Studies that did employ Parse's methodology have begun to appear. Parse (1990a) reported what she claimed was "the first study to fully use the emerging man-living-health research methodology" (p. 16). That study focused on the lived experience of hope in a sample of 10 persons. Parse maintained that hope is an appropriate phenomenon for study within the context of her theory because "it surfaces as a way of becoming in the human-environment interrelationship" (p. 12). Following Parse's lead, Mitchell (1990a), Smith (1990), Cody (1991), and Kelley (1991) also used the research methodology for their studies of diverse lived experiences. Mitchell reported the findings of her study of the meaning of taking life day-by-day as described by 10 elderly persons in Canada. Smith described the lived experience of struggling through a difficult time as reported by 10 unemployed persons. Cody developed a description of grieving a personal loss by means of dialogical engagement with three individuals who were grieving the loss of a close other through death and one individual who was grieving the loss of a close relationship. Kelley described the phenomenon of "struggling with going along in a situation you do not believe in" as lived by 40 members of the American Academy of Nursing.

Pragmatic Adequacy

Nursing Education

Use of the Theory of Human Becoming requires special education. This is because nursing practice based on the theory

> is a different kind of nursing. It is not offering professional advice and
> opinions stemming from the personal value system of the nurse. It is
> not a canned approach to cure. It is a subject-to-subject interrelation-
> ship, a loving, true presence with the other to promote health and the
> quality of life. (Parse, 1987, p. 169)

Consequently, the clinician must learn to avoid making judgments
about or labeling individuals' ways of being, thinking, or feeling. "It is,"
according to Parse (1992), "essential to go with the person where the
person is rather than attempting to judge, change, or control the person"
(p. 40).

Furthermore, the clinician must learn the interpersonal art of
being truly present with a person or group to practice nursing based on
the Theory of Human Becoming. True presence is grounded in the
belief that each person knows "the way" somewhere within himself or
herself. Parse (1992) described true presence as "a special way of 'being
with' in which the nurse bears witness to the person's or family's own
living of value priorities" (p. 40). Elaborating, Parse (1990b) stated:

> The true presence of the nurse is a nonroutinized, nonmechanical way
> of "being with" in which the nurse is authentic and attentive to
> moment-to-moment changes in meaning for the person or group. . . . .
> True presence is the sphere of the interhuman and this is where the
> nurse enters the person's world with an openness, a self-giving, and a
> strong knowledge base reflecting the [Theory of Human Becoming]
> . . . . Living a true presence with a person is placing the emphasis on
> the human-to-human interrelationship with the nurse valuing the per-
> son as coauthor freely choosing health. (p. 139)

Moreover, as pointed out in the significance section of this chapter,
nursing practice based on the Theory of Human Becoming requires considerable grounding in the basic tenets and vocabulary of existential
phenomenology and the use of that vocabulary in the theory. Indeed,
"one unfamiliar with existential phenomenology may initially have difficulty with Parse's terminology" (Phillips, 1987, p. 195).

Parse (1981) noted that various curricular patterns that incorporate
her theory could be developed. In a later publication, she pointed out
that a nursing curriculum should be based on educational theories of
the teaching-learning process and that the substantive content of the
curriculum should be nursing theories and frameworks. Elaborating,
she explained:

> Nursing theories and frameworks should not be the curriculum plan;
> the curriculum plan should be designed on an education theory since
> that comes from the science of education, but the substantive content
> to be taught is nursing science. (Parse, cited in Takahashi, 1992, p. 89)

Parse (1981) presented a detailed description of a master's degree program grounded in her theory. She specified the philosophy, program goals, level indicators, objectives, course content and sequence, teaching strategies, and evaluation plan. The program was designed to prepare for specialization in family health with role concentrations in teaching and nursing service administration.

Nursing Practice

Parse (1987) pointed out that "Practice is the empirical life of [a] theory, which means that the practice of one theory would be very different from the practice of another" (p. 166). Accordingly, she developed a methodology for practice that is directly derived from and consistent with the Theory of Human Becoming. The purpose or goal of nursing practice within that methodology is "the quality of life as perceived by the person and the family" (p. 167). She explained:

> What constitutes the quality of life for one individual or family may be very different from what constitutes the quality of life for another. The nurse respects each individual's or family's own view of quality and does not attempt to change that view to be consistent with his or her own view. (Parse, 1992, p. 39)

The practice methodology can be implemented in nurse-person or nurse-group participation situations. The methodology encompasses three dimensions and three processes that are directly derived from the three major nonrelational propositions (the principles) of the Theory of Human Becoming (Parse, 1981, 1987, 1992). The dimensions are illuminating meaning, synchronizing rhythms, and mobilizing transcendence. The processes, which are empirical activities, are explicating, dwelling with, and moving beyond.

The dimension of illuminating meaning is derived from the first principle of the theory: structuring meaning multidimensionally. That dimension refers to "shedding light through uncovering the what was, is, and will be, as it is appearing now" (1987, p. 167). Illuminating meaning occurs through the empirical activity of explicating, which is "a process of making clear what is appearing now through languaging" (1992, p. 39). Thus the nurse "in true presence with the person or family invites the person or family to relate the meaning of the situation" (1992, p. 39). In particular, illuminating meaning through explicating draws attention to the "unique ways in which generational and contemporary family interrelationships cocreate lived values. . . . [and focuses] on mobilizing family energies for structuring and languaging different meanings in light of family health possibilities" (1981, p. 81).

Parse claimed that "in telling about the meaning, persons share thoughts and feelings with themselves, the nurse, and others in a nurse-family situation. The process of explicating thoughts and feelings in itself sheds new light on the situation" (1992, p. 39) and "changes the meaning of a situation by making it more explicit" (1987, p. 168).

The dimension of synchronizing rhythms is derived from the second principle of the theory: cocreating rhythmical patterns of relating. It happens through the empirical activity of dwelling with, which is described as "giving self over to the flow of the struggle in connecting-separating" (1987, p. 167). Parse explained:

> Synchronizing rhythms happens in dwelling with the pitch, yaw, and roll of the interhuman cadence—the turning, spinning, and thrusting of human relationships. Pitch, yaw, and roll represent the ups and downs, the struggles, the moments of joy, the unevenness of day-to-day living. (1987, p. 168)

Parse explained that "the nurse in true presence stays with the person or family while the person or family describes . . . day-to-day living in the now moment. The nurse . . . does not try to calm uneven rhythms but rather goes with the rhythms set by the person or family" (1992, p. 39). Furthermore, she pointed out that synchronizing rhythms through dwelling with focuses on "illuminating the family patterns of interrelating in light of the changing value priorities in the family's living of health" (1981, p. 82).

Parse claimed that, through discussion, the nurse can lead the family "to recognize the harmony that exists within its own lived context. There is always a way to find the harmony in what appears to be the conflict in the spinning and turning of human relationships" (1987, p. 168). In addition, "family awareness of patterns of relating enhances opportunities for the changing of health patterns" (1981, p. 82).

The dimension of mobilizing transcendence is derived from the third principle of the theory: cotranscending with the possibles. That dimension is realized through the empirical activity of moving beyond, which is defined as "propelling toward the possibles in transforming" (1987, p. 167). Mobilizing transcendence, according to Parse, happens in true presence with the nurse "through moving beyond the meaning moment to what is not yet. It focuses on dreaming of the possibles and planning to reach for the dreams" (1987, p. 169).

Here the nurse "guides individuals and families to plan for the changing of lived health patterns—these patterns uncovered in the illuminating of meaning, synchronizing of rhythms, and mobilizing of transcendence" (1987, p. 169). "The moving beyond," then, "arises as the rhythmical dwelling of nurse with person or family erupts in explications of the situation which incarnate new meaning" (1992, p. 40). Parse claimed that mobilizing transcendence through moving beyond results in "mobilizing family energies in reflectively choosing shifts in viewpoints relative to the possibilities available in the changing health process" (1981, p. 82).

Parse (1987) pointed out that the middle-range theory propositions listed in Table 6–1 can serve as relatively concrete guides for nursing practice. The proposition "struggling toward goals" guides practice by focusing on "illuminating the process of revealing-concealing unique ways a person and family can mobilize transcendence in considering new dreams, to image new possibles" (p. 170). Elaborating, she explained:

> In a nurse-family process, members share their thoughts and feelings about a situation, which both tells and does not tell all they know in the continuous struggle to meet personal goals. In disclosing the significance of the situation, the meaning of it changes for the family members, thus for the family. (p. 170)

The proposition "creating anew . . ." guides practice by dealing with "illuminating ways of being alike and different from others in changing values" (p. 170). Here,

> in a nurse-family process, by synchronizing rhythms, the members uncover the opportunities and limitations created by the decisions made in choosing irreplaceable ways of being together. The choices of new ways of being together mobilizes transcendence. (p. 170)

The proposition "changing views emerge . . ." guides practice by focusing on "illuminating meaning of relating ways of being together as various changing perspectives shed different light on the familiar, which gives rise to new possibles (p. 170). In this case, family members

> relate their values through speech and movement; thus views change and through mobilizing transcendence ways of relating change. When changing views are talked about among family members new possibles are seen and thus the ways of relating among family members change. (p. 170)

Several reports dealing with the application of the Theory of Human Becoming have been published (Butler, 1988; Butler & Snodgrass, 1991; Liehr, 1989; Mitchell, 1986, 1988, 1990b; Mitchell & Copplestone, 1990; Mitchell & Pilkington, 1990; Rasmusson, Jonas, & Mitchell, 1991). Those publications provide initial evidence of the pragmatic adequacy of the theory. The theory is appropriate for such diverse nurse-person situations as elderly individuals, chronically mentally ill persons, homeless people, and surgical patients, as well as for nurse-family situations. The feasibility of implementing clinical protocols that reflect the theory by nurses who are fully grounded in the theory is evident, and clinicians have the legal ability to implement those protocols. How-

ever, the extent to which nursing practice based on the Theory of
Human Becoming is compatible with expectations for nursing practice
and the actual effects of its use have not been fully explored. In particular, the acceptance of Parse's practice methodology, which is a nontraditional form of nursing practice, by health care consumers requires
systematic scrutiny.

CONCLUSION

Parse has made a meaningful contribution to nursing knowledge
development by explicating a grand theory that focuses on the lived
experience of health. In addition, she has contributed distinctive methodologies for research and for practice that are consistent with her
theory. Widespread interest in Parse's work is attested to by the establishment of the International Parse Interest Group. Continued documentation of outcomes of the use of the Theory of Human Becoming is
needed, with special attention given to how the theory contributes to
patients' enhanced quality of life.

REFERENCES

Bandler, R., & Grinder, J. (1975). *The structure of magic I.* Palo Alto, CA: Science and Behavior Books.
Banonis, B. C. (1989). The lived experience of recovering from addiction: A phenomeno-logical study. *Nursing Science Quarterly, 2,* 37–43.
Buber, M. (1965). *The knowledge of man* (M. Friedman, Ed.). New York: Harper and Row.
Butler, M. J. (1988). Family transformation: Parse's theory in practice. *Nursing Science Quarterly, 1,* 68–74.
Butler, M. J., & Snodgrass, F. G. (1991). Beyond abuse: Parse's theory in practice. *Nursing Science Quarterly, 4,* 76–82.
Cody, W. K. (1991). Grieving a personal loss. *Nursing Science Quarterly, 4,* 61–68.
Coyne, A. B. (1981). Prologue. In R. R. Parse, *Man-Living-Health. A theory of nursing* (pp. vii–xii). New York: John Wiley & Sons.
Dilthey, W. (1961). *Pattern and meaning in history.* New York: Harper and Row.
Greene, M. (1978). *Landscapes of learning.* New York: Teachers College Press.
Heidegger, M. (1962). *Being and time.* New York: Harper and Row.
Holmes, C. A. (1990). Alternatives to natural science foundations for nursing. *International Journal of Nursing Studies, 27,* 187–198.
Jonas, C. M. (1992). The meaning of being an elder in Nepal. *Nursing Science Quarterly, 5,* 171–175.
Kelley, L. S. (1991). Struggling with going along when you do not believe. *Nursing Science Quarterly, 4,* 123–129.
Kempler, W. (1974). *Principles of gestalt family therapy.* Oslo: A. S. Nordales, Trykkert.
Liehr, P. R. (1989). The core of true presence: A loving center. *Nursing Science Quarterly, 2,* 7–8.
Merleau-Ponty, M. (1974). *Phenomenology of perceptions.* New York: Humanities Press.
Mitchell, G. J. (1986). Utilizing Parse's theory of man-living-health in Mrs. M.'s neighbor-hood. *Perspectives, 10*(4), 5–7.

Mitchell, G. J. (1988). Man-living-health. The theory in practice. *Nursing Science Quarterly, 1*, 120–127.

Mitchell, G. J. (1990a). The lived experience of taking life day by day in later life: Research guided by Parse's emergent method. *Nursing Science Quarterly, 3*, 29–36.

Mitchell, G. J. (1990b). Struggling in change: From the traditional approach to Parse's theory-based practice. *Nursing Science Quarterly, 3*, 170–176.

Mitchell, G. J., & Cody, W. K. (1992). Nursing knowledge and human science: Ontological and epistemological considerations. *Nursing Science Quarterly, 5*, 54–61.

Mitchell, G. J., & Copplestone, C. (1990). Applying Parse's theory to perioperative nursing. A nontraditional approach. *Association of Operating Room Nurses Journal, 51*, 787–798.

Mitchell, G. J., & Pilkington, B. (1990). Theoretical approaches in nursing practice: A comparison of Roy and Parse. *Nursing Science Quarterly, 3*, 81–87.

Nietzsche, F. (1968). *The will to power.* (W. Kaufmann, Ed.). New York: Vintage Books.

Nokes, K. M., & Carver, K. (1991). The meaning of living with AIDS: A study using Parse's theory of Man-Living-Health. *Nursing Science Quarterly, 4*, 175–180.

Parse, R. R. (1981). *Man-Living-Health: A theory of nursing.* New York: John Wiley & Sons.

Parse, R. R. (1987). *Nursing science: Major paradigms, theories, and critiques.* Philadelphia: W. B. Saunders.

Parse, R. R. (1990a). Parse's research methodology with an illustration of the lived experience of hope. *Nursing Science Quarterly, 3*, 9–17.

Parse, R. R. (1990b). Health: A personal commitment. *Nursing Science Quarterly, 3*, 136–140.

Parse, R. R. (1992). Human becoming: Parse's theory of nursing. *Nursing Science Quarterly, 5*, 35–42.

Parse, R. R., Coyne, A. B., & Smith, M. J. (1985). *Nursing research: Qualitative methods.* Bowie, MD: Brady Communications.

Phillips, J. R. (1987). A critique of Parse's Man-Living-Health theory. In R. R. Parse, *Nursing science: Major paradigms, theories, and critiques* (pp. 181–204). Philadelphia: W. B. Saunders.

Rasmusson, D. L., Jonas, C. M., & Mitchell, G. J. (1991). The eye of the beholder: Parse's theory with homeless individuals. *Clinical Nurse Specialist, 5*, 139–143.

Raths, L. E., Harmin, M., & Simon, S. B. (1978). *Values and teaching.* Columbus, OH: Charles E. Merrill.

Ray, M. A. (1990). Critical reflective analysis of Parse's and Newman's research methodologies. *Nursing Science Quarterly, 3*, 44–46.

Rogers, M. E. (1980). Nursing: A science of unitary man. In J. P. Riehl & C. Roy, *Conceptual models for nursing practice* (2nd ed., pp. 329–337). Norwalk, CT: Appleton-Century-Crofts.

Santopinto, M. D. A. (1989). The relentless drive to be ever thinner: A study using the phenomenological method. *Nursing Science Quarterly, 2*, 29–36.

Sarter, B. (1988). Philosophical sources of nursing theory. *Nursing Science Quarterly, 1*, 52–59.

Sartre, J-P. (1966). *Being and nothingness.* New York: Washington Square Press.

Schutz, A. (1967). On multiple realities. In M. Natanson (Ed.), *The problem of social reality: Collected papers* (Vol. 1, pp. 209–212). The Hague; Martinue Nijhoff.

Smith, M. C. (1990). Struggling through a difficult time for unemployed persons. *Nursing Science Quarterly, 3*, 18–28.

Takahashi, T. (1992). Perspectives on nursing knowledge. *Nursing Science Quarterly, 5*, 86–91.

Tillich, P. (1954). *Love, power and justice.* New York: Oxford University Press.

van den Berg, J. H. (1971). Phenomenology and metabletics. *Humanitas, 7*, 285.

Watzlawick, P. (1978). *The language of change.* New York: Basic Books.

White, L. A. (1938). Science is sciencing. *Philosophy of Science, 5*, 369–389.

Wondolowski, C., & Davis, D. K. (1988). The lived experience of aging in the oldest old: A phenomenological study. *The American Journal of Psychoanalysis, 48*, 261–270.

Wondolowski, C., & Davis, D. K. (1991). The lived experience of health in the oldest old: A phenomenological study. *Nursing Science Quarterly, 4*, 113–118.

ANNOTATED BIBLIOGRAPHY

Primary Sources

Parse, R. R. (1981). Caring from a human science perspective. In M. Leininger (Ed.), *Caring: An essential human need* (pp. 129–132). Thorofare, NJ: Slack.
Parse describes her ideas about caring from a human science perspective. She defines caring as risking being with someone toward a moment of joy. The chapter is a synopsis of Parse's presentation at the Third National Caring Conference held in Salt Lake City, Utah, in 1980.

Parse, R. R. (1981). *Man-Living-Health: A theory of nursing.* New York: Wiley. [Reprinted 1989. Albany, NY: Delmar]
This book contains Parse's original formulation of her theory, along with discussions of the use of the theory in nursing research, education, and practice.

Parse, R. E. (1987). Man-Living-Health theory of nursing. In R. R. Parse, *Nursing Science. Major paradigms, theories, and critiques* (pp. 159–180). Philadelphia: W. B. Saunders.
In this chapter, Parse specifies the philosophical assumptions, principles, concepts, and theoretical structures of the theory of Man-Living-Health. The author discusses the research and practice traditions in nursing. The practice methodology of Man-Living-Health and its dimensions and processes are described. Finally, an emerging research methodology consistent with the theory is presented.

Parse, R. E. (1989). Man-Living-Health: A theory of nursing. In J. P. Riehl-Sisca, *Conceptual models for nursing practice* (3rd ed., pp. 253–257). Norwark, CT: Appleton & Lange.
Parse presents an overview of her theory, including assumptions, principles, and theoretical structures. She also briefly describes her research and practice methodologies.

Parse, R. R. (1990). Health: A personal commitment. *Nursing Science Quarterly, 3,* 136–140.
Parse explains that health as a personal commitment is a view that evolves from her theory. She identifies implications for nursing practice and research related to her view of health, and explains how human beings move beyond the moment to change patterns of health through creative imagining, affirming self, and spontaneous glimpsing of the paradoxical. She also discusses the meaning of true presence.

Parse, R. R. (1992). Human becoming: Parse's theory of nursing. *Nursing Science Quarterly, 5,* 35–42.
Parse updates her theory and revises its language to be consistent with the change in name from man-living-health to human becoming. She also updates her research and practice methodologies. In addition, she presents the assumptions underpinning the research methodology for the first time.

Commentary by Parse and Others

Boyd, C. O. (1990). Critical appraisal of developing nursing research methods. *Nursing Science Quarterly, 3,* 42–43.
Boyd discusses Newman's and Parse's orientations to research and notes that both have contributed to the needed clarification of processes of analysis in qualitative research.

Bunting, S. (1993). *Rosemarie Parse: Theory of health as human becoming.* Newbury Park, CA: Sage.
Bunting presents an interpretation and analysis of Parse's theory of human becoming. Very brief reviews of her practice and research methodologies are included, along with a clinical example.

Cody, W. K. (1991). Multidimensionality: Its meaning and significance. *Nursing Science Quarterly, 4,* 140–141.
Cody discusses usages of the term multidimensionality. He notes that Parse cites Martha Rogers's original use of the concept of four-dimensionality as a contributing idea

to her theory of human becoming. He then describes Parse's use of multidimensionality.

DeFeo, D. J. (1990). Change: A central concern of nursing. *Nursing Science Quarterly, 3,* 88–94.

Drawing from Buddhism, existential philosophy, and modern developmental thought, DeFeo explores the concept of change as a fundamental, inevitable aspect of life and as a process of risking to choose. He also describes Parse's various usages of the concept.

Hall, B. A., & Parse, R. R. (1993). The theory-research-practice triad: Commentary [Hall]. Response [Parse]. *Nursing Science Quarterly, 6,* 10–12.

Hall comments on Parse's theory of human becoming and discusses two issues: The need to update theories and the consequences of not doing so due to death or retirement of the theorist and the differences in research procedures for theory that is proposed for predictive purposes versus theories that are more philosophical. Parse responds by noting that some nurse scholars are committed to update the original work of the major theorists and by explaining that the theory of human becoming does not lend itself to traditional approaches to theory testing.

Hickman, J. S. (1990). Rosemarie Rizzo Parse. In J. B. George (Ed.), *Nursing theories: The base for professional nursing practice* (3rd ed., pp. 311–332). Norwalk, CT: Appleton & Lange.

Hickman identifies Parse's academic and experiential credentials and describes and analyzes her theory.

Huch, M. H. (1991). Perspectives on health. *Nursing Science Quarterly, 4,* 33–40.

This article is the transcription of a panel discussion at the Nurse Theorist Conference sponsored by Discovery International and held in Pittsburgh, Pennsylvania in May 1989. Participants were Imogene King, Nola Pender, Betty Neuman, Martha Rogers, Afaf Meleis, and Rosemarie Parse. The discussion centered on the theorists' views of health.

Mitchell, G. J. (1990). A nurse responds [Letter to the editor]. *Holistic Nursing Practice,* 5(1), ix–x.

Donnelly, G. F. (1990). Editor's response. *Holistic Nursing Practice,* 5(1), x–xi.

Burkhardt, M. A., & Nagai-Jacobson, M. G. (1990). Authors' response. *Holistic Nursing Practice,* 5(1), xi–xii.

Mitchell expresses her thoughts upon reading the two articles by Nagai-Jacobson and Burkhardt in the May 1989 issue of *Holistic Nursing Practice.* Concerns regarding these authors' failure to credit Parse's work are raised.

Donnelly, who is the editor of the journal, reports that at the time of the writings of the articles by Nagai-Jacobson and Burkhardt, Parse's work had not been fully described in the nursing literature. In addition, the concepts described in the two articles are not exclusive to Parse's work as they have appeared in the works of scholars across many disciplines.

Burkhardt and Nagai-Jacobson maintain that the writing of their articles is based on their clinical experience, sharing with colleagues, and independent study and reading. They point out that the terminology used is derived from a synthesis of several sources, many of which predate publication of Parse's work.

Mitchell, G. J. (1992). Specifying the knowledge base of theory in practice. *Nursing Science Quarterly, 5,* 6–7.

Mitchell discusses the sources of knowledge used to guide practice. She argues for nursing knowledge contained in nursing models and theories, including Parse's theory. She presents a very brief overview of Parse's practice method.

Mitchell, G. J. (1993). Living paradox in Parse's theory. *Nursing Science Quarterly, 6,* 44–51.

Mitchell explores the historical development of paradox and its various forms and uses. She defines living paradox as a rhythmical shifting of views, the awareness of which arises through experiencing the contradiction of opposites in the day-to-day relating of value priorities while journeying to the not-yet. She claims that living paradox as specified in Parse's theory is a significant contribution to nursing and human science.

Mitchell, G. J., & Cody, W. K. (1992). Nursing knowledge and human science: Ontological and epistemological considerations. *Nursing Science Quarterly, 5,* 54–61.

Mitchell and Cody define and describe human science from Dilthey's perspective. They conclude that Parse's theory is not only congruent with, but goes beyond the human science perspective.

Parse, R. R. (1987). *Nursing science: Major paradigms, theories, and critiques.* Philadelphia: W. B. Saunders.

This edited book contains Parse's discussion of the characteristics of the totality and simultaneity paradigms, as well as papers by Parse, Roy, Orem, King, and Rogers. Critiques of the theorists' works also are included. The book is based on papers presented at the Nurse Theorist Conference sponsored by Discovery International and held in Pittsburgh, Pennsylvania in May 1985.

Phillips, J. R. (1987). A critique of Parse's man-living-health theory. In R. R. Parse, *Nursing Science: Major paradigms, theories, and critiques* (pp. 181–204). Philadelphia: W. B. Saunders.

Phillips discusses the coherence of Parse's work, the logical flow in the construction of the theory, and the symmetry and aesthetics in the relationships among its elements. He points out Parse's failure to clearly address the relationships of the concepts in the assumptions to Rogers's conceptual model and existential phenomenology. Other criticism on Parse's work includes a lack of testable propositions and its level of abstraction. Phillips suggests that Parse's work be considered a nursing model rather than a theory. In the present book, Parse's work is classified as a grand theory.

Pugliese, L. (1989). The theory of man-living-health: An analysis. In J. P. Riehl-Sisca, *Conceptual models for nursing practice* (3rd ed., pp. 259–265). Norwark, CT: Appleton & Lange.

Pugliese presents a brief critique of Parse's theory, including internal evaluation of its elements and external evaluation of its utility and significance.

Sarter, B. (1988). Philosophical sources of nursing theory. *Nursing Science Quarterly, 1,* 52–59.

Sarter identifies the philosophical roots of Parse's theory as a logically constructed and organized synthesis from Martha Rogers's conceptual system and existentialism.

Schumacher, L. P. (1986). Rosemarie Rizzo Parse: Man-Living-Health. In A. Marriner, *Nursing theorists and their work* (pp. 169–177). St. Louis: C. V. Mosby.

Lee, R. E., & Schumacher, L. P. (1989). Rosemarie Rizzo Parse: Man-Living-Health. In A. Marriner-Tomey, *Nursing theorists and their work* (2nd ed., pp. 174–186). St. Louis: C. V. Mosby.

In each edition, Parse's academic and experiential credentials are described and a rudimentary analysis of her theory is presented. A cursory critique of the theory is included.

Smith, M. C. (1991). Existential-phenomenological foundations in nursing: A discussion of differences. *Nursing Science Quarterly, 4,* 5–6.

Smith discusses the existential and phenomenological foundations of several nursing theories. She points out that Parse's theory includes the tenets of the unity or irreducible view of the person, health as an incarnation of the meaning of reality, patterns of relating that are health, health as transcendence, and the paradoxical nature of lived experiences of health.

Smith, M. C., & Hudepohl, J. H. (1988). Analysis and evaluation of Parse's theory of Man-Living-Health. *Canadian Journal of Nursing Research, 20*(4), 43–57.

The purpose of this article is to analyze Parse's theory of Man-Living-Health according to Fawcett's criteria for the analysis and evaluation of conceptual models in nursing. The analysis includes an historical evolution of Parse's work and a description of the basic assumptions and concepts. The evaluation consists of an examination of the comprehensiveness of the concepts and propositions, the logical congruence of the structure and substance, and the social significance and utility of the theory. The use of Fawcett's framework for nursing models was not appropriate for Parse's work, which is a grand theory.

Randell, B. P. (1992). Nursing theory: The 21st century. *Nursing Science Quarterly, 5,* 176–184.

This article is the transcription of a panel discussion at a conference sponsored by the University of California, Los Angeles, Neuropsychiatric Institute and Hospital and held in Los Angeles in September 1990. The participants were Dorothy Johnson, Betty Neuman, Dorothea Orem, Rosemarie Parse, Martha Rogers, and Callista Roy. Questions focused on the development of the theorists' works, the direction nursing theory will take in the 21st century, current research derived from the theorists' works, and the relationship of the theorists' works to the NANDA nursing diagnosis taxonomy.

Smith, M. J. (1988). Perspectives on nursing science. *Nursing Science Quarterly, 1,* 80–85.
This article is the transcription of a panel discussion at the Nurse Theorist Conference sponsored by Discovery International and held in Pittsburgh in May 1987. The panel was moderated by Mary Jane Smith; participants were Imogene King, Madeleine Leininger, Rosemarie Parse, Hildegard Peplau, Martha Rogers, Callista Roy, and Rozella Schlotfeldt. Questions focused on the issues of the uniqueness of theoretical frameworks, the phenomenon central to theoretical frameworks, and nursing diagnoses.

Takahashi, T. (1992). Perspectives on nursing knowledge. *Nursing Science Quarterly, 5,* 86–91.
This article is the transcription of a panel discussion at the Nurse Theorist Conference sponsored by Discovery International and held in Tokyo in May 1991. The panel was moderated by Hiroko Minami; participants were Imogene King, Rosemarie Parse, Hildegard Peplau, and Martha Rogers. Questions were related to the focus of each theorist's work, similarities and differences between the works, the use of nursing theories to structure curricula for nursing education, and the applicability of nursing models and theories in diverse cultures. The panel discussion provided an opportunity for considerable dialogue among the four theorists.

Winkler, S. J. (1983). Parse's theory of nursing. In J. J. Fitzpatrick & A. L. Whall, *Conceptual models of nursing: Analysis and application* (pp. 275–294). Bowie, MD: Brady.

Cowling, W. Richard III. (1989). Parse's theory of nursing. In J. J. Fitzpatrick & A. L. Whall, *Conceptual models of nursing: Analysis and application* (2nd ed., pp. 385–399). Norwalk, CT: Appleton & Lange.
In each edition of the book, the author describes Parse's theory, presents an analysis of the theory, and briefly discusses its relation to nursing research, education, and practice.

Practice

Balcombe, K., Davis, P., & Lim, E. (1991). A nursing model for orthopaedics. *Nursing Standard, 5*(49), 26–28.
The authors describe a framework for nursing practice based on Parse's theory. The framework acknowledges medical, paramedical, and nursing intervention, but emphasizes nursing intervention, especially the patient/nurse relationship. The patient's desired health status is of central importance, and the patient's definition of health becomes the reality from which the nurse must plan individual health education.

Butler, M. J. (1988). Family transformation: Parse's theory in practice. *Nursing Science Quarterly, 1,* 68–74.
Butler explains how the principles and practice dimensions of the theory of Man-Living-Health were used to change the health situation of a family facing the loss of the family patriarch who had experienced major neurosurgery. The value of theory-based nursing practice is discussed through a family situation.

Butler, M. J., & Snodgrass, F. G. (1991). Beyond abuse: Parse's theory in practice. *Nursing Science Quarterly, 4,* 76–82.
Butler and Snodgrass describe nursing practice with abused women and their families based on Parse's theory. A case study is included.

Cody, W. K., & Mitchell, G. J. (1992). Parse's theory as a model for practice: The cutting edge. *Advances in Nursing Science, 15*(2), 52–65.
Cody and Mitchell describe the use of Parse's theory in nursing practice and explicate the beliefs, values, and ethic of Parse's practice method. They review the results of

published and unpublished evaluation projects designed to determine the efficacy of the method and recommend additional evaluation projects.

Liehr, P. R. (1989). The core of true presence: A loving center. *Nursing Science Quarterly, 2*, 7–8.
Liehr describes the use of Parse's notion of true presence with a man who had had a heart transplant and was hospitalized 2 years later for a routine checkup that resulted in complications.

Magan, S. J., Gibbon, E. J., & Mrozek, R. (1990). Nursing theory applications: A practice model. *Issues in Mental Health Nursing, 11*, 297–312.
Based on the open system nursing principles of Parse, Newman, and Rogers, this article describes the implementation of nursing theory-based assessment and intervention strategies for hospitalized, chronically mentally ill patients. The authors discuss the empirical testing of the practice model.

Martin, M-L., Forchuk, C., Santopinto, M., & Butcher, H. K. (1992). Alternative approaches to nursing practice: Application of Peplau, Rogers, Parse. *Nursing Science Quarterly, 5*, 80–85.
The authors describe the use of works by Parse, Peplau, and Rogers in practice. They explain how theory-based practice differs from traditional practice and how nursing knowledge can guide practice. Tables display documentation from the perspective of each theorist's work.

Mattice, M., & Mitchell, G. J. (1991). Caring for confused elders. *The Canadian Nurse, 86*(11), 16–17.
Mattice and Mitchell discuss the use of Parse's theory in the care of confused older persons. They point out that when using Parse's theory, nurses realize that rather than telling others what they should experience, they seek to understand and be with patients as they experience life.

Mitchell, G. J. (1986). Utilizing Parse's theory of man-living-health in Mrs. M.'s neighborhood. *Perspectives, 10*(4), 5–7.
Mitchell describes how Parse's theory of Man-Living-Health guided the nursing care of a hospitalized elderly woman. The three dimensions in the practice methodology of Man-Living-Health are illustrated. The selected nursing interventions and the value of the theory in the care of the client are discussed.

Mitchell, G. J. (1988). Man-Living-Health. The theory in practice. *Nursing Science Quarterly, 1*, 120–127.
Mitchell outlines the Man-Living-Health theory. An examination of the theoretical assumptions, main themes, dimensions, and processes is presented. The author describes the application of the theory in the nursing care of an elderly person who was discharged from a rehabilitation unit to a home for the aged.

Mitchell, G. J. (1990). Struggling in change: From the traditional approach to Parse's theory-based practice. *Nursing Science Quarterly, 3*, 170–176.
Mitchell explains her struggle to change her practice from a traditional problem-based approach to being guided by Parse's theory. She identifies the benefits of the change as they relate to the client's perspective of enhanced quality of life and the nurse's perspective of professional practice.

Mitchell, G. J. (1991). Distinguishing practice with Parse's theory. In I. E. Goertzen (Ed.), *Differentiating nursing practice: Into the twenty-first century* (pp. 55–58). Kansas City, MO: American Academy of Nursing.
Mitchell explains how her practice changed when she began to apply Parse's theory and the results of an evaluation of the use of Parse's theory at St. Michael's Hospital in Toronto, Ontario, Canada (c.f. annotation in this section for Quiquero, A., Knights, D., & Meo, C. O. [1991]. Theory as a guide to practice: Staff nurses choose Parse's theory. *Canadian Journal of Nursing Administration, 4*(1), 14–16).

Mitchell, G. J. (1991). Human subjectivity: The cocreation of self. *Nursing Science Quarterly, 4*, 144–145.
Mitchell discusses subjectivity as the engagement of the unitary human being with-the-world and cites Parse's view of the human being as participant with the world in cocreation of self. She applies the notion of subjectivity to the nursing care of an elderly woman who had terminal cancer.

Mitchell, G. J. (1991). Nursing diagnosis: An ethical analysis. *Image: Journal of Nursing Scholarship, 23*, 99–103.
Mitchell identifies the ethical consequences of nursing diagnosis in terms of the principle "to do no harm" for both the patient and the nurse. She claims that human suffering is created through nursing actions that objectively judge and reduce human beings. She notes that Parse's theory is one approach that upholds the duty "to do no harm."

Mitchell, G. J. (1992). Parse's theory and the multidisciplinary team: Clarifying scientific values. *Nursing Science Quarterly, 5*, 104–106.
Mitchell explains how nurses have traditionally participated on multidisciplinary teams and how their participation is changing to reflect changes in nursing science. She comments that Parse's theory presents nurses with the opportunity to specify their unique contribution to human health and the quality of life.

Mitchell, G. J., & Copplestone, C. (1990). Applying Parse's theory to perioperative nursing: A nontraditional approach. *Association of Operating Room Nurses Journal, 51*, 787–798.
Perioperative nursing practice has traditionally focused on problem identification rather than on human relationships and life processes. In this article, the authors explain the use of Parse's theory to guide the perioperative nursing care of a client and his family.

Mitchell, G. J., & Pilkington, B. (1990). Theoretical approaches in nursing practice: A comparison of Roy and Parse. *Nursing Science Quarterly, 3*, 81–87.
The authors compare nursing practice as guided by Parse and Roy. They describe the practice methodologies for each approach, apply them to a nursing situation, and identify the opportunities and limitations of each. Opportunities offered by Parse's theory revolve around the nurse-person interrelationship, professional practice, and self-discovery. Limitations are changing traditional views about human beings and health. They note that being truly present to another requires energy, time, and devotion to the process.

Mitchell, G. J., & Santopinto, M. (1988). An alternative to nursing diagnosis. *The Canadian Nurse, 84*(11), 25–28.
The authors present their views on the limitations of the traditional nursing process and the use of nursing diagnosis which are grounded in the totality paradigm. In contrast, nursing care guided by Parse's theory is based on the simultaneity paradigm, which allows for a more dynamic approach. Using a care plan, the authors compare the traditional care based on nursing diagnosis with that of Parse's guide for practice based on emerging patterns of health.

Parse, R. R. (1991). Parse's theory of human becoming. In I. E. Goertzen (Ed.), *Differentiating nursing practice: Into the twenty-first century* (pp. 51–53). Kansas City, MO: American Academy of Nursing.
Parse provides a brief overview of her theory and explains how it can be applied in practice. She points out that the traditional nursing process of assessment, planning, diagnosis, implementation, and evaluation is inconsistent with her theory. She goes on to explain that the person shares with the Parse nurse a personal description of health and specifies paradoxical patterns of health and desires, as well as hopes in the situation.

Quiquero, A., Knights, D., & Meo, C. O. (1991). Theory as a guide to practice: Staff nurses choose Parse's theory. *Canadian Journal of Nursing Administration, 4*(1), 14–16.
The authors describe the changes that occurred in staff nurses' thoughts and actions when Parse's theory was used to guide practice on an acute care medical unit at St. Michael's Hospital in Toronto, Ontario, Canada. They concluded that Parse's theory led to a more humanistic way of nursing.

Rasmusson, D. L., Jonas, C. M., & Mitchell, G. J. (1991). The eye of the beholder: Parse's theory with homeless individuals. *Clinical Nurse Specialist, 5*, 139–143.
The authors describe how nursing practice with homeless persons in a community setting, in both individual and group encounters, was guided by Parse's theory. They explain how Parse's theory and practice method differ from traditional problem solving.

Smith, M. C. (1990). Pattern in nursing practice. *Nursing Science Quarterly, 3,* 57–59.
Smith traces the discussion of the concept of pattern in the nursing literature, starting with Martha Rogers and continuing with Parse's and Newman's notions of pattern. She notes that for Parse, patterns are rhythmical and paradoxical.

Smith, M. J. (1989). Research and practice application related to man-living-health: A theory of nursing. In J. P. Riehl-Sisca, *Conceptual models for nursing practice* (3rd ed., pp. 267–276). Norwark, CT: Appleton & Lange.
Smith describes the application of her findings from a study of the lived experience of rest (c.f. annotation for this paper in the Research section) in the nursing care of a family who is confronting a situation of unrest resulting from the addition of the husband's elderly mother to the household.

Sullivan, I. (1992). The nurse practitioner as healer: A process of interactive simultaneity. *Nurse Practitioner Forum, 3,* 226–227.
Sullivan describes how her idea of interactive simultaneity, which draws from Parse's theory, and her research on the healing activity of arctic and subarctic medicine women enhance contemporary clinical practice.

Administration

Mattice, M. (1991). Parse's theory of nursing in practice: A manager's perspective. *Canadian Journal of Nursing Administration, 4*(1), 11–13.
Mattice describes the nurse manager's participation in the application of Parse's theory at St. Michael's Hospital in Toronto, Ontario, Canada (c.f. annotation in the Practice section for Quiquero, A., Knights, D., & Meo, C. O. [1991]. Theory as a guide to practice: Staff nurses choose Parse's theory. *Canadian Journal of Nursing Administration, 4*(1), 14–16). She reports that the use of the theory favorably influenced the quality of care and nurse satisfaction and led to a more cohesive and humanistic nursing unit.

Parse, R. R. (1989). Parse's man-living-health model and administration of nursing service. In B. Henry, C. Arndt, M. Di Vincenti, & A. Marriner-Tomey (Eds.), *Dimensions of nursing administration* (pp. 69–74). Boston: Blackwell Scientific Publications.
Parse describes her theory and the associated practice methodology. She notes that the theory and methodology lead to a nontraditional administration of nursing services, with an emphasis on the administrator's openness and concern for the values of the practicing nurses. Parse identifies the administrative structures that would be required for use of her theory, including the philosophy of nursing, goals of nursing practice, and standards of practice.

Parse, R. R. (1989). The phenomenological research method: Its value for management science. In B. Henry, C. Arndt, M. Di Vincenti, & A. Marriner-Tomey (Eds.), *Dimensions of nursing administration* (pp. 291–296). Boston: Blackwell Scientific Publications.
Parse reviews the basic notions of the phenomenological research method and describes its use by administrators. She notes that the theory guiding management and administration of nursing services should govern the choice of a research method, so that a phenomenologic method would not be appropriate in some settings.

Research

Banonis, B. C. (1989). The lived experience of recovering from addiction: A phenomenological study. *Nursing Science Quarterly, 2,* 37–43.
Based on Rogers's conceptual system and Parse's theory of Man-Living-Health, this study uncovered a structural description of the experience of recovering from addiction. In the process of recovering from their addiction, three individuals described the rhythmical shifts of their lived experience. This study supports the value of the phenomenological method in nursing research as well as Parse's assumptions. Implications for nursing practice are discussed.

Cody, W. K. (1991). Grieving a personal loss. *Nursing Science Quarterly, 4,* 61–68.
Cody reports that the structure of the lived experience of grieving a personal loss is intense struggling in the flux of change while a shifting view fosters moving beyond

the now as different possibilities surface in dwelling with and apart from the absent presence and others in light of what is cherished.

Heine, C. (1991). Development of gerontological nursing theory. Applying the Man-Living-Health theory of nursing. *Nursing and Health Care, 12,* 184–188.

Heine describes the use of Parse's theory in gerontological nursing practice settings and for gerontological nursing research. She poses a research question—What is the structure of the lived experience of feeling restricted as experienced by institutionalized older adults?—and explains how Parse's research methodology could direct a study designed to answer the question.

Jonas, C. M. (1992). The meaning of being an elder in Nepal. *Nursing Science Quarterly, 5,* 171–175.

Jonas reports that the meaning of being an elder in Nepal is: cherishing necessities for survival intermingled with the rapture of celebration with important others, as diminishing familiar patterns expand moments of respite, while regard from others affirms self, and changing customs create comfort-discomfort as what-was unfolds into new possibles. She notes that the study findings are consistent with Parse's concepts of valuing, enabling-limiting, and transforming.

Kelley, L. S. (1991). Struggling with going along when you do not believe. *Nursing Science Quarterly, 4,* 123–129.

Kelley reports that she found the phenomenon of struggling with going along in a situation you do not believe in to be the predominant universal lived experience within the lives of outstanding nurses in the United States. The phenomenon is described as: justifiable yielding, as opposing views intensify personal convictions and compel disclosure while suffering consequences. Kelley states that the phenomenon is comparable to Parse's notion of valuing the powering of revealing-concealing.

Liehr, P. (1992). Prelude to research. *Nursing Science Quarterly, 5,* 102–103.

Liehr describes the thinking and observation that occur prior to formulating a research question. She provides two examples related to Parse's theory.

Mitchell, G. J. (1990). The lived experience of taking life day-by-day in later life: Research guided by Parse's emergent method. *Nursing Science Quarterly, 3,* 29–36.

Mitchell reports the findings of her study of the meaning of taking life day by day for a sample of individuals over age 75. The common concepts extracted from the data were: affirming self through interrelationships, glimpsing a diminishing now amidst expanding possibles, and the unburdened journey of moving beyond.

Nokes, K. M., & Carver, K. (1991). The meaning of living with AIDS: A study using Parse's theory of man-living-health. *Nursing Science Quarterly, 4,* 175–179.

Nokes and Carver report the findings of their qualitative descriptive study of persons with AIDS. Three themes related to the meaning of living with AIDS emerged: an abrupt shift in patterns of being give rise to changing priorities, fluctuating possibilities arise in the uncertainty of being with and away from close others, and changing hopes and dreams surface from the insights of suffering.

Parse, R. R. (1990). Parse's research methodology with an illustration of the lived experience of hope. *Nursing Science Quarterly, 3,* 9–17.

The purpose of this article is to describe the Parse research methodology and report the findings of a study using the emerging method to investigate the lived experience of hope for persons on hemodialysis. The structure of the lived experience is: hope is anticipating possibilities through envisioning the not-yet in harmoniously living the comfort-discomfort of everydayness while unfolding a different perspective of an expanding view.

Parse, R. R. (1993). The experience of laughter: A phenomenological study. *Nursing Science Quarterly, 6,* 39–43.

Parse reports the findings of her study of laughing in persons over 65. The structural definition of laughing was determined to be: laughing is a buoyant immersion in the presence of unanticipated glimpsings prompting harmonious integrity which surfaces anew through contemplative visioning. Parse notes that the definition is congruent with her theory and expands understanding of human experiences.

Parse, R. R., Coyne, A. B., & Smith, M. J. (1985). *Nursing research: Qualitative methods.* Bowie, MD: Brady.

This edited book contains a description of Parse's theory; chapters describing the phenomenological, ethnographic, and descriptive methods; and criteria for evaluation of qualitative research. The book also contains reports of studies using the various qualitative methods.

Phillips, J. R. (1990). New methods of research: Beyond the shadows of nursing science [Guest editorial]. *Nursing Science Quarterly, 3,* 1–2.
Phillips notes that Parse's research method (c.f. annotation in this section for Parse, R. R. [1990]. Parse's research methodology with an illustration of the lived experience of hope. *Nursing Science Quarterly, 3,* 9–17) addresses Bohm's notion of the implicate order and facilitates understanding of people's experiences rather than gathering data from them as objects.

Phillips, J. R. (1991). Human field research. *Nursing Science Quarterly, 4,* 142–143.
Although Phillips focuses his comments on Martha Rogers's work, he notes that the unity of opposites is evident in Parse's work through her principle of dealing with paradoxical rhythmical patterns.

Ray, M. A. (1990). Critical reflective analysis of Parse's and Newman's research methodologies. *Nursing Science Quarterly, 3,* 44–46.
Ray presents an analysis of Parse's research methodology. She points out that the method can facilitate development of new theory and, at the same time, expand the grand theory used to inform the research method.

Santopinto, M. D. A. (1989). The relentless drive to be ever thinner: A study using the phenomenological method. *Nursing Science Quarterly, 2,* 29–36.
The purpose of this study was to describe the lived experience of the relentless drive to be ever thinner. This lived experience is: a persistent struggle toward an imaged self lived through withdrawing-engaging.

Smith, M. C. (1990). Struggling through a difficult time for unemployed persons. *Nursing Science Quarterly, 3,* 18–28.
Smith reports the findings of a study using Parse's research methodology. She found that struggling through a difficult time is regarded by unemployed persons as sculpting new lifeways in turbulent change through affirming self while feeling expanded by assets and restricted by obstacles in the midst of grieving the loss of what was cherished.

Smith, M. J. (1989). Research and practice application related to man-living-health: A theory of nursing. In J. P. Riehl-Sisca, *Conceptual models for nursing practice* (3rd ed., pp. 267–276). Norwalk, CT: Appleton & Lange.
Smith describes the results of a study of the meaning of the lived experience of rest, using the phenomenological method. The findings revealed that rest for individuals in a structured confined situation is easy drifting through paradoxical swinging surfacing in deliberate picturing.

Wondolowski, C., & Davis, D. K. (1988). The lived experience of aging in the oldest old: A phenomenological study. *American Journal of Psychoanalysis, 48,* 261–270.
Based on Parse's Man-Living-Health theory, this phenomenological study uncovered ways in which the oldest old living in the community view the experience of aging. The investigation revealed that in a sample of 100 men and women, aged 80 to 101 years, aging is creating transfiguring in the presence of unfolding euphony enhanced by moments of transcent voyaging.

Wondolowski, C., & Davis, D. K. (1991). The lived experience of health in the oldest old: A phenomenological study. *Nursing Science Quarterly, 4,* 113–118.
The authors report the results of their phenomenological study of the lived experience of health for the oldest old. They found that health is regarded as an abiding vitality emanating through moments of rhapsodic reverie in generating fulfillment.

Doctoral Dissertations

Beauchamp, C. J. (1990). The structure of the lived experience of struggling with making a decision in a critical life situation, for a group of individuals with HIV. *Dissertation Abstracts International, 51,* 2815B.

Costello-Nickitas, D. M. (1990). The lived experience of choosing among life goals: A phenomenological study. *Dissertation Abstracts International, 50,* 3916B.

Dickerson, S. S. (1992). The lived experience of help seeking in spouses of cardiac patients. *Dissertation Abstracts International, 52,* 5758B.

Lemone, P. (1991). Transforming: Patterns of sexual function in adults with insulin-dependent diabetes mellitus. *Dissertation Abstracts International, 52,* 1354B.

Master's Theses

Baldwin-Donald, F. C. (1990). The lived experience of anger: An exploratory study. *Masters Abstracts International, 29,* 88.

Brennan, K. S. (1989). Integrating ambivalence: Living with the abortion experience. *Masters Abstracts International, 28,* 405.

Brown, L. L. (1991). Struggling in changing priorities. *Masters Abstracts International, 30,* 295.

Brunsman, C. S. (1988). A phenomenological study of the lived experience of hope in families with chronically ill children. *Master's Abstracts International, 26,* 416.

Cohen, D. (1990). A descriptive case study. One family's approach to a daughter's menarche: Illuminating the possibles. *Masters Abstracts International, 28,* 572.

Cutler, L. A. (1990). Assigning meaning to the lived experiences of women's menstrual cycles. *Masters Abstracts International, 28,* 572.

Donahue, D. M. (1991). Powerlessness and nurses' decision-making processes. *Masters Abstracts International, 30,* 94.

Hurren, D. A. (1989). Lived experience of caring for residents who verbalize concerns about death in a nursing home setting: A qualitative study. *Masters Abstracts International, 28,* 273.

Lavenia-Anderson, J. T. (1991). The lived experience of the spouse whose husband has cancer. *Masters Abstracts International, 30,* 96.

7

Peplau's Theory of Interpersonal Relations__

Hildegard Peplau's educational, clinical, and teaching experiences "led to an interest in clarifying what happens in a nurse-patient relationship" (Peplau, 1952, p. v). Peplau saw that both the nurse and the patient "participate in and contribute to [a] relationship and, further, that the relationship itself could be therapeutic" (Sills, 1989, p. ix). Those notions led to the formulation of what Peplau originally called "psychodynamic nursing" (1952) and later referred to as "a theory of interpersonal relations" (1992). The Theory of Interpersonal Relations was first taught to nursing students in 1948 and published by Peplau in 1952. Subsequently, she continued to discuss the theory and described its application to diverse clinical problems in a series of papers, many of which are now available in a volume edited by O'Toole and Welt (1989).

The one concept of the Theory of Interpersonal Relations and its dimensions are listed below. The concept and dimensions are described later in this chapter.

KEY CONCEPT___

Nurse-Patient Relationship	Phase of Exploitation
Phase of Orientation	Phase of Resolution
Phase of Identification	

ANALYSIS OF THE THEORY OF INTERPERSONAL RELATIONS

This section presents an analysis of Peplau's Theory of Interpersonal Relations. The analysis is based on Peplau's publications about her theory, drawing primarily from her 1952 book, *Interpersonal Relations in Nursing*, and her 1992 journal article, "Interpersonal Relations: A Theoretical Framework for Application in Nursing Practice."

Scope of the Theory

The central assertions of the Theory of Interpersonal Relations are that "nursing is a significant, therapeutic, interpersonal process" (Peplau, 1952, p. 16) and that "understanding of the meaning of the experience to the patient is required in order for nursing to function as an educative, therapeutic, maturing force" (Peplau, 1952, p. 41). O'Toole and Welt (1989) accurately classified the theory as middle-range. More specifically, the Theory of Interpersonal Relations is a middle-range descriptive classification theory. That categorization is supported by the fact that the theory is limited to a relatively specific and concrete taxonomy of phases of interpersonal relations, primarily between the nurse and the patient. The middle-range categorization is further supported by Peplau's own comments (1952; 1992; cited in Takahashi, 1992) regarding the scope of her theory. She stated:

> In this inquiry, we are interested in what happens when an ill person and a nurse come together to resolve a difficulty felt in relation to health. (1952, p. 18)

> The focus of my theory is on interaction phenomena and intrapersonal and interpersonal phenomena and it does not include, for instance, pathophysiology or biological phenomena and other aspects of the human experience. It is focused very specifically on interaction phenomena: person-to-person interaction. (Cited in Takahashi, 1992, p. 86)

> The theory of interpersonal relations does not provide explanations for [the] medical aspects of the patient's problems. . . . Concepts contained within interpersonal relations theory are relevant primarily as explanations of the personal behavior of nurse and patient in nursing situations and of psychosocial phenomena. Obviously, then, for the practice of nursing, a more comprehensive scope of theoretical constructs is needed. (1992, p. 13)

Context of the Theory

Metaparadigm Concepts and Proposition

Peplau (1965) alluded to the metaparadigm of nursing when she stated:

> It seems to me that interpersonal relations is the core of nursing. Basi-
> cally, nursing practice always involves a relationship between at least
> two real people—a nurse and a patient. . . . The way in which [the
> nurse] produces the effects of her teaching or of the application of a
> technical procedure has a good deal to do with the interaction
> between nurse and patient. (p. 274)

That statement indicates that the Theory of Interpersonal Relations is derived from the metaparadigm concepts *person* and *nursing. Person* encompasses the patient and the nurse, and nursing is the interpersonal process between the nurse and the patient. Moreover, Peplau's statement indicates that the most relevant metaparadigm proposition is *the [nursing] processes by which positive changes in [the patient's] health status are affected.*

Philosophical Claims

Peplau (1952; cited in Takahashi, 1992) has made several statements about human beings and behavior that represent philosophical claims:

1. The human being is reducible, one way or the other. (Cited in Takahashi, 1992, p. 88)
2. All human behavior is purposeful and goal seeking in terms of feelings of satisfaction and/or security. (1952, p. 86)
3. Human beings act on the basis of the meaning of events to them, that is, on the basis of their immediate interpretation of the climate and the performances that transpire in a particular relationship. (1952, pp. 283–284)
4. Each patient will behave, during any crisis, in a way that has worked in relation to crises faced in the past. (1952, p. 255)
5. The meaning of behavior of the patient to the patient is the only relevant basis on which nurses can determine needs to be met. (1952, pp. 226–227)
6. The interaction of nurse and patient is fruitful when a method of communication that identifies and uses common meanings is at work in the situation. (1952, p. 284)

In addition, Peplau (1952, 1992) identified several assumptions that represent the philosophical underpinnings for the Theory of Interpersonal Relations:

1. What goes on between people can be noticed, studied, explained, understood, and if detrimental changed. (1992, p. 14)
2. In every contact with another human being there is the possibility for the nurse of working toward common understandings and

goals; every contact between two human beings involves the possibility of clash of feelings, beliefs, ways of acting. (1952, p. xiii)

3. Every nurse-patient relationship is an interpersonal situation in which recurring difficulties of everyday living arise. (1952, p. xiii)

4. The nurse needs information about the patient's difficulties for the purpose of providing expert nursing care. Data from the patient about the immediate situation is a major source, superior to case history data, nursing history data, and other sources of information, which the nurse also uses. (1992, p. 14)

5. To encourage the patient to participate in identifying and assessing his problem is to engage him as an active partner in an enterprise of great concern to him. Democratic method applied to nursing requires patient participation. (1952, p. 23)

6. The kind of person each nurse becomes makes a substantial difference in what each patient will learn as he is nursed throughout his experience with illness. (1952, p. xii)

7. Fostering personality development in the direction of maturity is a function of nursing and nursing education; it requires the use of principles and methods that permit and guide the process of grappling with everyday interpersonal problems or difficulties. (1952, p. xii)

8. The professional and personal growth of the nurse requires changes in his or her own behavior. (1992, p. 14)

9. Nurses do not have the power to change the behavior of patients. (1992, p. 14)

10. Unwitting "illness-maintenance" by nurses is unacceptable behavior for a professional. (1992, p. 14)

11. The nursing process is educative and therapeutic when nurse and patient can come to know and to respect each other, as persons who are alike, and yet, different, as persons who share in the solution of problems. (1952, p. 9)

Sellers (1991) maintained that Peplau's theory "espouses the behaviorist philosophy of the medical model. Her [theory] exemplifies a mechanistic, deterministic, persistence . . . view" (p. 141). Peplau (1954/1989), however, rejected that characterization of her work by explicitly stating that her work is dynamic rather than mechanistic. Mechanistic theories, according to Peplau, are "largely partial, one-sided. [They] depend . . . on spectator observations made by an individual who presumes detachment from the individual studied" (p. 9). In contrast, as Peplau pointed out, dynamic theories require participant observation and consider data from both the nurse-observer and the patient, which are essential features of the Theory of Interpersonal Relations. Those features, along with scrutiny of Peplau's philosophical claims, indicate that the theory is most closely aligned with the *reciprocal interaction* worldview, with an emphasis on the elements of totality that are incorporated into that perspective. Indeed, Forchuk (1991a) indicated that Peplau's work reflects the totality worldview, and Sellers (1991) ultimately reached the same conclusion.

Conceptual Model

Harry Stack Sullivan's theory of interpersonal relations provided a strong conceptual base for Peplau's theory. She explained that she had studied Sullivan's work during the 1930s and 1940s and used it as a starting point for her thoery. Since 1948, however, her work has been "derived from extensive study of data from clinical work primarily with psychiatric patients" (Peplau, 1992, p. 13).

Peplau (1992) regards the person as a client or patient who as a human being merits "all of the humane considerations: respect, dignity, privacy, confidentiality, and ethical care" (p. 14). She went on to say that "patient-persons . . . have problems of one kind or another for which expert nursing services are needed or sought" (p. 14). She regards the nurse as a professional, a person with definable expertise. "That expert knowledge," according to Peplau, "pertains to the nature of phenomena within the purview of nursing and to the reliable interventions which have been research-tested and therefore have predictable, known outcomes" (p. 14).

Peplau has not devoted much attention to the environment, although she commented on the importance of culture on the formation of personality. In particular, she stated that "it is the interaction of cultural forces with the characteristic expression of a particular infant's biological constitution that determines personality" (Peplau, 1952, p. 163).

Health, according to Peplau (1952), "has not been clearly defined; it is a word symbol that implies forward movement of personality and other ongoing human processes in the direction of creative, constructive, productive, personal, and community living" (p. 12).

Peplau (1952) defined nursing as

> a significant, therapeutic, interpersonal process. It functions co-operatively with other human processes that make health possible for individuals in communities. In specific situations in which a professional health team offers health services, nurses participate in the organization of conditions that facilitate natural ongoing tendencies in human organisms. Nursing is an educative instrument, a maturing force, that aims to promote forward movement of personality in the direction of creative, constructive, productive, personal, and community living. (p. 16)

Consequently, the aim of professional nursing practice for Peplau (1992) is "to assist patients to become aware of and to solve their problems that interfere with constructive living" (p. 15).

Antecedent Knowledge

Peplau explictly acknowledged the influence of Harry Stack Sullivan and his followers on her ideas. In the preface to her 1952 book, she stated:

> the author wishes to express great indebtedness for indirect help gained through the written works of the late Dr. Harry Stack Sullivan and for direct assistance growing out of study with Dr. Erich Fromm, various members of the professional staff of the William Alanson White Institute of Psychiatry and of Chestnut Lodge. The Theory of Interpersonal Relations, as stated by Dr. Sullivan and under further development by these professional workers, is considered by the author to be one of the most useful theories in explaining observations made in nursing. This [book] has drawn heavily upon their contribution in order to make available to nurses in simpler form ideas that are of great value in understanding human behavior. (p. v).

Peplau (1987/1989) noted that the term "interpersonal relations" was coined by Jacob Moreno (1941), the psychiatrist who founded psychodrama, and was later defined and described by Sullivan (1953). She explained that although "Sullivan was a practicing psychoanalyst . . . his interpersonal constructs were drawn from both his psychiatric clinical work and from the social sciences available in the 1920s to 1950s" (1987/1989, p. 58). In a later publication, Peplau (1992) commented that Sullivan's theory of interpersonal relations drew more from theories in the social sciences than from psychoanalytical theories.

Peplau (1987/1989) noted that Sullivan defined interpersonal relations as "the study of what goes on between two or more people, all but one of whom may be completely illusory" (p. 58). She pointed out that the term is "interpersonal *relations*" rather than "interpersonal *relationships*." Relations, Peplau explained, "refers to connections, linkages, ties and bonds between things and people" (p. 58). She went on to explain that "In a nurse-patient relationship, and most particularly in psychiatric work, the aim of the nurse would be to study the interpersonal relations that go on (or went on) between a client and others, whether family, friends, staff, or the nurse" (p. 59).

Content of the Theory

A systematic analysis of Peplau's publications revealed that the Theory of Interpersonal Relations contains one concept: **Nurse-patient relationship.** Peplau (1992) explained that "the relationship is an interpersonal process. It has a starting point, proceeds through definable phases, and being time-limited, has an end point" (p. 14).

The nurse-patient relationship encompasses four phases, which represent the dimensions of the concept (Fig. 7–1). Peplau's discussion

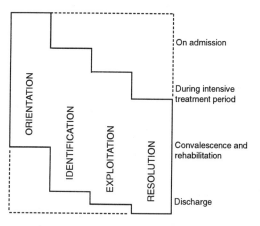

Figure 7–1. Overlapping phases in the nurse-patient relationship. (From *Interpersonal Relations in Nursing: A Conceptual Frame of Reference for Psychodynamic Nursing* (p. 21) by H. E. Peplau, 1952. New York: G.P. Putnam's Sons. Copyright 1991 by *Springer Publishing Company, Inc.*, New York 10012. Used by permission.)

of each phase encompasses a description of the developing interpersonal relationship between the nurse and the patient and the roles they assume (Fig. 7–2).The *phase of orientation* occurs as the patient has a felt need signifying a health problem and seeks assistance to clarify the problem. Peplau (1952) explained that the patient participates in the orienting phase by asking questions, by trying to find out what needs to be known in order to feel secure, and by observing ways in which professional people respond. The nurse participates in the orienting process by helping the patient to recognize and understand the health problem and the extent of need for assistance, to understand what professional services can offer, to plan the use of professional services, and to harness energy from tension and anxiety connected with felt needs.

Peplau (1992) pointed out that the orientation phase

> is especially important as it sets the stage for the serious work that is to follow. In this phase, for example, the patient begins to know the nurse's name, the nurse's purpose, the time to be made available, and the approach to the work. The nurse begins to know the patient as a person, his/her expectations of the nurse, and the patient's characteristic response patterns. It is the phase in which the nurse makes assessments of the patient's potentials, needs, and interests, and of the patient's inclination to experience fear or anxiety. (p. 14)

As can be seen in Figure 7–2, the nurse's initial role in the orientation phase is that of stranger acted out with the patient, who is also in the role of stranger. "A stranger," Peplau (1952) commented," is an individual with whom another individual is not acquainted" (p. 44). As the orientation phase progresses, the patient may assume the role of infant and, therefore, cast the nurse into a surrogate role, especially that of unconditional mother. Peplau (1965/1989) maintained that although the parental role may not be useful in some situations, "this surrogate

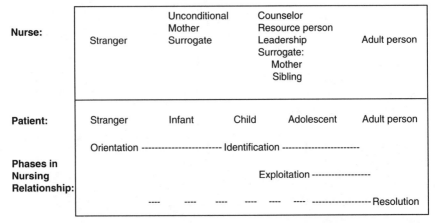

Nurse:	Stranger	Unconditional Mother Surrogate	Counselor Resource person Leadership Surrogate: Mother Sibling	Adult person
Patient:	Stranger	Infant	Child	Adolescent	Adult person

Orientation ---------------------- Identification -----------------------

Phases in Nursing Relationship:

Exploitation ------------------

---- ---- ---- ---- ---- ---- ------------------ Resolution

Figure 7–2. Phases and changing roles in the nurse-patient relationship. (From *Interpersonal Relations in Nursing: A Conceptual Frame of Reference for Psychodynamic Nursing* (p. 54) by H. E. Peplau, 1952. New York: G.P. Putnam's Sons. Copyright 1991 by *Springer Publishing Company, Inc.*, New York 10012. Used by permission.)

role may be the logical one for the nurse to fulfill . . . if the patient is acutely ill and requires continual mothering care" (1952, p. 55).

The *phase of identification* occurs as the patient learns how to make use of the nurse-patient relationship. During the identification phase, Peplau (1952) explained, the nurse and the patient come to know and to respect one another as persons who have like and different opinions about the ways of looking at a situation and in responding to events.

Peplau (1952) pointed out that during the identification phase, patients may respond "(1) on the basis of participation or interdependent relations with a nurse; (2) on the basis of independence or isolation from a nurse; [or] (3) on the basis of helplessness or dependence upon a nurse" (p. 33). She went on to say that the nurse-patient relationship may progress from one mode of response to another and that all three modes may be required to achieve goals.

Throughout this phase, the nurse uses professional education and skill to aid the patient to make full use of the relationship to solve the health problem. More specifically, the nurse may assume several roles, frequently moving from unconditional mother surrogate in response to the patient's roles of infant and child to counselor, resource person, leader, or surrogate in response to the patient's gradual assumption of the role of adolescent (Fig. 7–2). As a resource person, the nurse gives "specific, needed information that aids the patient to understand [the] health problem and the new situation" (Peplau, 1952, p. 21). As a counselor, the nurse listens to the patient review events that led up to hospitalization and feelings connected with these events. And as a leader, the nurse acts in a demographic rather than autocratic or laissez-faire manner. As a surrogate for mother, father, sibling, or other person, the nurse aids the patient by permitting reenactment and examination of older feelings about prior relationships.

The *phase of exploitation* occurs as the patient makes full use of available professional services. During this phase, "the main difficulty seems to be that of trying to strike a balance between a need to be dependent, as during serious illness, and a need to be independent, as following recovery" (Peplau, 1952, p. 38). The nurse's tasks during the exploitation phase are to understand what initiates shifts in the patient's behavior from dependence to independence and to guard against excessive exploitation on the patient's part. During the exploitation phase, the nurse continues in the roles of counselor, resource person, leader, or surrogate in response to the patient's role of adolescent (Fig. 7–2).

The *phase of resolution* occurs as the nurse helps the patient to organize actions so that he or she will want to be free for more productive social activities and relationships. Peplau (1952) pointed out that the patient's wish to terminate the relationship may not coincide with medical recovery. The central task of resolution, then, is the freeing of the patient to move on in life. Both nurse and patient must, of course, participate in the freeing process. As resolution occurs, both nurse and patient assume the role of adult person (Fig. 7–2).

Peplau (1952, 1965) identified several other roles that nurses might assume, including technical expert, consultant, teacher, tutor, socializing agent, safety agent, manager of the environment, mediator, administrator, recorder, observer, and researcher during various phases of the nurse-patient relationship. The role of technical expert may be assumed during any or all of the phases of the relationship. In that role, the nurse "understands various professional devices and manipulates them with skill and discrimination in the interest of the patient" (1952, p. 22). The role of teacher also may be assumed at any time during the nurse-patient relationship. That role is, according to Peplau, "a combination of all [other] roles" (1952, p. 48). In keeping with her focus on the patient, Peplau advocated a teaching style that "always proceeds from what the patient knows and it develops around his interest in wanting and being able to use additional medical information" (1952, p. 48). Although Peplau mentioned the other roles, she did not describe them.

Although nurses assume many different roles during their interactions with patients, they should not assume certain roles in which patients may try to cast them. In particular, Peplau (1965/1989) maintained that the roles of chum, friend, protagonist, and sex object are not useful ones for nurses to take.

Propositions

The descriptions of the nurse-patient relationship and the phases of that relationship constitute nonrelational propositions of the Theory of Interpersonal Relationships. Other nonrelational propositions about each phase of the nurse-patient relationship are as follows:

Phase of Orientation

Orientation is essential to full participation and to full integration of the illness event into the stream of life experiences of the patient. It is the only prevention against repressing or dissociating the event that a nurse can exercise on behalf of the patient. (Peplau, 1952, p. 23)

The patient needs to recognize and understand his difficulty and the extent of need for help. (Peplau, 1952, p. 22)

Seeking assistance on the basis of a need, felt but poorly understood, is often the first step in a dynamic learning experience from which a constructive next step in personal-social growth can occur. (Peplau, 1952, p. 19)

The patient needs assistance in recognizing and planning to use services that professional personnel can offer. (Peplau, 1952, p. 24)

Every patient needs to be assisted in harnessing energy that derives from tension and anxiety connected with felt needs, to [achieve] positive means for defining, understanding, and meeting productively the problem at hand. (Peplau, 1952, p. 26)

Orientation to the problem leads to expression of needs and feelings, older ones that are reactivated and new ones created by challenges in a new situation. (Peplau, 1952, p. 41)

Phase of Identification

Identification with a nurse who consistently symbolizes a helping person, providing abundant and unconditional care, is a way of meeting felt needs and overwhelming problems. When initial needs are met they are outgrown and more mature needs arise. (Peplau, 1952, p. 41)

When a nurse permits patients to express what they feel, and still get all of the nursing that is needed, then patients can undergo illness as an experience that reorients feelings and strengthens positive forces in personality. (Peplau, 1952, p. 31)

Phase of Exploitation

Exploiting what a situation offers gives rise to new differentiations of the problem and to the development and improvement of skill in interpersonal relations. New goals to be achieved through personal efforts can be projected. (Peplau, 1952, pp. 41–42)

Phase of Resolution

Movement from a hospital situation to participation in community life requires resolution of nurse-patient relations and the strengthening of

personality for new social interdependent relationships. When resolution occurs on the basis of lacks in a situation needs are intensified
and become longings that, together with unclear meanings of the
event itself, limit the possibility of integration of the total experience.
(Peplau, 1952, p. 42)

The stage of resolution implies the gradual freeing from identification
with helping persons and the generation and strengthening of ability
to stand more or less alone. These outcomes can be achieved only
when all of the earlier phases are met in terms of "psychological mothering": unconditional acceptance in a sustaining relationship that provides fully for need-satisfaction; recognition of and responses to
growth cues, however trivial, as and when they come from the patient;
shifting of power from the nurse to the patient as he becomes willing
to delay gratification of his wishes and to expend his own efforts in
achieving new goals. (Peplau, 1952, pp. 40–41)

Still other nonrelational propositions characterize the four phases.
Those propositions assert:

Four clearly discernible phases in the relationship . . . are to be
thought of as interlocking.

[The four phases] can be recognized; they enter into every total nursing situation.

Each phase is characterized by overlapping roles or functions in relation to health problems as nurse and patient learn to work co-opera-
tively to resolve difficulties. (Peplau, 1952, p. 17)

The interlocking and overlapping nature of the phases of the nurse-
patient relationship, which can be seen in Figures 7–1 and 7–2, is especially evident in the following nonrelational propositions:

Initially, the patient functions in relation to overlapping situations.
That is, he is pulled toward being home where he is sure of familiar
responses and he is drawn toward remaining in the hospital and solving the emergent problem. (Peplau, 1952, p. 29)

The phase of exploitation overlaps identification and resolution, the
terminal phase of the nurse-patient relationship. Orientation over-
lapped the previous social or home situation. The phase under discussion represents all prior ones and an extension of the self of the
patient into the future. It is characterized by an intermingling of needs
and a shuttling back and forth. (Peplau, 1952, p. 38)

Inasmuch as the theory contains just one concept, there are no relational propositions.

EVALUATION OF THE THEORY OF INTERPERSONAL RELATIONS

This section presents an evaluation of Peplau's Theory of Interpersonal Relations. The evaluation is based on the results of the analysis of the theory as well as on publications by others who have used or commented on this nursing theory.

Significance

The metaparadigmatic origin of the Theory of Interpersonal Relations was easily inferred from Peplau's work, although she never explicitly addressed that underpinning of the theory. Peplau did, however, explicitly identify several philosophical claims undergirding the theory, and others were extracted from her publications.

Peplau has always been especially explicit about the conceptual base for her theory, citing Sullivan's theory of interpersonal relations and the publications of his work as the major source of antecedent knowledge. In fact, it is difficult to discern exactly where Sullivan's theory leaves off and Peplau's theory begins. Inasmuch as Peplau (1969) regards nursing as an applied science, the lack of a clear distinction between the theories is not surprising.

Peplau also acknowledged the contributions of Sullivan's followers to her thinking, although she mentioned only Erich Fromm by name. She did, however, provide an extensive bibliography for the many topics she addressed in her 1952 book, including anxiety, child development, communication, conflict, frustration, guilt, illness as an event, leadership, learning, motivation, needs, parental roles, personality, psychopathology, therapeutic methods, and general methods.

The special significance of the Theory of Interpersonal Relations lies in its contributions to understanding the phases of the nurse-patient relationship. "That knowledge," as Sills (1978) pointed out, "helped give nursing's moral aspirations a concrete basis which narrowed the gap between the ideal and the real" (p. 123).

A special feature of the theory is its broad applicability in most, if not all, clinical areas of nursing. Speaking to the significance of her theory, Peplau (1992) stated that the theory is important because "the behavior of the nurse-as-a-person has significant impact on the patient's well-being and the quality and outcome of nursing care" (p. 14). Another special feature is the enduring nature of the theory. In 1978, Sills noted that a literature review spanning the then 25 years since the publication of Peplau's book revealed that the theory, with no revisions, was still useful. The theory continues to be useful more than 40 years later, as documented by the recent literature cited in the annotated bibliography at the end of this chapter, as well as the reprinting of Peplau's 1952 book by Macmillan Education Ltd. (London) in 1989 and by Springer Publishing Company in 1991.

Furthermore, Peplau (1992; cited in Takahashi, 1992) pointed out that interpersonal relations theory has led to development of various interviewing techniques and psychotherapeutic modalities, including counseling, psychotherapy, family therapy, and group therapy. In addition, she claimed that "advanced psychiatric nursing gained considerable impetus from this theory, as did the clinical specialist movement, particularly in psychiatric nursing" (1992, p. 18).

Internal Consistency

All elements of Peplau's work are congruent. The Theory of Interpersonal Relations is logically derived from Peplau's philosophical claims and from the conceptual model, which is based on Sullivan's (1953) theory of interpersonal relations.

The Theory of Interpersonal Relations demonstrates semantic clarity. Peplau provided a clear and concise description of the concept nurse-patient relationship and clear descriptions of the four phases of the nurse-patient relationship.

The theory demonstrates partial semantic consistency. Peplau's (1952) original work contained the four distinct phases of the nurse-patient relationship. Forchuk (1991b), however, combined the phases of identification and exploitation into one phase that she labeled the *working phase*. Peplau implied her agreement with that classification when she cited Forchuk's publication and used her list of the phases in her 1992 article. Although Peplau apparently has agreed with Forchuk's (1991b) revision of the four phases of the nurse-patient relationship to three phases, it is completely clear that the phases of identification and exploitation make up the working phase.

There are no concept redundancies. One area of confusion does, however, exist. It is unclear whether the various roles assumed by the nurse are associated with particular phases of the nurse-patient relationship or are taken on during all four phases. The former situation is evident in Figure 7–2, but the latter situation is introduced by the following statement:

> *During orientation as well as during the other three phases* in the total relationship four interlocking nursing functions may operate: (1) The nurse may function in the role of resource person, . . . (2) A nurse may function in a counseling relationship, . . . (3) The patient may cast the nurse into roles, such as surrogate for mother, father, sibling, . . . (4) The nurse also functions as a technical expert, ... (Peplau, 1952, pp. 21–22) [Italics added]

The analysis of Peplau's theory revealed structural consistency. The Theory of Interpersonal Relations is a logical product of deduction from Sullivan's interpersonal theory and induction from Peplau's clinical observations. O'Toole and Welt (1989) commented:

> Peplau's method of theory development is both inductive and deductive. . . . The process of combining induction (observation and classification) with deduction (the application of known concepts and processes to data) provides a creative nonlinear approach to the formation of ideas: one that uses the data of practice, as well as extant theories, as the basis of those formulations. (p. 355)

Parsimony

The analysis presented in this chapter yielded a parsimonious structure for the Theory of Interpersonal Relations that consists of one concept with four dimensions and several nonrelational propositions. In contrast, Forchuk (1991b) regards the Theory of Interpersonal Relations as "quite complex . . . due to the many concepts, subconcepts, and . . . sub-subconcepts that are interrelated" (pp. 54–55). Indeed, her analysis of Peplau's work yielded a complicated structure that combined what is regarded in this book as the metaparadigm concepts (person, environment, health, and nursing); the middle-range theory concept of nurse-patient relationship and its dimensions (the phases of the nurse-patient relationship); and several other concepts and subconcepts (i.e., dimensions). Those concepts and their dimensions are communication, with the dimensions of verbal communication and nonverbal communication; pattern integration; roles; thinking, with the dimensions of preconceptions and self-understanding; learning; competencies; and anxiety.

Furthermore, O'Toole and Welt (1989) claimed that loneliness, anxiety, self, hallucinations, thought disorders, focal attention, and learning are "major concepts that form the backbone of Peplau's interpersonal theory" (p. xvi). Repeated readings of Peplau's publications indicated that the additional concepts identified by Forchuk and by O'Toole and Welt are either an integral part of the description of the phases of the nurse-patient relationship or clinical situations for which the Theory of Interpersonal Relations is especially appropriate. Hence, here they are not regarded as central concepts of the theory.

Testability

The Theory of Interpersonal Relations is testable by means of a clinical methodology developed by Peplau (1952). She explained that "observation, communication, and recording are all interlocking performances in interpersonal relations that make it possible for nurses to study what is happening in their contacts with patients" (p. 309).

The purpose of observation, within the context of the Theory of Interpersonal Relations, "is the identification, clarification, and verification of impressions about the interactive drama, of the pushes and pulls in the relationship between nurse and patient, as they occur" (Peplau, 1952, p. 263). The specific data to be collected are "(a) the observer's behavior, (b) the behavior of the observed, and (c) the interaction phenomena—what goes on between them" (Peplau, 1992, pp. 14–15). Participant-observation is the main data collection technique.

One aim of communication is "the selection of symbols or concepts that convey both the reference, or meaning in the mind of the individual, and referent, the object or actions symbolized in the concept" (Peplau, 1952, p. 290). Another aim is "the wish to struggle toward the development of common understanding" for words between two or more people (p. 290). Hence, the words the nurse chooses when communicating with patients are extremely important. Peplau (1952) advised using the principles of clarity and continuity as guides to the selection of words. With regard to clarity, she stated:

> Words and sentences used are clarifying events when they occur within the frame of reference of common experiences of both or all participants, or when their meaning is established or made understandable as a result of joint and sustained effort of all parties concerned. (p. 290)

Clarity is promoted, therefore, when the nurse and the patient discuss their preconceptions about the meaning of words and work toward a common understanding. Clarity is achieved "when the meaning [of a word] to the patient is expressed and talked over and a new view is expanded in awareness" (p. 291).

Continuity in communication, Peplau explained,

> occurs when language is used as a tool for the promotion of coherence or connections of ideas expressed and leads to discrimination of relationships or connections among ideas and the feelings, events, or themes conveyed in those ideas. (p. 290)

Thus, continuity is promoted "when the nurse is able to pick up threads of conversation that the patient offers in the course of a conversation and over a longer period such as a week and when she aids the patient to focus and to expand these threads" (p. 293).

Recording is the written record of the communication between nurse and patient. In effect, the written record represents the data collected through participant-observation. The aim of recording is to capture the exact wording of the interaction between the nurse and the patient. Peplau (1952) suggested using a form that permits verbatim recording of the nurse's observations of the patient when initially approached; the nurse's opening remarks, feelings, and thoughts about the patient; the patient's responses; and the nurse's responses. She also commented that tape recorders and nonparticipant observation by another nurse may be used to record interactions.

Data can be organized in terms of the identification, exploitation, and resolution phases of the nurse-patient relationship and are analyzed with reference to the nurse's hypotheses, which are formulated from first impressions or hunches about the patient. Analysis of the data ultimately yields inferences about the pattern integrations, that is, the connections or linkages, in interpersonal relations. Drawing from Sullivan (1953), Peplau (1987/1989, 1992) identified five dimensions of relations. Those dimensions are:

- Nature (patterns, themes, and variations)
- Origin (history)
- Function (intent, motive, expectation, aim, goal, or purpose)
- Mode (form, style, and method)
- Integrations (patterns of linkages with others' behaviors)

Thus "nurses observe the ways in which patients transform energy into patterns of action that bring satisfaction or security in the face of a recurring problem" (Peplau, 1952, p. 309).

The clinical methodology yields qualitative data. Quantitative data related to the Theory of Interpersonal Relations can be collected by using instruments developed by Methven and Schlotfeldt (1962), Spring and Turk (1962), La Monica (1981), and Forchuk, Beaton, Bethune, Crawford, Ide, and Voorberg (1986).

The Social Interaction Inventory, developed by Methven and Schlotfeldt (1962), measures the nature and type of verbal responses nurses give in emotion-laden practice situations. A scale developed by Spring and Turk (1962) contains categories of verbal behavior evident in psychiatric nurse therapists' communications with their patients and yields a therapeutic behavior score. La Monica (1981) developed an instrument designed to measure empathy, which she defined as "a central focus and feeling with and in the client's world. [Empathy] involves accurate perception of the client's world by the helper, communication of this understanding of the client, and the client's perception of the helper's understanding" (p. 398). The Relationship Form, devised by Forchuk et al. (1986; Forchuk & Brown, 1989), measures the progress of the nurse-patient relationship through the four phases delineated by Peplau. The Stages of Learning Form, also developed by Forchuk et al. (1986; Forchuk & Voorberg, 1991), measures the eight stages of learning outlined by Peplau (1963). Those stages are observe, describe, analyze, formulate, validate, test, integrate, and utilize.

Empirical Adequacy

Forchuk and Brown's (1989) report of instrument development work provides direct evidence of the empirical adequacy of the Theory of Interpersonal Relations. Their findings indicated that each phase of the nurse-patient relationship could be documented on the basis of the nurse's and the patient's behaviors. The findings also indicated that "when the nurse can accurately assess the phase of the relationship, appropriate interventions within Peplau's theory are more likely to be selected" (p. 33). Additional evidence of empirical adequacy comes from Forchuk and Voorberg's (1991) report of the evaluation of a community mental health program based on Peplau's theory, a psychiatric rehabilitation model, and case management. They reported that within the initial 2-year period of the program, the problem identification phase of the nurse-patient relationship was most common, and that just 13 percent of the 91 clients had not moved beyond the orientation phase. In addition, the clients demonstrated progress in the stages of learning, with 78 percent at the second stage (describe), and almost 8 percent at the fourth stage (formulate) and another 8 percent at the fifth stage (validate).

Additional evidence of empirical adequacy comes from Lund and Frank's (1991) research. They found that psychiatric patients' and nurses' perceptions of the extent of medication noncompliance were similar. The investigators commented that the study results supported Peplau's theory in that "the nurses . . . adequately implemented their assessment skills during the initial orientation phase of the nurse-patient relationship" (p. 7).

The work of other investigators who cited Peplau provides indirect evidence of empirical adequacy. Hays's (1961) exploratory study was designed to identify and describe the phases and steps of experiential teaching of a concept of anxiety to patients. Analysis of nurse-patient group interactions yielded three phases: orientation, concept teaching, and evaluation. Garrett, Manuel, and Vincent (1976) identified various sources of stress experienced by student nurses, including physical care of patients, interpersonal relations with clinical instructors, academic pressures, and personal problems with family members and boyfriends.

A review of the literature revealed no other publications reporting the results of tests of the Theory of Interpersonal Relations. Consequently, although Peplau's (1952) work "influenced the interpersonal nature and direction of clinical work and studies" (Sills, 1977, p. 203), there is very little evidence of its empirical adequacy. That situation may be due to the tendency to *assume* the adequacy of theories that are an integral part of the history of nursing theory development. As O'Toole and Welt (1989) commented,

> Peplau's theoretical ideas . . . have become a part of the collective culture of the discipline of nursing. Many commonly understood and assumed ideas basic to nursing stem from her work. As we accumulate knowledge, we tend to lose sight of the individual contributions of the originators of that knowledge. In other words, it becomes knowledge in the public domain. For historical and intellectual reasons, it is extremely important to credit and evaluate those early contributions in light of their relevance to our discipline today. It is apparent . . . that Peplau's [theory] continue[s] to be germane to our research and practice. (p. 365)

Clearly, systematic research designed to test the validity of the four phases of the nurse-patient relationship as originally described by Peplau (1952) and their generalizability to diverse clinical situations is needed to determine the empirical adequacy of the theory.

Pragmatic Adequacy

Nursing Education

The task of nursing education, according to Peplau (1952), "is the gradual development of each nurse as a person who *wants* to nurse patients in a helpful way" (p. xiii). More specifically, the central task of nursing education is "the fullest development of the nurse as a person who is aware of how she functions in a situation" (p. xii). Additional tasks include "release of human interest in others who are in difficulty, liberation of emotional and intellectual capacity for making choices, [and] development of nurses as persons whose enlightened self-interest will lead to no other choice but productive relations with all kinds of patients, students, [and] citizens" (p. xii).

Special education is required for application of the Theory of Interpersonal Relations. Nurses must learn to "have control over the signals (stimuli, messages, inputs, cues) that they send to a patient" because the nurses' behaviors "serve as stimuli for evoking behavioral changes by patients" (Peplau, 1992, p. 14). Nurses must also learn "to identify human problems that confront patients, the degrees of skill used to meet situations, and be able to develop with patients the kinds of relationships that will be conducive to improvement in skill" (Peplau, 1952, p. xv).

Peplau (1952) maintained that students must engage in productive learning so that they may grow and expand their personalities. She pointed out that as students grow, however, they may experience "frustrations, conflicts, and anxieties as older patterns of behavior are foregone and more productive, new ones are developed" (p. xvi).

Furthermore, graduate nurses must accept responsibility for continued learning. Peplau (1952) stated:

> While the basic school can do much to foster the development of students as useful, productive persons, each graduate nurse can also take on the responsibility for expanding her own insight into the effects of life experiences on personality functioning and for planning steps that will lead to a mode of life that is more creative and more productive. (p. xvii)

The importance of basic and continuing education is underscored by the following comment:

> What each nurse becomes—as a functioning personality—determines the manner in which she will perform in each interpersonal contact in every nursing situation. The extent to which each nurse understands her own functioning will determine the extent to which she can come to understand the situation confronting the patient and the way he sees it. Positive, useful nursing actions flow out of understanding of the situation. (Peplau, 1952, p. xii)

Nursing Practice

The purpose of nursing practice "is to promote favorable changes in patients" (Peplau, 1992, p. 13). The purpose is accomplished through the nurse-patient relationship. Within that relationship, the nurse's major function is to study the interpersonal relations between the patient/client and others. Such study, Peplau (1987/1989) explained,

> enables identification of those human responses and patterns that are problematic in terms of health. In other words, while a client is describing an event, incident, relationship or dilemma, the nurse in that situation would be studying what was happening. Such study would include observing, noticing gestures and body movements, listening, and hearing the facts and data being presented. During this study process the nurse would also begin to notice relations and to generate inferences or to apply theory as professionally oriented intellectual operations, in order privately to interpret the data. (p. 59)

The task of nursing service, according to Peplau (1952), is "concern for the patient" (p. xiii). The operationalization of that task is evident in the following five characteristics of professional nursing practice:

1. The focus of professional nursing is the patient.
2. The nurse uses participant observation rather than spectator observation.

3. The nurse is aware of the various roles she assumes in the nurse-patient relationship.
4. Professional nursing is primarily investigative, with emphasis on observation and collection of data that are made available to the patient, rather than task-oriented.
5. Professional nursing is grounded in the use of theory. (Peplau, 1965/1989)

The Theory of Interpersonal Relations is implemented primarily through interpersonal techniques, which Peplau (1992) defined as "verbal interventions used by nurses during nurse-patient relationships aimed at accomplishing problem resolution and competence development in patients" (p. 18). Those techniques, Peplau explained,

> rest on a one-way focus; the nurse's interests are the concerns and the development of the patient, rather than on having a reciprocal, social relationship. Such techniques are primarily verbal and investigative. In order for both to understand the patient's dilemmas, the nurse uses comments and questions to force the patient to think, to respond, and to use those capacities that will produce the necessary data. In this process, the nurse privately uses theory to interpret observations and to guide the patient's work in formulating his/her own interpretations of personal experience. (p. 18)

Evidence of the pragmatic adequacy of the Theory of Interpersonal Relations is accruing. Survey results indicate that the theory is widely used. Martin and Kirkpatrick's (cited in Forchuk, 1991b) survey, which was conducted at a Canadian tertiary care psychiatric hospital, revealed that Peplau's theory was the most frequently used of 17 different nursing theories to guide staff nurses' practice. In addition, Hirschmann (1989) found that one-half of the 165 psychiatric nurses she surveyed in the United States used Peplau's theory to guide their clinical practice.

Peplau (1992) claimed that the theory "is useful in all areas of nursing practice, . . . especially in psychiatric nursing, because psychiatric patients, generally, have problems with communication and in relatedness to people" (p. 13). Clinical problems that are particularly amenable to application of the Theory of Interpersonal Relations include anxiety, loneliness, learning, the self-system, and paratactic distortions and hallucinations (O'Toole & Welt, 1989; Peplau, 1992).

There is, however, a question regarding the applicability of the theory with children. As can be seen in Figure 7–2, the nurse-patient relationship ends with both nurse and patient assuming the role of adult person. Peplau did not discuss the role that would be assumed by the patient if he or she were a child.

Furthermore, although emphasis is placed on the interpersonal relationship between the nurse and the patient, the theory may also be applied to relationships between the nurse and family members, the nurse and other nurses, the instructor and student, the administrator and staff nurse, and the nurse and other members of the health care team (Peplau, 1952, 1992).

The Theory of Interpersonal Relations does not, as Peplau (1992; cited in Takahashi, 1992) has clearly noted, deal with the medical or physiological aspects of the patient's problems. The theory may, however, "be useful when nurses use health teaching to help patients understand [the medical] aspects of their health problem" (1992, p. 13).

The feasibility of implementing clinical protocols that reflect the theory is evident. Peplau (1969) characterized the encounter between the professional nurse and the patient as "a very fluid interaction" (p. 34). She explained that the professional nurse uses four steps in those interactions: (1) observation, (2) interpretation of the observations, (3) responses using theory-based interventions, and (4) evaluation of the effects of the interventions. She went on to say that continuing evaluations by professional nurses

> lead to standardization of practices in relation to observation of known phenomena. Such standardized practices can then be developed into manuals for technical nursing practice. . . . Thus, technical nursing has to do with known or standardized nursing practices as these have been evolved by professional nurses through repeated use of the four steps described in relation to . . . nursing [interactions]. (pp. 34–35)

Thus a practice protocol should encompass what to observe, what to do as a consequence of the observation, and a rationale for that action. Furthermore, Peplau (1965/1989) maintained that practice protocols should meet the following four criteria:

1. The situation should be structured so that the patient is clear about the nurse's intentions.
2. The nurse should behave like an expert.
3. The nurse should show appreciation for what the patient is up against.
4. The nurse should provide opportunities for the patient to check the meaning of experiences.

A review of the literature revealed a few specific protocols for nursing practice based on the Theory of Interpersonal Relations. Morrison (1992) described the development and successful use of a practice protocol based on Peplau's phases of the nurse-patient relationship, including the various roles assumed by nurses; Bowen's family systems theory; and the nursing process steps of assessment, diagnosis, planning, implementation, and evaluation. The protocol was designed to guide clinical nurse specialist practice in an inpatient psychiatric unit. Furthermore, Forchuk and her colleagues (1989) described a practice protocol that incorporated Peplau's theory and case management. That protocol was used successfully by the staff of a community mental health promotion program for the nursing care of chronically mentally ill clients who lived in boarding homes.

In addition, Peplau (1955, 1962, 1963) developed specific protocols that reflect the Theory of Interpersonal Relations for such clinical problems as anxiety, loneliness, and learning. For example, she described the following technique to abate severe anxiety in patients:

1. Encourage the patient to identify the anxiety as such. This is done by having all personnel help [the patient] recognize what he is experiencing at the point when he is actually anxious.
2. Encourage the patient to connect the relief-giving patterns that he uses to the anxiety which requires such relief. The nursing personnel focus their efforts on maintaining the patient's awareness of the anxiety and connecting it to his anxiety-relieving behavior.
3. Encourage the patient to provide himself and the nurse with data descriptive of situations and interactions which go on immediately before an increase in anxiety is noticed.
4. Encourage the patient to formulate from the descriptive data the probably immediate, situational causes for the increase in his anxiety. (1962, pp. 53–54)

Clinicians have the legal ability to implement practice protocols derived from the Theory of Interpersonal Relations. In fact, Peplau (1952) maintained that "the nursing profession has legal responsibility for the effective use of nursing and for its consequences to patients" (p. 6). In a later publication, Peplau (1985) commented that "advances in professional practice have, in part, been the result of a sensible balance between self-regulation and external controls" (p. 141). She went on to express her concern that "the privilege of self-regulation is being given away or taken away" (p. 141) and urged nurses to guard against further erosion of self-regulation.

The extent to which nursing practice based on the Theory of Interpersonal Relations is compatible with expectations for nursing practice is beginning to be explored. Bristow and Callaghan (1991) found that the application of Peplau's theory significantly improved nurses' use of the nursing process 3 months after its implementation in a large psychiatric hospital in England. Staff nurse satisfaction, however, changed very little and patient satisfaction decreased. Commenting on their findings, Bristow and Callaghan stated:

Patient satisfaction is adversely affected, perhaps because of the increasing administrative tasks of the [theory] which take nurses away from patients. As the [theory] emphasises the partnership between the nurse and the patient, the added responsibility expected from the patient may invoke an increase in stress. Patients whose very problems may stem from difficulties in assuming responsibilities for their activities of living may see this stress as a deterioration in their health and thus in their satisfaction with nursing care. (p. 40)

CONCLUSION

Peplau proposed her Theory of Interpersonal Relations more than four decades ago. "She was," as Kerr (1990) pointed out, "the first nurse theorist to delineate psychiatric/mental health nursing as an interpersonal process governed by lawful principles" (p. 5). Yet the theory extends beyond psychiatric/mental health nursing and greatly enhances understanding of the nature and substance of interpersonal relations between *all* nurses and patients. Furthermore, the theory is a very useful perspective of the verbal communications between the nurses and the patient. Most important, as Peplau (1992) noted, "the theory assists nurses in their personal growth and in the promotion of growth and understanding in their patients" (p. 18). Peplau's work, then, clearly represents a major contribution to nursing knowledge development.

More evidence of the empirical adequacy of the Theory of Interpersonal Relations is, however, needed. As Kerr (1990) noted, "the task remains for us to develop [and test] theoretical models that define how we are to use acquired interpersonal skills to effect greater degrees of mental health in our clients" (p. 5). Thus continued documentation of the outcomes of the use of the Theory of Interpersonal Relations is required, with special attention given to the ways in which its utilization promotes favorable changes in patients, as well as the precise nature and stability of those favorable changes.

REFERENCES

Bristow, F., & Callaghan, P. (1991). Using Peplau's model in affective disorders. *Nursing Times, 87*(18), 40–41.

Forchuk, C. (1991a). A comparison of the works of Peplau and Orlando. *Archives of Psychiatric Nursing, 5,* 38–45.

Forchuk, C. (1991b). Peplau's theory: Concepts and their relations. *Nursing Science Quarterly, 4,* 54–60.

Forchuk C., Beaton, S., Bethune, J., Crawford, L., Ide, L., & Voorberg, N. (1986, August). *A marriage between Peplau and case management: Instrument development.* Paper presented at the Nursing Theory Congress, "Theoretical Pluralism: Direction for a Practice Discipline," Toronto, Ontario, Canada. (Audio cassette recording)

Forchuk, C., Beaton, S., Crawford, L., Ide, L., Voorberg, N., & Bethune, J. (1989). Incorporating Peplau's theory and case management. *Journal of Psychosocial Nursing and Mental Health Services, 27*(2), 35–38.

Forchuk, C., & Brown, B. (1989). Establishing a nurse-client relationship. *Journal of Psychosocial Nursing and Mental Health Services, 27*(2), 30–34.

Forchuk, C., & Voorberg, N. (1991). Evaluation of a community mental health program. *Canadian Journal of Nursing Administration, 4*(2), 16–20.

Garrett, A., Manuel, D., & Vincent, C. (1976). Stressful experiences identified by student nurses. *Journal of Nursing Education, 15*(6), 9–21.

Hays, D. (1961). Teaching a concept of anxiety. *Nursing Research, 10,* 108–113.

Hirschmann, M. (1989). Psychiatric and mental health nurses' beliefs about therapeutic paradox. *Journal of Child Psychiatric Nursing, 2*(1), 7–13.

Kerr, N. J. (1990). Editor's corner. *Perspectives in Psychiatric Care, 26*(4), 5–6.

La Monica, E. L. (1981). Construct validity of an empathy instrument. *Research in Nursing and Health, 4,* 389–400.

Lund, V. E., & Frank, D. I. (1991). Helping the medicine go down: Nurses' and patients' perceptions about medication compliance. *Journal of Psychosocial Nursing and Mental Health Services, 29*(7), 6–9.

Methven, D., & Schlotfeldt, R. M. (1962). The social interaction inventory. *Nursing Research, 11,* 83–88.

Moreno, J. (1941). Psychodrama and group psychotherapy. *Sociometry,9,* 249–253.

Morrison, E. G. (1992). Inpatient practice: An integrated framework. *Journal of Psychosocial Nursing and Mental Health Services, 30*(1), 26–29.

O'Toole, A. W., & Welt, S. R. (Eds.). (1989). *Interpersonal theory in nursing practice. Selected works of Hildegard E. Peplau.* New York: Springer.

Peplau, H. E. (1952). *Interpersonal relations in nursing. A conceptual frame of reference for psychodynamic nursing.* New York: G. P. Putnam's Sons. Reprinted 1989. London: Macmillan Education. [Reprinted 1991. New York: Springer.]

Peplau, H. E. (1955). Loneliness. *American Journal of Nursing, 55,* 1476–1481.

Peplau, H. E. (1962). Interpersonal techniques: The crux of psychiatric nursing. *American Journal of Nursing, 62,* 50–54.

Peplau, H. E. (1963). Process and concept of learning. In S. Burd & M. Marshall (Eds.), *Some clinical approaches to psychiatric nursing* (pp. 333–336). New York: Macmillan.

Peplau, H. E. (1965). The heart of nursing: Interpersonal relations. *The Canadian Nurse, 61,* 273–275.

Peplau, H. E. (1969). Theory: The professional dimension. In C. M. Norris (Ed.), *Proceedings. First nursing theory conference* (pp. 33–46). Kansas City, KS: University of Kansas Medical Center Department of Nursing Education.

Peplau, H. E. (1985). Is nursing's self-regulatory power being eroded? *American Journal of Nursing, 85,* 140–143.

Peplau, H. E. (1989). Interpersonal relationships in psychiatric nursing. In A. W. O'Toole & S. R. Welt (Eds.), *Interpersonal theory in nursing practice. Selected works of Hildegard E. Peplau* (pp. 5–20.). New York: Springer. (Original work presented in 1954.)

Peplau, H. E. (1989). Interpersonal relationships: The purpose and characteristics of professional nursing. In A. W. O'Toole & S. R. Welt (Eds.), *Interpersonal theory in nursing practice. Selected works of Hildegard E. Peplau* (pp. 42–55.). New York: Springer. (Original work presented in 1965.)

Peplau, H. E. (1989). Interpersonal constructs for nursing practice. In A. W. O'Toole & S. R. Welt (Eds.), *Interpersonal theory in nursing practice. Selected works of Hildegard E. Peplau* (pp. 56–70.). New York: Springer. (Original work published in 1987.)

Peplau, H. E. (1992). Interpersonal relations: A theoretical framework for application in nursing practice. *Nursing Science Quarterly, 5,* 13–18.

Sellers, S. C. (1991). A philosophical analysis of conceptual models of nursing. *Dissertation Abstracts International, 52,* 1937B. (University Microfilms No. AAC9126248)

Sills, G. M. (1977). Research in the field of psychiatric nursing 1952–1977. *Nursing Research, 26,* 201–207.

Sills, G. M. (1978). Hildegard E. Peplau: Leader, practitioner, academician, scholar, and theorist. *Perspectives in Psychiatric Care, 16,* 122–128.

Sills, G. M. (1989). Foreword. In A. W. O'Toole & S. R. Welt (Eds.), *Interpersonal theory in nursing practice. Selected works of Hildegard E. Peplau* (pp. ix–xi). New York: Springer.

Spring, F. E., & Turk, H. (1962). A therapeutic behavior scale. *Nursing Research, 11*, 214–218.

Sullivan, H. S. (1953). *The interpersonal theory of psychiatry.* (H. S. Perry & M. L. Gawel, Eds.). New York: Norton.

Takahashi, T. (1992). Perspectives on nursing knowledge. *Nursing Science Quarterly, 5,* 86–91.

Annotated Bibliography

Primary Sources

O'Toole, A. W., & Welt, S. R. (Eds.). (1989). *Interpersonal theory in nursing practice: Selected works of Hildegard E. Peplau.* New York: Springer.
This book contains reprints of many of Peplau's published and unpublished papers, along with commentaries and a summary of her work by the editors.

Peplau, H. E. (1952). *Interpersonal relations in nursing.* New York: G. P. Putnam's Sons. [Reprinted 1989 London: Macmillan Education Ltd.; Reprinted 1991 New York: Springer]
Peplau describes her theory of interpersonal relations and explains the stages of the nurse-patient relationship.

Peplau, H. E. (1963). A working definition of anxiety. In S. F. Burd & M. A. Marshall, *Some clinical approaches to psychiatric nursing* (pp. 323–327). New York: Macmillan.
In this chapter, Peplau provides a definition of anxiety and discusses its manifestations, causes, and effects.

Peplau, H. E. (1963). Process and concept of learning. In S. F. Burd & M. A. Marshall, *Some clinical approaches to psychiatric nursing* (pp. 333–336). New York: Macmillan.
Peplau illustrates steps in the learning process that nurses utilize to acquire knowledge about a patient situation. Perceptual and thinking processes associated with each learning step are outlined. Finally, the author presents examples of statements nurses can use to facilitate the development of the learning process in the patient.

Peplau, H. E. (1963). Interpersonal relations and the process of adaptation. *Nursing Science, 1,* 272–279.
Using two examples, Paplau illustrates how the phases of adaptation take place. The author defines adaptation as a process by which a new pattern of behaviors evolves in response to a new condition in the psychosocial environment of the person. The need to study the concepts and processes of adaptation in order to advance nursing science is discussed.

Peplau, H. E. (1964). *Basic principles of patient counseling.* Philadelphia: Smith, Kline and French Laboratories.
Peplau describes the major principles of counseling, developed through ward studies at state psychiatric hospitals in the 1950s and 1960s.

Peplau, H. E. (1965). The heart of nursing: Interpersonal relations. *The Canadian Nurse, 61,* 273–275.
Peplau reflects on the several features that the profession of nursing wants to emphasize and proposes that the central force of nursing needs to be clearly identified. According to Peplau, interpersonal relations is the core of nursing, and the nurse-patient relationship serves as the vehicle within which a nurse carries on many important sub-roles in her work role. The beginning development of a science of interpersonal relations is reported.

Peplau, H. E. (1992). Interpersonal relations: A theoretical framework for application in nursing practice. *Nursing Science Quarterly, 5,* 13–18.
Peplau discusses the major features of her theory. She explains the development of the theory and its use in practice. She claims that her theory is among the most useful for understanding nurse-patient interactions.

Welt, S. R., & O'Toole, A. W. (1989). Hildegard E. Peplau: Observations in brief. *Archives of Psychiatric Nursing, 3,* 254–264.
This article presents collected and edited excerpts from Peplau's work, letters, and lectures. A variety of concepts such as worry, nursing practice, jealousy, powerlessness, learning, control, and dependency in psychiatric patients, as well as the problems confronting psychiatric nurses, are addressed. Peplau's thoughts on manic depressive illness, sibling relations, and aging are also described.

Commentary by Peplau and Others

Adams, T. (1991). Paradigms in psychiatric nursing. *Nursing (London), 4*(35), 9–11.
Adams identifies and describes various paradigms used for psychiatric nursing practice in the United Kingdom, including the medico-custodial, the interpersonal, and the holistic. He points out that Peplau developed the interpersonal paradigm.

Aggleton, P., & Chalmers, H. (1990). Peplau's developmental model. *Nursing Times, 86*(2), 38–40.
The authors describe the similarities between Peplau's work and the nursing process. The phases of initial orientation, identification, exploitation, and resolution are examined, and the use of a clinical example illustrates the main roles that the nurse can take to facilitate growth and development.

Belcher, J. R., & Fish, L. J. B. (1980). Hildegard E. Peplau. In Nursing Theories Conference Group, J. B. George (Chairperson), *Nursing theories: The base for professional nursing practice* (pp. 73–89). Englewood Cliffs, NJ: Prentice-Hall.

Belcher, J. R., & Fish, L. J. B. (1985). Hildegard E. Peplau. In J. B. George (Ed.), *Nursing theories: The base for professional nursing practice* (2nd ed., pp. 50–68). Englewood Cliffs, NJ: Prentice-Hall.

Belcher, J. R., & Fish, L. J. B. (1990). Hildegard E. Peplau. In J. B. George (Ed.), *Nursing theories: The base for professional nursing practice* (3rd ed., pp. 43–60). Norwalk, CT: Appleton & Lange.
Belcher and Fish identify Peplau's academic and experiential credentials and describe and analyze her theory.

Blake, M. (1980). The Peplau developmental model for nursing practice. In J. P. Riehl & C. Roy, *Conceptual models for nursing practice* (2nd ed., pp. 53–59). New York: Appleton-Century-Crofts.
Blake presents a brief review of the elements of Peplau's theory.

Bradley, J. C., & Edinberg, M. A. (1986). *Communication in the nursing context* (2nd ed.). Norwalk, CT: Appleton and Lange.
In discussing communication and its theoretical nursing base, the authors identify Peplau's contribution to the definition of the therapeutic interpersonal process. In addition, they describe King's work, which they claim supports and builds on Peplau's framework.

Carey, E. T., Rasmussen, L., Searcy, B., & Stark, N. L. (1986). Hildegard E. Peplau: Psychodynamic nursing. In A. Marriner, *Nursing theorists and their work* (pp. 181–195). St. Louis: C. V. Mosby.

Carey, E. T., Noll, J., Rasmussen, L., Searcy, B., & Stark, N. L. (1989). Hildegard E. Peplau: Psychodynamic nursing. In A. Marriner-Tomey, *Nursing theorists and their work* (2nd ed., pp. 203–218). St. Louis: C. V. Mosby.
Carey and her coauthors describe Peplau's academic and experiential credentials and present a rudimentary analysis of her theory. They also include a cursory critique of the theory.

Field, W. E., Jr. (1979). *The psychotherapy of Hildegard E. Peplau.* New Braunfels, TX: PSF Productions.
Field presents Peplau's principles of psychotherapy. He notes that the contents of the book were gleaned directly from Peplau's spoken words in lectures.

Forchuk, C. (1991). A comparison of the works of Peplau and Orlando. *Archives of Psychiatric Nursing, 5,* 38–45.

Forchuk comments that Peplau and Orlando have had a great impact on past and current mental health nursing practice. She compares and critiques their works, pointing out that Peplau places a greater emphasis on the development of the individual, whereas Orlando focuses on the immediate needs of the client.

Forchuk, C. (1991). Peplau's theory: Concepts and their relations. *Nursing Science Quarterly, 4*, 54–60.

Forchuk describes the concepts and propositions of Peplau's theory.

Gregg, D. E. (1978). Hildegard E. Peplau: Her contributions. *Perspectives in Psychiatric Care, 16*, 118–121.

Gregg describes Peplau's career and many contributions through her teaching, consultation, writing, professional organization activities, and governmental advisory endeavors.

Iveson-Iveson, J. (1982). A two-way process. *Nursing Mirror, 155*(18), 52.

The author reviews the assumptions underlying Peplau's work and presents the phases of the interpersonal relationship between the patient and the nurse. A brief description of the criticism of Peplau's theory is provided.

Johnston, R. L. (1982). Individual psychotherapy: Relationship of theoretical approaches to nursing conceptual models. In J. J. Fitzpatrick, A. L. Whall, R. L. Johnston, & J. A. Floyd, *Nursing models and their psychiatric mental health applications* (pp. 37–68). Bowie, MD: Brady.

Johnston discusses several theories of individual psychotherapy from nursing and other disciplines. She includes a description of Peplau's theory.

Kerr, N. (1990). Editor's corner. *Perspectives in Psychiatric Care, 26*(4), 5–6.

Kerr points out that Peplau was the first nurse theorist to delineate psychiatric/mental health nursing as an interpersonal process governed by lawful principles.

Lego, S. (1980). The one-to-one nurse-patient relationship. *Perspectives in Psychiatric Care, 18*, 67–89.

Lego presents a review of the theory and practice of psychiatric nursing from 1946 to 1974. The issue of nurses doing psychotherapy is examined. The author discusses the history and trends of psychiatric nursing, critically assessing the theory, practice, and published research reported by psychiatric nurses. A summary of patterns from the literature that have provided a direction for the one-to-one relationship in psychiatric nursing is presented. An overview of Peplau's theory is included.

McBride, A. B. (1986). Present issues and future perspectives of psychosocial nursing. Theory and research. *Journal of Psychosocial Nursing and Mental Health Services, 24*(9), 27–32.

McBride examines the developments in nursing and, in particular, in psychosocial nursing. An overview of nursing theorists' contributions to nursing and the increasing need for nurses to engage in research activities are presented. Theoretical and research influences on the development of psychosocial nursing are described. She notes that both Orlando and Peplau were prime movers in the development of psychosocial nursing practice. She goes on to address the importance of research as a means for theory development.

McGilloway, F. (1980). The nursing process: A problem solving approach to patient care. *International Journal of Nursing Studies, 17*, 79–80.

McGilloway notes that Peplau and Orlando made early attempts to analyze nursing actions and recognized that nursing intervention is an interpersonal process.

Morse, J. M., Anderson, G., Bottorff, J. L., Yonge, O., O'Brien, B., Solberg, S. M., & McIlveen, K. H. (1992). Exploring empathy: A conceptual fit for nursing practice? *Image: Journal of Nursing Scholarship, 24*, 273–280.

Morse and her coauthors examine the efficacy of empathy in clinical settings. They note that Peplau, in her 1952 book, introduced the term "empathy" to nursing through her description of the process by which maternal emotions are transmitted to infants. The authors conclude that empathy, which was uncritically adopted from psychology, is a poor fit for the clinical realities of nursing practice.

Osborne, O. (1984). Intellectual traditions in psychiatric nursing. *Journal of Psychosocial Nursing and Mental Health Services, 22*(11), 27–32.

Osborne explained that the study of psychiatric nursing textbooks used for undergraduate nursing students and published since the late 1920s has revealed three distinct intellectual traditions: the psychiatrists, the collaborative, and the psychiatric
nurse. The author emphasizes Peplau's contribution in the tradition of psychiatric
mental health nursing theorizing. The influence of higher education for nurses, dein-
stitutionalization, and the movement toward community mental health on the contents of psychiatric textbooks is presented. The author discusses the need for a theory
unique to psychiatric nursing.

Pearson, A., & Vaughan, B. (1986). *Nursing models for practice*. Rockville, MD: Aspen.
The authors outline the beliefs and values on which Peplau's views are based. Survival of the organism, helping individuals in a forward movement of personality, and
influencing social policy constitute nursing goals. For the therapeutic interpersonal
process to take place, Peplau believes that nurses need to acquire a knowledge base
and specific skills. The authors present the four phases a patient moves through,
which correspond to the four phases of the nursing process. Finally, the nursing process is illustrated in two patient case studies.

Peplau, H. E. (1969). Theory: The professional dimension. In C. M. Norris (Ed.), *Proceedings. First Nursing Theory Conference* (pp. 33–46). Kansas City, KS: University of Kansas Medical Center Department of Nursing Education. [Reprinted in Nicoll, L. H.
(Ed.). (1986). *Perspectives on nursing theory* (pp. 455–466). Boston: Little, Brown; and
Nicoll, L. H. (Ed.). (1991). *Perspectives on nursing theory* (2nd ed., pp. 501–512). Philadelphia: J. B. Lippincott.]
The use of established concepts and processes and the development of knowledge
from observations in nursing situations are described in this paper. As suggested by
Peplau, the use of known concepts and processes requires considerable development
of intellectual competencies in professional nurses through collegiate education. In
addition, the author discusses the need to organize a nomenclature for nursing phenomena. Peplau emphasizes the need for nursing to clarify the parameters of the profession and claim its unique knowledge.

Peplau, H. E. (1978). Psychiatric nursing: Role of nurses and psychiatric nurses. *International Nursing Review, 25*, 41–47.
Peplau differentiates the roles of nurses in psychiatric settings from those of psychiatric nurses. Specific issues such as nursing education and theoretical frameworks as
guiding psychiatric nursing practice are discussed. The author presents three main
schools of thought on mental illness and their relevancy to nursing. Peplau describes
the organization and services of community mental health centers and addresses the
issues pertaining to the role of the nurse in the multidisciplinary team.

Peplau, H. E. (1982). Foreword. In J. J. Fitzpatrick, A. L. Whall, R. L. Johnston, & J. A. Floyd,
Nursing models and their psychiatric mental health applications (p. vii). Bowie, MD:
Brady.
Peplau points out that the work described in the book reflects the intellectual ferment
taking place during the transition from medically oriented nursing care toward
nurse-directed nursing practice.

Peplau, H. E. (1982). Some reflections on earlier days in psychiatric nursing. *Journal of
Psychosocial Nursing and Mental Health Services, 20*(8), 17–24.
This paper presents Peplau's thoughts on the historical evolution of psychiatric nursing over the last century. The author presents the changes in education, the development of school affiliations, the generation of theories of mental illnesses, the practice of psychiatric nursing, the conditions under which patients were hospitalized,
and the introduction of therapies for the treatment of violent patients. The contribution of nurses' efforts to psychiatric nursing from 1882 to 1942 is discussed.

Peplau, H. E. (1985). Is nursing's self-regulatory power being eroded? *American Journal of
Nursing, 85*, 140–143.
Concerned about the danger for the nursing profession to loose control over the privilege of self-regulation, Peplau examines how external controls exercise rule-making
powers that have an impact on nursing. Factors such as economic gain, maintenance
of status, protection of territory, and power needs have motivated other professions
to gain control over nursing practice. Nursing's efforts toward self-regulation include
advanced practice and the establishment of state boards of nursing.

Peplau, H. E. (1985). Help the public maintain mental health: Hildegard Peplau, EdD, RN [Interview]. *Nursing Success Today, 2*(5), 30–34.
    In this interview, Peplau discusses her decision to specialize in psychiatric nursing and to develop graduate psychiatric nursing programs. Reflections on the public's perceptions of psychiatric nurses and on the need to market psychiatric nurses' services to the public are presented.

Peplau, H. E. (1986). Hildegard Peplau: Grande dame of psychiatric nursing [Interview]. *Geriatric Nursing, 7*, 328–330.
    This article presents Peplau's biography and contribution to psychiatric nursing.

Peplau, H. E. (1987). Nursing science: A historical perspective. In R. R. Parse, *Nursing science. Major paradigms, theories, and critiques* (pp. 13–29). Philadelphia: W. B. Saunders.
    In this chapter, Peplau reviews the historical evolution of nursing. Criteria by which to judge that nursing is a science are examined. Finally, the author discusses the nature of nursing science and the need for nursing to further develop its science.

Peplau, H. E. (1988). The art and science of nursing: Similarities, differences, and relations. *Nursing Science Quarterly, 1*, 8–15.
    Peplau suggests definitions of art and science as they apply to nursing practice. Nursing as an act has three major components: medium, process, and product. The science of nursing consists of systematized knowledge. Peplau points out that both nursing's art and science are essential in the performance of mission and work. Although the two concepts differ in their orientation, the author believes that a balanced movement between art and science is transcended by experienced and expert nurses.

Peplau, H. E. (1989). Future directions in psychiatric nursing from the perspective of history. *Journal of Psychosocial Nursing and Mental Health Services, 27*(2), 18–28.
    This article features an historical overview of psychiatric nursing since the first organized training school in psychiatric nursing in 1882. The author discusses the social, economic, professional, and organizational factors that produced profound changes in the practice and education of psychiatric nursing. Concerned with a movement toward a service economy, high technology, and the new social arrangement in families and institutions, Peplau presents the challenges facing psychiatric nurses and proposes future directions for psychiatric nursing.

Peplau, H. E. (1992). Notes on Nightingale. Guidelines for caring then and now. In F. Nightingale, *Notes on nursing: What it is, and what it is not* (Commemorative edition, pp. 48–57). Philadelphia: J. B. Lippincott. (Original work published in 1859).
    Peplau discusses the influence of Nightingale's work on her theory of interpersonal relations and describes the difficulty she faced in getting her 1952 book published. She also notes that both her own and Nightingale's ideas must be subject to judgments of history.

Reed, P. G., & Johnston, R. L. (1983). Peplau's nursing model: The interpersonal process. In J. J. Fitzpatrick & A. L. Whall, *Conceptual models of nursing: Analysis and application* (pp. 27–46). Bowie, MD: Brady.

Reed, P. G., & Johnston, R. L. (1989). Peplau's nursing model: The interpersonal process. In J. J. Fitzpatrick & A. L. Whall, *Conceptual models of nursing: Analysis and application* (2nd ed., pp. 49–67). Norwalk, CT: Appleton & Lange.
    The authors describe Peplau's theory, present an analysis of the theory, and briefly discuss its relation to nursing research, education, and practice.

Sills, G. M. (1978). Hildegard E. Peplau: Leader, practitioner, academician, scholar, and theorist. *Perspectives in Psychiatric Care, 16*, 122–128.
    Sills describes Peplau's major contributions to nursing and her commitment to the development and testing of her theory. Finally, Peplau's impact on the author's career is conveyed.

Smith, M. J. (1988). Perspectives on nursing science. *Nursing Science Quarterly, 1*, 80–85.
    This article is the transcription of a panel discussion at the Nurse Theorist Conference sponsored by Discovery International and held in Pittsburgh in May 1987. The panel was moderated by Mary Jane Smith; participants were Imogene King, Madeleine Leininger, Rosemarie Parse, Hildegard Peplau, Martha Rogers, Callista Roy, and Roz-

ella Schlotfeldt. Questions focused on the issues of the uniqueness of theoretical frameworks, the phenomenon central to theoretical frameworks, and nursing diagnoses.

Smoyak, S. (1990). Interview with Hildegard E. Peplau. *New Jersey Nurse, 20*(5), 10–11, 14.
   In this interview, Peplau describes her career and background, and reflects on her contributions toward graduate education in psychiatric nursing. Her thoughts about the need for nursing to recognize the importance of specialties are expressed.

Takahashi, T. (1992). Perspectives on nursing knowledge. *Nursing Science Quarterly, 5,* 86–91.
   This article is the transcription of a panel discussion at the Nurse Theorist Conference sponsored by Discovery International that was held in Tokyo in May 1991. The panel was moderated by Hiroko Minami; participants were Imogene King, Rosemarie Parse, Hildegard Peplau, and Martha Rogers. Questions were related to the focus of each theorist's work, similarities and differences between the theories, the use of nursing theories to structure curricula for nursing education, and the applicability of the theories in diverse cultures. The panel discussion provided an opportunity for considerable dialogue among the four theorists.

Torres, G. (1986). *Theoretical foundations of nursing.* Norwalk, CT: Appleton-Century-Crofts.
   Torres presents a brief description and an evaluation of Peplau's theory. She also describes the application of the theory within the context of the nursing process framework of assessment, diagnosis, planning, implementation, and evaluation.

Whall, A. L. (1980). Congruence between existing theories of family functioning and nursing theories. *Advances in Nursing Science, 3*(1), 59–67.
   Whall examines the relationship between specific family theories and the nursing theories of King, Peplau, and Rogers. According to Whall, Peplau's approach to nursing theory is congruent with the psychoanalytic approach to family functioning, King's theory is consistent with the approach of communicationists, and Rogers' work is the closest to the family systems approach. The author discusses the need to reformulate existing theories in terms of nursing theory.

Practice

Beeber, L. S. (1989). Enacting corrective interpersonal experiences with the depressed client: An intervention model. *Archives of Psychiatric Nursing, 3,* 211–217.
   In an attempt to protect the self from anxiety associated with the need for tenderness, the depressed patient enacts particular interpersonal phenomena designed to create distance and control intimacy. A theoretical framework using Sullivan and Peplau explains these phenomena in the context of the therapeutic nurse-patient relationship and guides specific responses by the nurse to create a corrective interpersonal experience. Case material illustrates these processes.

Beeber, L., Anderson, C. A., & Sills, G. M. (1990). Peplau's theory in practice. *Nursing Science Quarterly, 3,* 6–8.
   The authors explain that Peplau espouses the view that effectiveness in interpersonal relationships is a legitimate concern in professional nursing practice. They identify the four key elements in Peplau's work as: mutuality, phasic relatedness, the anxiety gradient, and uniqueness. They also present a case study of a 42-year-old man who is HIV-positive.

Bird, J. (1992). Helping Billy move on. *Nursing Times, 88*(31), 42–44.
   Bird describes how she established a therapeutic relationship with a 45-year-old man with a long history of psychiatric problems. She explains the progress of the relationship through Peplau's four phases of the nurse-patient relationship.

Day, M. W. (1990). Anxiety in the emergency department. *Point of View, 27*(3), 4–5.
   Day explains the use of Peplau's concepts for determining a patient's anxiety when in the emergency department. Peplau's work can guide nursing interventions to meet the patient's needs as well as provide a framework to evaluate the patient's responses to the interventions.

Forchuk, C., Beaton, S., Crawford, L., Ide, L., Voorberg, N., & Bethune, J. (1989). Incorporating Peplau's theory and case management. *Journal of Psychosocial Nursing and Mental Health Services, 27*(2), 35–38.
> The authors identify the similarities between Peplau's theory of the nurse-patient relationship and the case management model. They describe a combined Peplau/case management model that provides a framework for the delivery of comprehensive permanent follow-up for the chronic mental health client.

Martin, M-L., Forchuk, C., Santopinto, M., & Butcher, H. K. (1992). Alternative approaches to nursing practice: Application of Peplau, Rogers, Parse. *Nursing Science Quarterly, 5,* 80–85.
> The authors describe the use of works by Parse, Peplau, and Rogers in practice. They explain how theory-based practice differs from traditional practice and how nursing knowledge can guide practice. Tables display documentation from the perspective of each theorist's work.

Morrison, E. G. (1992). Inpatient practice: An integrated framework. *Journal of Psychosocial Nursing and Mental Health Services, 30*(1), 26–29.
> Morrison describes the complexity of the clinical nurse specialist's responsibilities, and maintains that they require specialized knowledge in psychiatric-mental health nursing and systems concepts. She compares the steps of the nursing process (assessment, diagnosis, planning, implementation, evaluation) with Peplau's phases of the nurse-patient relationship. A case study demonstrating the integration of Bowen's family systems theory with Peplau's theory and the nursing process is included.

Nordel, D., & Soto, A. (1980). Peplau's model applied to primary nursing in clinical practice. In J. P. Riehl & C. Roy, *Conceptual models for nursing practice* (2nd ed., pp. 60–73). New York: Appleton-Century-Crofts.
> The authors identify the similarities between Peplau's theory and primary nursing. They describe the phases of the nurse-patient relationship in four case studies.

Nyatanga, B. (1989). Method in their madness. *Nursing Times, 85*(4), 46–48.
> Nyatanga describes the application of Peplau's work on a psychiatric ward. Reflections on nursing practice in this setting are described.

O'Brien, D., & Smith, A. (1991). In search of destiny. *Nursing Times, 87*(20), 26–28.
> The authors describe a comprehensive nursing care plan for a depressed young woman based on Peplau's theory.

Peplau, H. E. (1953). Themes in nursing situations: Power. *American Journal of Nursing, 53,* 1221–1223.
> Peplau bases the importance of recognizing themes in interpersonal situations on four main reasons: themes describe what takes place in the interaction, they allow economical communication to transpire, they provide a basis for comparing one situation with others, and lastly, they allow nurses to use reasoning skills. Using power as a first theme, the author explains how power expressed by nurses in some of their relationships with psychiatric patients can have negative consequences.

Peplau, H. E. (1953). Themes in nursing situations: Safety. *American Journal of Nursing, 53,* 1343–1346.
> Concerned with the recurring themes in the patient's past and present relationships with people, Peplau discusses the needs for nurses to recognize whether safety can be used constructively in a psychotherapeutic nurse-patient experience. The exclusive focus on safety and security by everyone relating to a patient may become an obstacle rather than an aid to recovery. The author challenges psychiatric nursing care and encourages nurses to have a voice in determining policies that influence nursing practices.

Peplau, H. E. (1955). Loneliness. *American Journal of Nursing, 55,* 1476–1481.
> Based on clinical observations, the author describes the phenomenon of loneliness often present in psychiatric patients. Using several examples, Peplau illustrates the roots and manifestations of loneliness in psychiatric patients as well as their efforts to overcome it. The patterns of living of lonely patients and the author's recommendations for guiding nursing care are described.

Peplau, H. E. (1960). Talking with patients. *American Journal of Nursing, 60,* 964–967.
> Peplau maintains that for verbal interchanges with patients to be productive, the

nurse must be aware of her own verbal patterns before deciding to talk with patients. She also maintains that the focus in the nurse-patient relationship will be on the patient's needs and difficulties. Peplau identifies communication skills nurses must have in order to assess the patient's experience.

Peplau, H. E. (1962). Interpersonal techniques: The crux of psychiatric nursing. *American Journal of Nursing, 62*, 50–54.
Peplau distinguishes between general practitioners (psychiatric nurses) and practitioners (psychiatric nursing) by the level of clinical specialized functions. The emphasis of psychiatric nursing is on the counseling and psychotherapeutic role, and psychiatric nurses focus on technical expertness and on managerial, socializing-agent, and health teaching activities. Interpersonal techniques useful in relation to specific problems and the benefits of integrating these techniques in basic schools of nursing are addressed.

Peplau, H. E. (1964). Psychiatric nursing skills and the general hospital patient. *Nursing Forum, 3*(2), 28–37.
Peplau explains how the appreciation of behavioral science theories is relevant to all nursing situations. Drawing from a philosophy of patient care widely used by psychiatric nurses, Peplau demonstrates the benefits of integrating psychiatric nursing skills in the care of patients hospitalized in general hospitals.

Peplau, H. E. (1965). The nurse in the community mental health program. *Nursing Outlook, 13*(11), 68–70.
Based on a need for expert clinical supervision of public health nurses in community mental health, Peplau describes a program in which clinical supervisors would foster staff development. Several areas in which supervision is necessary are addressed. These include the nurse's intellectual and assessment skills, the nurse's techniques with respect to direct services to mentally ill patients, and the relationships between the nurse's work and the total mental health effort within a community.

Peplau, H. E. (1965). Specialization in professional nursing. *Nursing Science, 3*, 268–287.
Peplau discusses the trend toward specialization in nursing. Specialization could follow several classification systems, namely, the area of practice, an anatomical taxonomy, the chronology of the patient population, the acuity and length of patients' illnesses, subroles of the staff nurse's work role, professional services, and clinical services. Inasmuch as clinical practice is the center of nursing, Peplau emphasizes the need for clinical specialists. The knowledge base, working title, education, and roles of the clinical specialist, as well as the problems in developing programs for these experts, are addressed.

Peplau, H. E. (1966). Nurse-doctor relationships. *Nursing Forum, 5*(1), 60–75.
The social, economic, and educational factors that played a major role in changing the working relation between nurses and physicians are discussed.

Peplau, H. E. (1967). The work of psychiatric nurses. *Psychiatric Opinion, 4*(1), 5–11.
Peplau describes the clinical practice of psychiatric nurses in relation to four processes: observation, interpretation, interventions, and supervisory review. Categories of psychiatric nurses' work patterns are presented.

Peplau, H. E. (1967). Interpersonal relations and the work of the industrial nurse. *American Association of Industrial Nurses Journal, 15*(10), 7–12.
Peplau uses interpersonal and behavioral sciences theories to help the industrial nurse understand the relationship between various employees, the nurse, and the work environment. The effects of interpersonal phenomena on the workers' behaviors and their relation to health problems are presented. She suggests that the nurse adopt an investigative approach in the form of situational counseling in all nursing situations.

Peplau, H. E. (1968). Psychotherapeutic strategies. *Perspectives in Psychiatric Care, 6*, 264–289.
Peplau discusses the areas in which psychotherapeutic strategies are developed. First, behavioral interactions within the ward milieu between patients and staff should provide stimuli to the development of new behaviors. Second, verbal tactics should be used by nurses to force change in the use of language and thought in patients.

Peplau, H. E. (1969). Professional closeness as a special kind of involvement with a patient, client, or family group. *Nursing Forum, 8,* 342–360.
Peplau defines professional closeness as an essential element of nursing care. Distinct from the other types of closeness, professional closeness focuses exclusively on the interests, concerns, and needs of the patient. Peplau discusses Sullivan's theorem of reciprocal emotion to guide the nurse toward an awareness of her own needs. Specific nursing behaviors indicative of successful professional closeness are outlined. The relevancy of the affective involvement in the nurse-patient situation is addressed.

Peplau, H. E. (1985). The power of the dissociative state [Interview]. *Journal of Psychosocial Nursing and Mental Health Services, 23*(8), 31–32.
In this interview, Peplau recalls an event that occurred hours before a nursing administrator set a fire at a large psychiatric institution in the late 1940s. Peplau explains how the panic episode she experienced when she encountered the administrator produced a dissociative state and how she experienced the empathic transmission of anxiety.

Peplau, H. E. (1986). The nurse as counselor. *Journal of American College of Health, 35,* 11–14.
Peplau discusses counseling as one aspect of college nursing practice. Specific requirements essential to ensure counseling competence for work with college students are outlined. Peplau presents three clinical choices suggestive of different levels of psychosocial and psychiatric assessment. Major health problems of college students necessitating counseling are described.

Peplau, H. E. (1987). Interpersonal constructs for nursing practice. *Nurse Education Today, 7,* 201–208.
Drawing from Sullivan's work, Peplau presents the definition of interpersonal relations and its major theoretical constructs. Specific features in relations such as empathic linkages, gestural messages, and patterns and variations are outlined. Inasmuch as the focus of nursing practice is on the problematic patterns in intrapersonal, interpersonal, and system phenomena, the author describes the many patterns of behaviors psychiatric patients demonstrate. Recommendations for nursing research, education, and practice are given.

Peplau, H. E. (1987). Psychiatric skills: Tomorrow's world. *Nursing Times, 83*(1), 29–33.
Challenges in health care require that psychiatric nurses learn new skills to keep pace with the developments in psychiatric services. In this paper, Peplau examines the basic skills most relevant to psychiatric nurses. Implications of the movement toward community health on the need for further refinement and expansion of psychiatric nursing skills are discussed.

Runtz, S. E., & Urtel, J. G. (1983). Evaluating your practice via a nursing model. *Nurse Practitioner, 8*(3), 30, 32, 37–40.
The authors describe the use of Orem's and Peplau's works as an evaluative tool to guide nursing practice in the primary care setting. Specifically, the authors illustrate how Orem's Self-Care Framework and Peplau's theory can be instrumental in planning, implementing, and evaluating the care of patients with different health care problems in the ambulatory setting.

Stark, M. (1992). A system for delivering care. *British Journal of Nursing, 1,* 85–87.
Stark describes the nursing care provided at Maudsley Hospital in London, England. The ward on which the author works bases nursing care on Peplau's and Maslow's theories and uses primary nursing as the care delivery model. Stark presents a case study of a 41-year-old woman with a history of depression.

Thomas, M. D., Baker, J. M., & Estes, N. J. (1970). Anger: A tool for developing self-awareness. *American Journal of Nursing, 70,* 2586–2590.
Through a nurse-patient interaction, the authors illustrate the process of anger. Guidelines for therapeutic nursing interventions with the angry patient are offered.

Thompson, L. (1986). Peplau's theory: An application to short-term individual therapy. *Journal of Psychosocial Nursing and Mental Health Services, 24*(8), 26–31.
Thompson describes the phases of the nurse-client relationship to guide and analyze the therapeutic process in specific clinical situations involving short-term individual therapy.

Williams, C. A. (1989). Perspectives on the hallucinatory process. *Issues in Mental Health Nursing, 10,* 99–119.
Drawing from Peplau's, Rector's, and Field's works, Williams explores the literature related to hallucination and presents clinical observations. Foundations for recommendations for assessment and intervention with the hallucinating client are provided. The author addresses issues related to clinical research with psychiatric clients and identifies the need for further research with the hallucinating patient.

Education

Peplau, H. E. (1951). Toward new concepts in nursing and nursing education. *American Journal of Nursing, 51,* 1475–1477.
Peplau describes the importance of understanding one's own behavior in order to help others identify felt difficulties and the application of principles of human relations as functions of psychodynamic nursing. The teaching method used by school personnel to train student nurses and its influence on their learning is addressed. The clinical instructor's pattern of relations and the instructor-student relationship serve as a basis for the development of students' patterns of behavior in interpersonal situations. The contents of the article were adapted from the introduction to Peplau's 1952 book.

Peplau, H. E. (1956). An undergraduate program in psychiatric nursing. *Nursing Outlook, 4,* 400–410.
Peplau describes the Rutgers University School of Nursing undergraduate program, including the specific teaching devices and the educative strategies developed to prepare students to become staff nurses in psychiatric facilities.

Peplau, H. E. (1963). Foreword. In S. F. Burd & M. A. Marshall, *Some clinical approaches to psychiatric nursing* (pp. vii–ix). New York: Macmillan.
Peplau addresses the causes of the nursing shortage in psychiatric settings and, in particular, the insufficient preparation nurses receive about psychiatric nursing within their basic nursing education programs. The benefits of higher education for psychiatric nurses are discussed.

Research

Bristow, F., & Callaghan, P. (1991). Using Peplau's model in affective disorders. *Nursing Times, 87*(18), 40–41.
Bristow and Callaghan report the findings of their study of the introduction of Peplau's theory on a unit at a large psychiatric hospital in London, England. They found that use of Peplau's theory resulted in improved use of the nursing process, little change in staff satisfaction, and decreased patient satisfaction.

Elms, R. R., & Leonard, R. C. (1966). Effects of nursing approaches during admission. *Nursing Research, 15,* 39–48.
This study examined the effectiveness of an experimental approach, congruent with Orlando's and Peplau's works, in relieving distress experienced by patients during an elective admission to a general hospital. Although the somatic and subjective indicators of distress failed to show consistent differences between the experimental and control groups, they indicate that a patient-centered nursing approach is more apt to alleviate distress than approaches that emphasize technical tasks. The authors discuss the need for instrument development and for testing theories.

Forchuk, C. (1992). The orientation phase of the nurse-client relationship: How long does it take? *Perspectives in Psychiatric Care, 28,* 7–10.
Forchuk reports the results of a study dealing with the length of the orientation phase of the nurse-patient relationship with clients with chronic mental illness. She found that the orientation phase was related to the number and length of hospitalizations and that a return to the orientation phase can be triggered by a change of staff or by the client's worsening paranoia or depression.

Forchuk, C., & Brown, B. (1989). Establishing a nurse-client relationship. *Journal of Psychosocial Nursing and Mental Health Services, 27*(2), 30–34.

Forchuk and Brown describe the development of an instrument, based on Peplau's work, to measure the phases of the nurse-client relationship. Preliminary results from the validity and reliability testing of the Relationship Form are reported.

Forchuk, C., & Voorberg, N. (1991). Evaluation of a community mental health program. *Canadian Journal of Nursing Administration, 4*(2), 16–20.
Forchuk and Voorberg report the results of an evaluation of a community mental health program guided by Peplau's theory. Instruments used (Relationship Form and Stage of Learning Form) were directly derived from Peplau's work. They found that problem identification was the most common phase of the nurse-patient relationship for clients after 2 years and that clients progressed in their problem-solving abilities.

Garrett, A., Manuel, D., & Vincent, C. (1976). Stressful experiences identified by student nurses. *Journal of Nursing Education, 15*(6), 9–21.
The purpose of this study was to identify and compare the experiences considered stressful by nursing students completing their sophomore, junior, and senior levels of collegiate study. Academic pressures, personal problems with boyfriends and family, clinical problems with physical care of patients, and problems with interpersonal relationships with clinical instructors were most stressful.

Hays, D. (1961). Teaching a concept of anxiety. *Nursing Research, 10,* 108–113.
Hays reports that her study yielded a pattern of teaching that evolved when a nurse facilitated the application of the concept of anxiety to experiences described in group discussions by six schizophrenic patients over 12 sessions. The author identifies three phases of experiential teaching and discusses the need for further research.

Hirschmann, M. (1989). Psychiatric and mental health nurses' beliefs about therapeutic paradox. *Journal of Child Psychiatric Nursing, 2*(1), 7–13.
Hirschmann reports that half of the 165 American psychiatric nurses surveyed indicated that they used Peplau's theory as a basis for their practice.

La Monica, E. (1981). Construct validity of an empathy instrument. *Research in Nursing and Health, 4,* 389–400.
La Monica describes the development and psychometric testing of an instrument designed to measure empathy. She comments that Peplau, among several other nurse scholars, considers empathy to be a necessary component in nurse behaviors.

Lund, V. E., & Frank, D. I. (1991). Helping the medicine go down: Nurses' and patients' perceptions about medication compliance. *Journal of Psychosocial Nursing and Mental Health Services, 29*(7), 6–9.
Lund and Frank note that the nurse's approach in implementation of the role of facilitator of clients' medication compliance was influenced by Peplau's theory. They found that nurses and patients have similar perceptions of the estimated frequency of medication compliance. Nurses and patients differed, however, in reasons given for noncompliance.

Madden, B. P. (1990). The hybrid model for concept development: Its value for the study of therapeutic alliance. *Advances in Nursing Science, 12*(3), 75–87.
The investigator noted that the definition of therapeutic alliance as "a process that emerges within a provider-client interaction in which both the client and the provider are (1) actively working toward the goal of developing client health behaviors chosen for consistency with the client's current health status and life style, (2) focusing on mutual negotiation to determine activities to be carried out toward that goal, and (3) using a supportive and equitable therapeutic relationship to facilitate that goal" (p. 85) is consistent with Peplau's and Travelbee's perspectives, as well as with Orlando's notion of the primacy of the nurse-client relationship.

Methven, D., & Schlotfeldt, R. M. (1962). The social interaction inventory. *Nursing Research, 11,* 83–88.
The authors describe the development, refinement, and testing of an instrument designed to determine the nature of verbal responses nurses tend to give in emotion-ladened situations typically encountered in nursing practice. Peplau's work was used to analyze the response types given by the nurses. According to the authors, the Social Interaction Inventory can be useful in assessing verbal communication skills of nursing students and nurse practitioners. The data indicated that some practicing nurses lack skill in communicating effectively with patients who are anxious.

Ramos, M. C. (1992). The nurse-patient relationship: Theme and variations. *Journal of Advanced Nursing, 17,* 496–506.
Ramos reports the findings of her analysis of critical incidents describing nurses' perceptions of their relationships with patients. The study addresses characteristics of relationships in the tradition developed by Orlando and Peplau. The analysis revealed that close relationships, described as modified social relationships, were common.

Sills, G. M. (1977). Research in the field of psychiatric nursing 1952–1977. *Nursing Research, 28,* 201–207.
Sills reviews 25 years of psychiatric nursing research. She points out that Peplau's work influenced the interpersonal nature and direction of clinical work and studies at Teachers College, Columbia University in the 1950s.

Spring, F. E., & Turk, H. (1962). A therapeutic behavior scale. *Nursing Research, 11,* 214–218.
The purpose of Spring and Turk's study was to develop an objective scale, consistent with Peplau's work, in order to assess the observed interaction of nurses with patients. Validity and reliability data for the instrument are described.

Topf, M., & Dambacher, B. (1979). Predominant source of interpersonal influence in relationships between psychiatric patients and nursing staff. *Research in Nursing and Health, 2,* 35–43.
In the discussion of their study findings, Topf and Dambacher commented that nurses should not expect to establish rapport with psychiatric patients as quickly as they might in other interpersonal situations. They pointed out that Peplau had maintained that the prolonged time required for rapport with a psychiatric patient reflects the patient's need to reestablish basic trust.

Vogelsang, J. (1990). Continued contact with a familiar nurse affects women's perceptions of the ambulatory surgical experience: A qualitative-quantitative design. *Journal of Post-Anesthesia Nursing, 5,* 315–320.
Vogelsang reports the findings of her practice-based study of the impact of continued contact with a familiar nurse from preadmission procedures through postoperative awakening in the postanesthesia care unit (PACU). The study was guided by Peplau's theory. The continued contact group was ready to go home when discharged from the ambulatory surgery unit significantly more often than the women who received standard nursing care. The continued contact group also expressed greater satisfaction with nursing care than the standard care group.

Whitley, G. G. (1988). A validation study of the nursing diagnosis anxiety. *Florida Nursing Review, 3*(2), 1–7.
The study was designed to test NANDA's diagnosis of Anxiety, which was based on Peplau's work. Results indicated that 4 defining characteristics of anxiety were identified as critical, 24 were acceptable, and 1 was discarded. None of the personal or professional characteristics were significant. Whitley discusses the implications of a taxonomy of validated diagnoses on nursing.

Whitley, G. G. (1992). Concept analysis of anxiety. *Nursing Diagnosis, 3,* 107–116.
Whitley presents an analysis of the concept of anxiety.

Doctoral Dissertations

Forchuk, C. (1992). The orientation phase of the nurse-client relationship: Testing Peplau's theory. *Dissertation Abstracts International, 53,* 2245B.

Peden, A. R. (1992). The process of recovering in women who have been depressed. *Dissertation Abstracts International, 52,* 5193B.

Ramos, M. C. N. (1992). Empathy within the nurse-patient relationship. *Dissertation Abstracts International, 52,* 5193B.

CHAPTER

8

Watson's Theory of Human Caring_____

Jean Watson planned to write a textbook presenting an integrated curriculum for a baccalaureate nursing curriculum. Instead, she developed a novel structure for basic nursing processes (Watson, 1979). That work solved some of Watson's conceptual and empirical problems about nursing and formed the foundation for the science and art of human caring. As Watson went on to solve other conceptual problems, as well as philosophical problems about nursing, the Theory of Human Caring was developed and formalized (Watson, 1985). This chapter presents an analysis and evaluation of that theory.

The concepts of the Theory of Human Caring and their dimensions are listed below. Each concept is defined and described later in this chapter.

KEY CONCEPTS_____

Transpersonal Caring	Sensitivity to Self and
Self	Others
Phenomenal Field	Helping-Trusting, Human
Actual Caring Occasion	Care Relationship
Intersubjectivity	Expressing Positive and
Carative Factors	Negative Feelings
Humanistic-Altruistic	Creative Problem-Solving
System of Values	Caring Process
Faith-Hope	

Transpersonal Teaching-Learning Supportive, Protective, and/or Corrective Mental, Physical, Societal, and Spiritual Environment	Human Needs Assistance Existential-Phenomenological-Spiritual Forces

ANALYSIS OF THE THEORY OF HUMAN CARING

This section presents an analysis of Watson's theory. The analysis is based on Watson's publications about her theory, especially her 1979 book, Nursing: The Philosophy and Science of Caring, and her 1985 book, Nursing: Human Science and Human Care: A Theory of Nursing.

Scope of the Theory

The Theory of Human Caring focuses on the human component of caring and the moment-to-moment encounters between the one giving care and the one cared for. Watson (1989b) claimed that her theory encompasses the whole of nursing; the emphasis is, however, placed on the interpersonal process between the caregiver and the care recipient.

The theory consists of a description of transpersonal caring and a taxonomy of interventions referred to as carative factors. It is, therefore, appropriately categorized as a middle-range descriptive classification theory.

Context of the Theory

Metaparadigm Concepts and Proposition

Watson did not identify the linkage between the metaparadigm of nursing and her theory. A review of her publications, however, led to the conclusion that the Theory of Human Caring focuses on the metaparadigm concepts person and nursing. The metaparadigm proposition of interest is the [nursing] processes by which positive changes in [the person's] health status are affected.

Philosophical Claims

The analysis of Watson's work revealed that the theory is based on a metaphysical, spiritual-existential, and phenomenological orientation that draws on Eastern philosophy. Watson (1989b) regards her theory as metaphysical. She explained that "it goes beyond the rapidly emerging existential-phenomenological approaches in nursing, to perhaps a higher level of abstraction and sense of personhood, incorporating the concept of the soul and transcendence" (p. 221). Accordingly, Watson's evolving ideas and ideals, which are the result of reflective thinking, "are concerned with spirit rather than matter, flux rather than form, inner knowledge and power, rather than circumstance" (p. 219).

Watson's philosophical claims take the form of values and assumptions about those values. Her values about human care are expressed throughout the 1985 book. Those values are:

1. Deep respect for the wonder and mysteries of life.
2. Acknowledgement of a spiritual dimension to life and internal power of the human care process.
3. The power of humans to grow and change.
4. Nonpaternalistic values related to human autonomy and freedom of choice.
5. A high regard and reverence for the subjective-internal world of the person.
6. A high value on how the person, including the patient and the nurse, perceives and experiences health-illness conditions.
7. Emphasis on helping a person to gain more self-knowledge, self-control, and readiness for self-healing, regardless of the health-illness condition.
8. A high value on the relationship between the person and the nurse, with the nurse viewed as a coparticipant in the human care process.
9. Human caring is the moral ideal of nursing, with the goal of protection, enhancement, and preservation of human dignity. (pp. 34–35, 73)

Eleven assumptions related to human care values were identified by Watson (1985):

1. Care and love are the most universal, the most tremendous, and the most mysterious of cosmic forces: they comprise the primal and universal psychic energy.
2. Often these needs are overlooked; or we know people need each other in loving and caring ways, but often we do not behave well toward each other. If our humanness is to survive, however, we need to become more caring and loving to nourish our humanity and evolve as a civilization and live together.
3. Since nursing is a caring profession, its ability to sustain its caring ideal and ideology in practice will affect the human development of civilization and determine nursing's contribution to society.
4. As a beginning we have to impose our own will to care and love upon our own behavior and not on others. We have to treat ourselves with gentleness and dignity before we can respect and care for others with gentleness and dignity.

5. Nursing has always held a human-care and caring stance in regard to people with health-illness concerns.
6. Caring is the essence of nursing and the most central and unifying focus for nursing practice.
7. Human care, at the individual and group level, has received less and less emphasis in the health care delivery system.
8. Caring values of nurses and nursing have been submerged. Nursing and society are, therefore, in a critical situation today in sustaining human care ideals and a caring ideology in practice. The human care role is threatened by increased medical technology, bureaucratic-managerial institutional constraints in a nuclear age society. At the same time there has been a proliferation of curing and radical treatment cure techniques often without regard to costs.
9. Preservation and advancement of human care as both an epistemic and clinical endeavor is a significant issue for nursing today and in the future.
10. Human care can be effectively demonstrated and practiced only interpersonally. The intersubjective human process keeps alive a common sense of humanity; it teaches us how to be human by identifying ourselves with others, whereby the humanity of one is reflected in the other.
11. Nursing's social, moral, and scientific contributions to humankind and society lie in its commitment to human care ideals in theory, practice and research. (pp. 32–33).

Watson's philosophical claims are consistent with humanism (Sellers, 1991). Indeed, Watson (1985) explicitly rejected the mechanistic, reductionistic view of the world in favor of a human science perspective. She stated, "The context [of the theory] is humanitarian and metaphysical. It incorporates both the art and science of nursing. Science is emphasized in a human science context" (p. 76). Taken together, Watson's philosophical claims and her discussion of human science indicate that the Theory of Human Becoming is most closely aligned with the *reciprocal interaction* worldview.

Conceptual Model

The conceptual model from which Watson's theory was derived is not explicit, but it can be inferred from her publications. It clearly reflects the metaphysical, spiritual, existential, and phenomenological orientation of her philosophical claims. The model comprises descriptions of human life, health, and nursing that provide a conceptual base for the Theory of Human Caring.

Watson's description of human life is based on her definition of the soul. "The concept of the soul," according to Watson (1985) "refers to the *geist*, spirit, inner self, or essence of the person, which is tied to a greater sense of self-awareness, a higher degree of consciousness, an inner strength, and a power that can expand human capacities and allow a person to transcend his or her usual self" (p. 46).

With regard to human life, Watson (1985) stated:

> My conception of life and personhood is tied to notions that one's soul possesses a body that is not confined by objective space and time. The lived world of the experiencing person is not distinguished by external and internal notions of time and space, but shapes its own time and space, which is unconstrained by linearity. Notions of personhood, then, transcend the here and now, and one has the capacity to coexist with past, present, future, all at once. . . . The individual spirit of a person or of collective humanity may continue to exist throughout time, keeping alive a higher sense of humankind. . . . [Thus,] human life is defined as (spiritual-mental-physical) being-in-the-world, which is continuous in time and space. (pp. 45–47)

Watson differentiated between health and illness. Her view of health underscores the entire individual in the physical, social, esthetic, and moral realms. Accordingly, "Health refers to unity and harmony within the mind, body, and soul. Health is also associated with the degree of congruence between the self as perceived and the self as experienced" (Watson, 1985, p. 48).

Illness, according to Watson, is not necessarily disease, although it can lead to disease. She explained, "Illness is subjective turmoil or disharmony with a person's inner self or soul at some level or disharmony within the spheres of the person. . . . Illness connotes a felt incongruence within the person such as an incongruence between the self as perceived and the self as experienced. A troubled inner soul can lead to illness, and illness can produce disease" (Watson, 1985, p. 48).

Watson (1985) maintained that nursing is a human science. Human science, which focuses on the whole person, contrasts with natural science, which reduces phenomena to their parts. She explained:

> The mandate for nursing within science as well as within society is a demand for cherishing of the wholeness of human personality. It is thus that I regard nursing as a human science and the human care process in nursing as a significant humanitarian and epistemic act that contributes to the preservation of humanity. (p. 29)

The goal of nursing, according to Watson (1985) "is to help persons gain a higher degree of harmony within the mind, body, and soul which generates self-knowledge, self-reverence, self-healing, and self-care processes while increasing diversity" (p. 49). Watson went on to say that nursing is directed toward "finding meaning in one's own existence and experiences, discovering inner power and control, and potentiating instances of transcendence and self-healing" (p. 74).

The process of nursing is human-to-human caring. The individual patient is regarded as the agent of change. The nurse can function as a coparticipant through the human care process, but the "personal, internal mental-spiritual mechanisms of the person [allow] the self to be healed through various internal or external means, or without external agents, [and] through an intersubjective interdependent process wherein both persons may transcend self and usual experiences" (Watson, 1985, p. 74).

Watson (1985) identified several premises that can be considered conceptual model-level propositions. The premises are:

1. A person's mind and emotions are windows to the soul. Nursing care can be and is physical, procedural, objective, and factual, but at the highest level of nursing the nurses' human care responses, the human care transactions, and the nurses' presence in the relationship transcend the physical and material world, bound in time and space, and make contact with the person's emotional and subjective world as the route to the inner self and the higher sense of self.

2. A person's body is confined in time and space, but the mind and soul are not confined to the physical universe. One's higher sense of mind and soul transcends time and space and helps to account for notions like collective unconscious, causal past, mystical experiences, parapsychological phenomena, a higher sense of power, and may be an indicator of the spiritual evolution of human beings.

3. A nurse may have access to a person's mind, emotions, and inner self indirectly through any sphere—mind, body or soul—provided the physical body is not perceived or treated as separate from the mind and emotions and higher sense of self (soul).

4. The spirit, inner self, or soul (geist) of a person exists in and for itself. The spiritual essence of the person is related to the human ability to be free, which is an evolving process in the development of humans. The ability to develop and experience one's essence freely is limited by the extent of others' ability to "be." The destiny of one's being (humankind's destiny) is to develop the spiritual essence of the self and in the highest sense, to become more God-like. However, each person has to question his or her own essence and moral behavior toward others, because if people are dehumanized at a basic level, for example, a human care level, that dehumanizing process is not capable of reflecting humanity back upon itself.

5. People need each other in a caring, loving way. Love and caring are two universal givens. . . . These needs are often overlooked, or even though we know we need one another in a loving and caring way, we do not behave well toward each other. If our humanness is to survive, we need to become more loving, caring, and moral to nourish our humanity, advance as a civilization, and live together.

6. A person may have an illness that is "completely hidden from our

eyes." To find solutions it is necessary to find meanings. A person's human predicament may not be related to the external world as much as to the person's inner world as he or she experiences it. (pp. 50–51)

Antecedent Knowledge

Watson (1985, 1988b, 1989a) noted that her theory developed from her own values and beliefs about the person and life, which were inspired at least in part by experiences in New Zealand, Australia, Indonesia, Malaysia, The Republic of China, Thailand, India, and Egypt. She also acknowledged and cited the contributions to her thinking made by many noted scholars. She stated that she drew on the work of Carl Rogers (1959) for her definition of the self, and she used Mumford's (1970) notion of the human center as a starting point for the transpersonal process. Other ideas were stimulated by the works of Giorgi (1970), Whitehead (1953), de Chardin (1967), Kierkegaard (1846/1941), Taylor (1974), and Gadow (1980, 1984). Watson also acknowledged the contributions of Marcel, although she did not cite any of his works. In addition, she acknowledged the tenets of Eastern philosophy but did not cite specific scholars or publications.

Content of the Theory

Analysis of several chapters of Watson's 1985 book revealed that the main concepts of the Theory of Human Caring are *transpersonal caring* and *carative factors*.

Transpersonal Caring

Transpersonal caring is defined as "human-to-human connectedness . . . [whereby] each is touched by the human center of the other" (Watson, 1989a, p. 131). The concept has four components or dimensions: *self, phenomenal field, actual caring occasion of the patient and the nurse*, and *intersubjectivity*.

Watson (1985) identified various forms of the *self*: the self as it is, the ideal self that the person would like to be, and the spiritual self, which is synonymous with the geist or soul or essence of the person, and which is the highest sense of self. Quoting Rogers (1959, p. 200), she defined the self as

the organized consistent conceptual gestalt composed of perceptions of the characteristics of the "I" or "me" and the perceptions of the relationships of the "I" or "me" to others and to various aspects of life, together with the values attached to those perceptions. It is a fluid and changing gestalt, a process, but at any moment a specific entity. (p. 55)

The *phenomenal field* is made up of the "totality of human experience (one's being-in-the-world). [It] is the individual's frame of reference that can be known only to the person" (Watson, 1985, p. 55). Watson explained that the phenomenal field, which is the person's subjective reality, determines perceptions and responses in given situations in conjunction with the objective conditions or external reality.

The *actual caring occasion* of the patient and the nurse is the event when the caregiver and the recipient of care come together. Elaborating, Watson (1985) stated that this occasion "involves action and choice both by the nurse and the individual. The moment of coming together in a caring occasion presents the two persons with the opportunity to decide how to be in the relationship—what to do with the moment" (p. 59).

Intersubjectivity is not defined directly, but it is described through the adjective, transpersonal, in the concept *transpersonal caring*. Watson (1985) stated:

> Transpersonal refers to an intersubjective human-to-human relationship in which the person of the nurse affects and is affected by the person of the other. Both are fully present in the moment and feel a union with the other. They share a phenomenal field which becomes part of the life history of both and are coparticipants in becoming in the now and the future. Such an ideal of caring entails an ideal of intersubjectivity, in which both persons are involved. (p. 58)

Watson (1989a) further explained that the "intersubjective human flow from one to the other has the potential to allow the caregiver to become the care receiver" (p. 128).

Carative Factors

The second main concept of the Theory of Human Caring is **carative factors.** Carative factors are nursing interventions or caring processes. It should be noted that Watson (1985) finds the term "intervention" harsh, mechanical, and inconsistent with her ideas and ideals, but she used that term to describe carative factors for pedagogical purposes. The 10 carative factors identified by Watson (1979, 1985) are:

1. Formation of a humanistic-altruistic system of values
2. Instillation of faith-hope
3. Cultivation of sensitivity to one's self and to others
4. Development of a helping-trusting, human care relationship
5. Promotion and acceptance of the expression of positive and negative feelings

6. Systematic use of a creative problem-solving caring process
7. Promotion of transpersonal teaching-learning
8. Provision for a supportive, protective, and/or corrective mental, physical, societal, and spiritual environment
9. Assistance with gratification of human needs
10. Allowance for existential-phenomenological-spiritual forces

The first and most basic carative factor focuses on the development of a value system over the period of one's lifetime. A humanistic-altruistic value system, according to Watson (1979), "is a qualitative philosophy that guides one's mature life. It is the commitment to and satisfaction of receiving through giving. It involves the capacity to view humanity with love and to appreciate diversity and individuality" (p. 11). Watson (1989b) maintained that human caring is grounded on universal humanistic and altruistic values. Furthermore, she claimed that the best professional care is promoted when the nurse subscribes to such a value system.

The second carative factor underscores the therapeutic effects of faith and hope in both the carative and the curative process. Watson (1979) pointed out that the nurse must instill in the other person a sense of faith and hope about the treatment and the nurse's competence.

The third carative factor emphasizes the need to recognize one's feelings and to experience those feelings as a foundation for empathy with others. The development of sensitivity to self and others plays a part in the nurse's development of self, the ability to utilize the self with others, and the ability to give holistic care.

The fourth carative factor underscores the need to develop an effective interpersonal relationship with the one cared for. This is accomplished when the nurse views the other person as a separate thinking and feeling being. Watson (1979) maintained that the attitudinal processes of congruence, or genuineness, empathy, and nonpossessive warmth are essential elements of the helping-trusting relationship. She further maintained that a helping-trusting relationship is a basic element of high-quality nursing care.

The fifth carative factor highlights the importance of the expression of both positive and negative feelings and the nurse's acknowledgment and acceptance of those feelings in the self and in others.

The sixth carative factor focuses attention on the nursing process. Watson (1979, 1989b) views the nursing process as a creative problem-solving process encompassing assessing, planning, intervening, and evaluating. She pointed out that the process requires the "full use of self and all domains of knowledge, including empirical, aesthetic, intuitive, affective, and ethical knowledge" (1989b, p. 230).

The seventh carative factor highlights the processes used by both the nurse and the one cared for in the situation of health teaching. Both persons are regarded as coparticipants in the process of learning. Scanning, formulating, appraising, planning, implementing, and evaluating facilitate data gathering, decision making, and feedback as teaching and learning occur.

The eighth carative factor focuses attention on the external conditions or factors undergirding a supportive, protective, or corrective environment. Those factors are provision of comfort, privacy, safety, and clean aesthetic surroundings. Watson (1979) linked the provision of such an environment with the quality of holistic health care.

The ninth carative factor emphasizes the nurse's role in helping others in their activities of daily living as well as in fostering growth and development. Watson (1979, 1989b) identified and hierarchically ordered the needs she regarded as most relevant to nursing as human caring. The need for survival encompasses needs for food and fluid, elimination, and ventilation. The functional need includes activity-inactivity and sexuality. The integrative need is made up of achievement and affiliation needs. Finally, the growth-seeking need encompasses intrapersonal and interpersonal needs, spiritual development, and self-actualization.

The last carative factor underscores the separateness and identity of each person and the personal, subjective experience of each. Moreover, that factor emphasizes the importance of appreciating and understanding the inner world of each person and the meaning each one finds in life, as well as helping others find meaning in life. "Dealing with another as he or she *is* and in relation to what he or she would *like* to be or could be is," according to Watson (1979), "a matter of existential-phenomenological [and spiritual] concern for the nurse who practices the science of [human] caring" (p. 205).

Propositions

The definitions and descriptions of transpersonal caring and its dimensions and of carative factors are nonrelational propositions. Other nonrelational propositions represent an elaboration of the concept *transpersonal caring*. That concept is further defined and described in terms of relationships and transactions. A transpersonal caring relationship, according to Watson (1985),

> connotes a special kind of human care relationship—a union with another person—high regard for the whole person and their being-in-the-world. Caring, in this sense, is viewed as the moral ideal of nursing where there is the utmost concern for human dignity and preservation of humanity. Human care can begin when the nurse enters into the

life space or phenomenal field of another person, is able to detect the other person's condition of being (spirit, soul), feels this condition within him- or herself, and responds to the condition in such a way that the recipient has a release of subjective feelings and thoughts he or she had been longing to release. As such, there is an intersubjective flow between the nurse and patient. (p. 63)

The transactions or processes of transpersonal caring are viewed as both science and art. Watson (1985) explained:

Transpersonal human care and caring transactions are those scientific, professional, ethical, yet esthetic, creative and personalized giving-receiving behaviors and responses between two people (nurse and other) that allow for contact between the subjective world of the experiencing persons (through physical, mental, or spiritual routes or some combination thereof). (p. 58)

The following propositions underscore the emphasis Watson (1985) places on the art of the transpersonal caring process.

The art of transpersonal caring in nursing as a moral ideal is a means of communication and release of human feelings through the coparticipation of one's entire self in nursing. (p. 70)

Collectively, the art of transpersonal caring allows humanity to move towards greater harmony, spiritual evolution and perfection. (p. 70)

The more the art of transpersonal caring in nursing advances the kinder and more helpful feelings for the human, the more we can define ideal caring with reference to its content and subject matter of nursing. (p. 70)

The transpersonal caring process is largely art because of the way it touches another person's soul and feels the emotion and union with another, the goal being the movement of the person toward a higher sense of self and a greater sense of harmony within the mind, body, and soul. (p. 71)

Transpersonal caring transactions can, according to Watson (1985), expand human capacities and offer new opportunities to both the nurse and the patient. She explained that when the caring occasion is transpersonal and allows for the presence of the geist or spirit of both the nurse and the patient,

the event expands the limits of openness and has the ability to expand the human capacities. It thereby increases the range of certain events that could occur in space and time at the moment as well as in the future. The moment of the caring occasion becomes part of the past life history of both persons and presents both with new opportunities. (p. 59)

Elaborating on the expansion of human capacities through transpersonal caring, Watson (1988b) stated:

> Transpersonal caring expands the limits of openness and accesses the higher human spirit or field consciousness, therefore it has the capacity to expand human consciousness, transcend the moment, and potentiate healing. (p. 176)

Elaborating on consciousness in a brief overview of her theory, Watson (1992) recently stated, "Human caring-healing become relational, connected, transpersonal, and intersubjective, thereby opening up a higher energy field-consciousness that has metaphysical, spiritual, transcendent potentialities" (p. 1481). She went on to identify the following transpersonal caring-healing human field-consciousness phenomena:

> The whole caring-healing consciousness is contained in a single caring moment.
> The one caring and the one-being-cared-for are interconnected; caring-healing process is connected with other humans and to the higher energy of the universe.
> The caring-healing consciousness of the nurse is communicated to the one-being-cared-for.
> Caring-healing consciousness exists through time and space and is dominant over physical illness. (p. 1481)

Still other nonrelational propositions describe the taxonomy of *carative factors* as both hierarchical in nature, whereby each preceding factor contributes to the next one, and interacting to promote holistic nursing care. The hierarchical nature of the carative factors is evident in the following propositions:

> Faith-hope builds on and draws from a humanistic-altruistic value system to promote holistic professional care and produce positive health. The formation of a humanistic-altruistic value system and the instillation of faith-hope complement each other and further contribute to the third carative factor—the cultivation of sensitivity to one's self and to others. (Watson, 1979, p. 16)

> The development of a helping-trusting relationship [as well as the promotion and acceptance of the expression of positive and negative feelings] depends on the [first three] carative factors. (Watson, 1979, p. 23)

The interactive nature of the carative factors is evident in other propositions:

> Obviously all the factors interact for a holistic approach to understanding and studying nursing care. (Watson, 1979, p. 23).

> Promoting interpersonal teaching-learning . . . interacts with other carative factors in order to promote holistic health care. (Watson, 1979, p. 78)

> Practice of the carative factor assistance with the gratification of human needs, combined with the other carative factors, helps gratify higher order needs and provides the essence of what nursing ultimately seeks for quality health care. (Watson, 1979, p. 106)

The two major concepts of the theory of human caring are linked in a relational proposition asserting that *transpersonal caring* is accomplished through utilization of the *carative factors*. More specifically, Watson (1989b) explained that "Transpersonal caring is the full actualization of the carative factors in a human-to-human transaction" (p. 232).

EVALUATION OF THE THEORY OF HUMAN CARING

This section presents an evaluation of Watson's Theory of Human Caring. The evaluation is based on the results of the analysis of the theory as well as on publications by others who have used or commented on this nursing theory.

Significance

Although Watson did not explicity identify the metaparadigm concepts and proposition addressed by her theory, the metaparadigmatic origins could be inferred from her publications. She did, however, explicate the philosophical claims and conceptual orientation for the theory. Although she did not label the conceptual model content presented in the analysis section of this chapter as such, it was possible to extract components of a conceptual model from her writings. It must be noted, however, that the division of statements into philosophical claims and conceptual model seen in the analysis section required certain arbitrary decisions.

The significance of the Theory of Human Caring lies in the theory's contributions to understanding a process that nurses can use to effect positive changes in patients' health states. The theory is a comprehensive description of a form of caring that can be used by nurses as they interact with patients, or in Watson's terminology, the ones cared for, the care receivers.

The significance of the Theory of Human Caring also lies in Watson's rejection of people as objects. Instead, she embraces an orientation that emphasizes "new caring-healing possibilities associated with both the art and science of transpersonal caring-healing and transcendent views of persons in health and illness" (Watson, 1988b, p. 176). Watson's orientation leads to a form of nursing that "attends to the human center of both the one caring and the one being cared for" (p. 177).

A special feature of the theory is the attention given to the spiritual aspects of human existence and the soul. Another special feature of the Theory of Human Caring is the potential for personal growth by nurses as they engage in transpersonal caring relationships. Furthermore, through establishment of intersubjectivity, the caregiver can become the care receiver. Watson (1989a) explained:

> The one who is cared for (with expanded aesthetic caring processes) can experience a release of subjective feelings and thoughts that had been longing and wishing to be released or expressed. . . . Thus, both care provider and care receiver are coparticipants in caring; the release can potentiate self-healing and harmony in both. The release can also allow the one who is cared for to be the one who cares, through the reflection of the human condition that in turn nourishes the humanness of the care provider. (pp. 131–132)

Watson explicitly acknowledged and cited much of the knowledge she drew on from other disciplines, although she did not cite specific sources of adjunctive knowledge from Eastern philosophy. Sarter's (1988) philosophical analysis of Watson's theory revealed influences from Vedic, Hindu, and Buddhist philosophies. In addition, Sarter noted that Watson's portrayal of harmony among body, mind, and soul "may have been indirectly derived from some Eastern source such as Taoism" (p. 57).

Overall, the orientation that undergirds the Theory of Human Caring is a relatively new way of thinking about the world in Western society. That orientation is, however, in keeping with efforts that nurses have been making for several years to advance a science that reflects the complexities of human life. It is likely that not all members of nursing's scientific and clinical communities will agree with the orientation that guided Watson's work, but she should not be faulted for her efforts.

Internal Consistency

Sarter's (1988) philosophical analysis of the Theory of Human Caring raised a question regarding internal consistency. She pointed out that although Watson would undoubtedly describe her work as congruent with a holistic perspective, elements of dualism are evident. She identified dualism in Watson's distinctions between body, mind, and soul; objective and subjective experience; and health and illness. According to Sarter, "whenever Watson speaks of harmony among various aspects of human life, there is an implicit dualism" (p. 56).

Similarly, Mitchell and Cody (1992) noted that Watson presented inconsistent views of human beings. They pointed out that although Watson claimed that people are irreducible wholes, she also referred to several selves (real, inner, ideal) as distinct entities; to the mind, body, spirit, and soul; to physical, emotional, and spiritual spheres; and to the "I" and the "me." Watson (1992) apparently has attempted to overcome the charge of dualism and more effectively convey her idea of a holistic being by using the term "human mindbodyspirit" in a recent brief overview of her theory (p. 1481).

Mitchell and Cody (1992) also pointed out that Watson violated her claim that human beings are free to self-determine and choose. They explained:

> First, there are references to the nurse's helping, integrating, and "correcting" the patient's condition to increase harmony and to try to find meaning in the situation. Second, Watson maintains that "*ideally* [italics added], a person should have the opportunity for self-determination of the meaning of a health-illness experience *before professionals make decisions* [italics added] about treatments and interventions" (1985, p. 66). (p. 58)

Furthermore, although Watson claimed allegiance to the human science perspective, her distinction between the person's experience of the world and the world as it actually is, as well as her suggestion of incongruities between the person and nature, are inconsistent with the human science view that humans cannot be separated from their experienced worlds (Mitchell & Cody, 1992). In addition, Watson emphasized the metaphysical, spiritual realm, which Mitchell and Cody noted is inconsistent with the human science view that the lived experience is the "primal foundation of human knowledge" (p. 58).

Semantic clarity is evident in the definitions and descriptions Watson provided for the concepts of the theory and most of their dimensions. There is, however, some confusion about the precise definition of intersubjectivity because that term is defined only in conjunction with transpersonal caring.

Semantic consistency is evident in the consistent use of most terms. One area of potential confusion is, however, evident in the interchangeable use of the terms "transpersonal caring" and "human care relationship" throughout Watson's (1985) book and the subsequent discussion of the *components* of transpersonal caring as self, phenomenal field, actual caring occasion, and intersubjectivity (pp. 60–61) and the *concepts* of the human care relationship as phenomenal field, actual caring occasion, and transpersonal caring (p. 73). Another area of potential confusion is Watson's introduction of the hyphenated terms caring-healing (1988b), human caring-healing (1992), transpersonal caring-healing (1988b), caring-healing consciousness (1988b), and transpersonal caring-healing human field-consciousness (1992).

Evaluation of the structural consistency of the Theory of Human Caring revealed no evidence of contradictions in propositions. Moreover, the one relational proposition provides the necessary link between transpersonal caring and the carative factors.

Parsimony

Analysis of the Theory of Human Caring revealed that it is elegant in its simplicity and relative economy of words. Several readings of Watson's works were, however, required to identify the two main concepts and the propositions. Although Watson (1985) provided what she called a structural overview of the theory, she did not distinguish between the conceptual and theoretical elements of her work when she identified the subject matter, values, goals, agent of change, interventions, perspective, context, approach, and method. Moreover, the concepts and propositions of the theory were not listed explicitly in the subject matter section of the overview. Rather, Watson stated that the primary subject matter of the theory includes (1) nursing, (2) mutuality of person/self within a context of intersubjectivity, (3) the human care relationship, (4) health-illness, (5) environment, and (6) the universe.

Testability

The Theory of Human Caring is testable. In fact, Watson (1985) has presented a methodology for studying the theory. She maintained that the "optimal method for studying the theory is . . . through field study that is qualitative in design . . . a phenomenological-existential methodology" (p. 76). She then explained the method of empirical phenomenology and presented examples of descriptive phenomenological analysis and transcendental or depth phenomenology, the latter expressed in poetry. To her credit, Watson cautioned that a method should not supersede the research question. Thus although she encouraged investigators to consider "creative-paradigm transcending" (p. 76) methods that are consistent with human science, rather than methods that are more consistent with natural and medical sciences, she was not dogmatic about a particular method. This is an especially important point to consider as investigators struggle to identify the best ways to not only describe human life and human conditions from a human science perspective but also to further develop theories so that predictions may be made with some degree of certainty about the effects of nursing interventions on human life and human conditions from a human science perspective.

Holmes (1990) has questioned the generalizability of Watson's research methodology:

> Unfortunately, Watson adumbrates only one case [in her 1985 book], which concerns experiences of grief and loss among Aboriginal

people in Western Australia, and it requires a considerable leap of imagination to transpose the technique into other settings, particularly complex, urbanized ones. Nevertheless, it must be regarded as a courageous attempt to explore the phenomenological epoche as a practical tool for health care purposes, and is a powerful stimulus to innovation. (pp. 192–193)

Although a research methodology for the Theory of Human Caring has been proposed, the concepts and propositions of the theory have not yet been described in an empirically measurable manner. Moreover, no specific instruments associated with the theory have been published. Ykema (1991), however, presented a research proposal that included the development of a Caring Behaviors Assessment tool. She claimed that the instrument items are congruent with the carative factors. Furthermore, Stanfield (1992) developed the Caring Behaviors Assessment instrument, which is based on Watson's carative factors. Acknowledging the need for further work, Watson (1989b) stated, "The cognitive factors and the human process of caring need to be further delineated, expanded, and researched" (p. 227). In particular, operational definitions need to be developed for transpersonal caring and the 10 carative factors so that human caring can be observed in the real world of clinical practice.

Another approach to testing the Theory of Human Caring involves illustrations of human care and caring through art, metaphor, and poetry. Some examples of those forms of expression have been published (Krysl & Watson, 1988; Watson, 1990b).

Empirical Adequacy

The carative factors are grounded in a firm base of adjunctive philosophical and empirical knowledge that is described in detail in Watson's 1979 book. The outcomes of transpersonal caring through the carative factors, however, have not yet been fully documented empirically.

Clayton (1989) noted that although the findings of her phenomenological study of the caring transactions among four elderly person-nurse dyads were congruent with Watson's theory, more research is needed. Elaborating, she maintained that:

Key philosophical and moral ideals associated with the human-to-human caring process need to be further delineated. Additional exemplar cases need to be explored wherein events preceding and following caring transactions can be investigated. Caring needs of diverse populations and caring behaviors of nurses need study to determine goodness of fit. The spiritual dimension, a foundation to Watson's theory, has been scantily studied in nursing. Watson's ten carative factors need to be examined. (p. 251)

Some empirical studies have begun to provide evidence regarding the validity of the carative factors. Schindel Martin (1990) based her master's thesis research on Watson's carative factors and conducted a phenomenological study directed toward identification of the nursing acts that reflected instillation of faith-hope in a sample of seven patients undergoing long-term hemodialysis. She claimed that the findings supported Watson's theory and underscored the importance of the nurse-client interpersonal relationship. In another qualitative study, Schindel Martin (1991) used Watson's theory to guide an exploration of the experiences of adults with polycystic kidney disease. She focused on the subjects' expressions of their positive and negative thoughts about their kidney disease and discussed the implications of her findings for nursing practice within the context of Watson's theory.

Lemmer's (1991) study of parental perceptions of caring following a perinatal death was guided by five of Watson's carative factors: instillation of faith-hope, cultivation of sensitivity to one's self and others, development of a helping-trust relationship, promotion and acceptance of the expression of positive and negative feelings, and allowance for existential-phenomenological factors. Forrest (1991) pointed out that Lemmer's results "support Watson's (1985) theory of nursing and the growing body of literature on caring in nursing" (p. 491).

Swanson (1991) described the inductive derivation and validation of a middle-range theory of caring that encompasses five caring processes: knowing, being with, doing for, enabling, and maintaining belief. She discussed the parallels between those processes and Watson's carative factors and then noted that her theory "provides a meaningful base for why the carative factors . . . may be perceived as nurturing or helpful by nursing clients" (p. 165).

Burns (1991) found striking similarities between the elements of spirituality identified by her study participants and the description of spirituality found in Watson's theory. On the basis of her phenomenological study findings, Burns recommended that the Theory of Human Caring "needs to be expanded to include the study of the components of spirituality, particularly the depth experience, as it occurs in the everyday living of persons" (p. 151).

The Center for Human Caring at the University of Colorado fosters "the study, teaching, and practice of human caring" (Watson, 1990a, p. 47). Additional research conducted by Center-sponsored scholars and other investigators is needed to establish or refute the validity of the Theory of Human Caring.

Pragmatic Adequacy

Nursing Education

A commitment to transpersonal caring, according to Watson (1988b), is a moral ideal and a standard for nursing care. The delivery of nursing care based on the Theory of Human Caring requires considerable education to better understand the expanded view of nursing, science, person, and health-illness that is reflected in the theory (Watson, 1990b). In fact, Watson (1988a) proposed that professional nursing education be at the postbaccalaureate level of the Doctorate of Nursing (ND), and such a program was established at the University of Colorado in 1990 (Watson & Phillips, 1992).

The nature of human life, according to Watson (1988a), is the subject matter of nursing. Hence nursing education focuses on clarification of the values and views regarding human life. A moral context for nursing education that emphasizes a way of being as a caring professional is required. In particular, a curriculum based on the Theory of Human Caring acknowledges caring as a moral ideal and incorporates philosophical theories of human caring, health, and healing. The humanities, social-biomedical science, and human caring content and process are regarded as core areas of content.

Six areas of knowledge that are needed to engage in human care have been identified (Watson, 1989b):

1. Knowledge of human behavior and human responses to actual or potential health problems.
2. Knowledge and understanding of individual needs.
3. Knowledge of how to respond to others' needs.
4. Knowledge of our strengths and limitations.
5. Knowledge of the meaning of the situation for the person.
6. Knowledge of how to comfort, offer compassion and empathy. (p. 227)

In addition, Watson (1988a) claimed that new approaches to studying the concepts of caring are needed, such as courses using art, music, literature, poetry, drama, and movement to facilitate understanding of responses to health and illness as well as to new caring-healing modalities. Thus considerable change in the typical curriculum of most schools of nursing would be required.

The curriculum of the ND program at the University of Colorado serves as an exemplar. The 4-year curriculum of that program is made up of a clinical sciences core, a clinical arts and humanities caring core, a discipline-specific human caring nursing core, a health professional and ethical foundation core, and a 1 calendar year full-time professional practice residency (Watson & Phillips, 1992).

Nursing Practice

Human caring, according to Watson (1990b), is required when curing is possible, but especially when curing has failed. Drawing on Gaut's (1983) philosophical analysis of caring, Watson (1989b) noted that the provision of human care through application of the carative factors requires "an intention, caring values, knowledge, a will, a relationship, and actions" (p. 227). Elaborating on actions, Watson (1989b) explained that the provision of human care "requires enabling actions—that is, actions that allow another to solve problems, grow, and transcend the here and now, actions that are related to general and specific knowledge of caring and human responses" (p. 227).

Holistic nursing practice based on the Theory of Human Caring requires the integration of all 10 carative factors. Watson (1979) explained, "No one factor can be effective alone. The student nurse and the practicing nurse must continue to integrate the factors that effect positive health care" (p. 214).

Nursing practice based on the Theory of Human Caring is not necessarily easy. Indeed, Watson (1989a) pointed out that human caring, "with its need for ethics, emotions, compassion, knowlege, wisdom, intentions, and so on, is always fragile and threatened because it requires a personal, social, moral, and spiritual engagement of self and a commitment to one*self* and to others' *self* and dignity" (p. 129). Thus "a radical transformation of traditional professional relationships" is required (p. 132). Furthermore, nurses must continuously "question and be open to new possibilities" (Watson, 1992, p. 1481).

Despite the potential difficulty in using the Theory of Human Caring, evidence of its utility is beginning to emerge. Jones (1991) based her AIDS educational model for preadolescents on Watson's theory. More specifically, she developed a comprehensive teaching guide for AIDS education based on the carative factors. Jones maintained that "caring may be the key link in helping to educate preadolescents about AIDS in all settings: schools, community, clinic[s,] and hospitals" (p. 596).

In addition, Lyne and Waller (1990) described the Denver Nursing Project in Human Caring (DNPHC), which is a nurse-managed center devoted to the care of persons with human immunodeficiency virus (HIV) infections. Nursing practice at the DNPHC is based on Watson's philosophy and science of human caring, and care is delivered through the carative factors. The personal and professional growth experienced by one of the authors as a result of working at the DNPHC was described, but the acceptability and influence of Theory of Human Caring–based nursing care on the HIV-positive clients and their significant others remains to be documented.

Sithichoke-Rattan (1989) found that Watson's theory provided an appropriate framework for understanding the nursing care of preterm infants and their parents. She pointed out, however, that the effects of actual nursing care based on Watson's theory must be determined in various areas of nursing practice.

Aucoin-Gallant (1990) described the use of the carative factors in nursing practice. Although empirical evidence was not offered, the author claimed benefits for both caregivers and care receivers, stating that "when incorporated into a treatment plan, the factors can help clients and their families develop a sense of responsibility and control over illness-induced stress. For nurses, the [theory] can be a source of motivation and job satisfaction" (p. 35).

Collectively, those publications provide initial evidence of the pragmatic adequacy of the Theory of Human Becoming. The theory is appropriate for various clinical problems. Furthermore, the feasibility of implementing clinical protocols is evident, and clinicians have the legal ability to implement nursing actions based on the carative factors. The extent to which carative factors–based actions are compatible with expectations for nursing practice and the effects of those actions on care receivers and caregivers requires further consideration.

CONCLUSION

Watson has made a substantial contribution to nursing by explicating a new form of nursing care. Her work clearly reflects her commitment "to preserve and restore the human mindbodyspirit in theory and practice" (Watson, 1992, p. 1481).

Evidence of the empirical and pragmatic adequacy of the Theory of Human Caring is beginning to accrue. Investigators and clinicians need to continue to compile evidence so that the validity of the theory and its utility in nursing practice can be fully determined.

In closing, Walker (1989) raised a particularly intriguing issue regarding Watson's notion of caring: "That is whether caring is equally the moral ideal for all helping relationships: minister-sinner, doctor-patient, therapist-client. If so, then Watson's work is relevant to all these relationships not just nurse-patient ones" (p. 154). As Walker pointed out, this point requires clarification so the distinctive contribution of Watson's work to nursing knowledge and the possible contribution of that work to the knowledge base of other disciplines can be determined.

REFERENCES

Aucoin-Gallant, G. (1990). La théorie du caring de Watson. Une approache existentielle-phénoménologique et spirituelle des soins infirmiers. *The Canadian Nurse, 86*(11), 32–35.

Burns, P. (1991). Elements of spirituality and Watson's theory of transpersonal caring: Expansion of focus. In P. L. Chinn (Ed.), *Anthology on caring* (pp. 141–153). New York: National League for Nursing.

Clayton, G. M. (1989). Research testing Watson's theory: The phenomena of caring in an elderly population. In J. P. Riehl-Sisca, *Conceptual models for nursing practice* (3rd ed., pp. 245–252). Norwalk, CT: Appleton and Lange.

de Chardin, T. (1967). *On love.* New York: Harper and Row.

Forrest, D. (1991). Commentary [on "Parental perceptions of caring following perinatal bereavement."] *Western Journal of Nursing Research, 13,* 491–492.

Gadow, S. (1980). Existential advocacy: Philosophical foundation of nursing. In S. Spicker & S. Gadow (Eds), *Nursing images and ideals: Opening dialogue with the humanities* (pp. 79–101). New York: Springer.

Gadow, S. (1984, March). *Existential advocacy as a form of caring: Technology, truth, and touch.* Paper presented to the Research Seminar Series: The Development of Nursing as a Human Science. University of Colorado School of Nursing, Denver.

Gaut, D. A. (1983). Development of a theoretically adequate description of caring. *Western Journal of Nursing Research, 5,* 313–324.

Giorgi, A. (1970). *Psychology as a human science.* New York: Harper and Row.

Holmes, C. A. (1990). Alternatives to natural science foundations for nursing. *International Journal of Nursing Studies, 27,* 187–198.

Jones, S. B. (1991). A caring-based AIDS educational model for pre-adolescents: Global health human caring perspective. *Journal of Advanced Nursing, 16,* 591–596.

Kierkegaard, S. (1941). *Concluding unscientific postscript* (New ed., H. J. Patton, Trans.). Princeton, NJ: Princeton University Press. (Original work published in 1846)

Krysl, M., & Watson, J. (1988). Existential moments of caring: Facets of nursing and social support. *Advances in Nursing Science, 10*(2), 12–17.

Lemmer, C. M., Sr. (1991). Parental perceptions of caring following perinatal bereavement. *Western Journal of Nursing Research, 13,* 475–493.

Lyne, B. A., & Waller, P. R. (1990). The Denver Nursing Project in Human Caring: A model for AIDS nursing and professional education. *Family and Community Health, 13,* 78–84.

Mitchell, G. J., & Cody, W. K. (1992). Nursing knowledge and human science: Ontological and epistemological considerations. *Nursing Science Quarterly, 5,* 54–61.

Mumford, L. (1970). *The myth of the machine: The pentagon of power.* New York: Harcourt Brace Jovanovich.

Rogers, C. R. (1959). A theory of therapy, personality, and interpersonal relationships as developed in the client-centered framework. In S. Koch (Ed.), *Psychology: A study of a science* (Vol. 3, pp. 184–256). New York: McGraw-Hill.

Sarter, B. (1988). Philosophical sources of nursing theory. *Nursing Science Quarterly, 1,* 52–59.

Schindel Martin, L. J. (1990). A phenomenological study of faith-hope in aging clients undergoing long-term hemodialysis. *Masters Abstracts International, 28,* 583.

Schindel Martin, L. (1991). Using Watson's theory to explore the dimensions of adult polycystic kidney disease. *American Nephrology Nurses' Association Journal, 18,* 493–496.

Sellers, S. C. (1991). A philosophical analysis of conceptual models of nursing. *Dissertation Abstracts International, 52,* 1937B. (University Microfilms No. AAC9126248)

Sithichoke-Rattan, N. (1989). A clinical application of Watson's theory. *Pediatric Nursing, 15,* 458–462.

Stanfield, M. H. (1992). Watson's caring theory and instrument development. *Dissertation Abstracts International, 52,* 412B.

Swanson, K. M. (1991). Empirical development of a middle-range theory of caring. *Nursing Research, 40,* 161–165.

Taylor, R. (1974). *Metaphysics.* Englewood Cliffs, NJ: Prentice-Hall.

Walker, L. O. (1989). Book review of Watson, J. (1985). *Nursing: Human science and human care. A theory of nursing. Nursing Science Quarterly, 2,* 153–154.

Watson, J. (1979). *Nursing: The philosophy and science of caring.* Boston: Little, Brown.

Watson, J. (1985). *Nursing: Human science and human care: A theory of nursing.* Norwalk, CT: Appleton-Century-Crofts. Reprinted 1988. New York: National League for Nursing.

Watson, J. (1988a). Human caring as moral context for nursing education. *Nursing and Health Care, 9,* 422–425.

Watson, J. (1988b). New dimensions of human caring theory. *Nursing Science Quarterly, 1,* 175–181.

Watson, J. (1989a). Human caring and suffering: A subjective model for health sciences. In R. L. Taylor & J. Watson (Eds.), *They shall not hurt. Human suffering and human caring* (pp. 125–135). Boulder, CO: Colorado Associated University Press.

Watson, J. (1989b). Watson's philosophy and theory of human caring in nursing. In J. P.

Riehl-Sisca, *Conceptual models for nursing practice* (3rd ed., pp. 219–236). Norwalk, CT: Appleton and Lange.

Watson, J. (1990a). Human caring: A public agenda. In J. S. Stevenson & T. Tripp-Reimer (Eds.), *Knowledge about care and caring. State of the art and future developments* (pp. 41–48). Kansas City, MO: American Academy of Nursing.

Watson, J. (1990b). Transpersonal caring: A transcendent view of person, health, and nursing. In M. E. Parker (Ed.), *Nursing theories in practice* (pp. 277–288). New York: National League for Nursing.

Watson, J. (1992). Window on theory of human caring. In M. O'Toole (Ed.), *Miller-Keane encyclopedia & dictionary of medicine, nursing, & allied health* (5th ed., p. 1481). Philadelphia: W. B. Saunders.

Watson, J., & Phillips, S. (1992). A call for educational reform: Colorado nursing doctorate model as exemplar. *Nursing Outlook, 40,* 20–26.

Whitehead, A. N. (1953). *Science and the modern world.* Cambridge: Cambridge University Press.

Ykema, M. (1991, April). *Importance of nurse caring behaviors as perceived by post-myocardial infarction patients and ICU nurses: A comparison.* Paper presented at the Samaritan Health Service Fourth Annual Nursing Research Conference, Phoenix, AZ.

ANNOTATED BIBLIOGRAPHY

Primary Sources

Watson, J. (1979). *Nursing: The philosophy and science of caring.* Boston: Little, Brown. [Second printing, 1985. Boulder, CO: Colorado Associated University Press.]
Watson presents the 10 carative factors and discusses the underlying philosophical premises and empirical evidence for each factor.

Watson, J. (1981). Some issues related to a science of caring for nursing practice. In M. Leininger (Ed.), *Caring: An essential human need* (pp. 61–67). Thorofare, NJ: Slack.
Watson discusses her ideas about caring and identifies the carative factors. The chapter is from a presentation at the First National Caring Conference, held in Salt Lake City, Utah, in 1978. The content is drawn from Watson's book, *Nursing: The philosophy and science of caring,* which had not been published at the time of the conference.

Watson, J. (1985). *Nursing: Human science and human care.* Norwalk, CT: Appleton-Century-Crofts. [Second printing, 1988. Boulder, CO: Colorado Associated University Press. Third printing, 1988. New York: National League for Nursing.]
Watson presents her theory of human caring in considerable detail. Her chapter on methodology includes the results of one study using the method of descriptive phenomenology and another study using the method of transcendental or depth phenomenology.

Watson, J. (1988). New dimensions of human caring theory. *Nursing Science Quarterly, 1,* 175–181.
Watson discusses the changing nature of nursing. She maintains that shifting directions toward a new consciousness of human caring and healing guide and direct nursing's future and offer a hopeful paradigm for the future of health care. She claims that a moral ideal of human caring that raises new questions and reverses the traditional medical treatment model is emerging. Watson introduces a caring ethic in relation to transpersonal caring theory that allows for new epistemologies and ontologies of being, such as evolution of consciousness and transcendence.

Watson, J. (1989). Watson's philosophy and theory of human caring in nursing. In J. P. Riehl-Sisca, *Conceptual models for nursing practice* (3rd ed., pp. 219–236). Norwalk, CT: Appleton & Lange.
Watson describes her theory of human caring and the philosophical assumptions upon which the theory is based.

Watson, J. (1990). Transpersonal caring: A transcendent view of person, health, and nursing. In M. E. Parker (Ed.), *Nursing theories in practice* (pp. 277–288). New York: National League for Nursing.
> Watson discusses applications of the theory of human caring and presents examples of caring found in poetry and art.

Watson, J. (1992). Window on theory of human caring. In M. O'Toole (Ed.), *Miller-Keane encyclopedia & dictionary of medicine, nursing, & allied health* (5th ed., p. 1481). Philadelphia: W. B. Saunders.
> Watson provides a very brief overview of her theory.

Commentary by Watson and Others

Bennett, P. M., Porter, B. D., & Sloan, R. S. (1989). Jean Watson: Philosophy and science of caring. In A. Marriner-Tomey, *Nursing theorists and their work* (2nd ed., pp. 164–173).
> Porter, B. D., & Sloan, R. S. (1986). Jean Watson: Philosophy and science of caring. In A. Marriner, *Nursing theorists and their work* (pp. 160–168). St. Louis: C. V. Mosby.
> In each edition, the authors describe Watson's academic and experiential credentials and present a rudimentary analysis of her theory. They also include a cursory critique of the theory.

Boyd, C., & Mast, D. (1989). Watson's model of human care. In J. J. Fitzpatrick & A. L. Whall, *Conceptual models of nursing: Analysis and application* (2nd ed., pp. 371–383). Norwalk, CT: Appleton & Lange.
> Boyd and Mast describe Watson's theory, present an analysis of the theory, and briefly discuss its relation to nursing research, education, and practice.

Brenner, P. (1986). Disseminating care research literature. *Journal of Nursing Administration, 16*(1), 26–27.
> Concerned with nursing service administrators' involvement in care research, Brenner examined key nursing reports published in a leading nursing administration journal. Based on Watson's and Leininger's works, a content analysis of 63 articles and two reports reviewed revealed that care was never used as the major independent or dependent variable but rather appeared as an intervening variable related to job satisfaction and/or job stability. The need for research on care is addressed.

Cohen, J. A. (1991). Two portraits of caring: A comparison of the artists, Leininger and Watson. *Journal of Advanced Nursing, 16*, 899–909.
> Cohen explores the themes of caring presented by Watson and Leininger, along with their views of the nature of nursing, use of theory development strategies, and their contributions to nursing knowledge development.

Mitchell, G. J., & Cody, W. K. (1992). Nursing knowledge and human science: Ontological and epistemological considerations. *Nursing Science Quarterly, 5*, 54–61.
> Mitchell and Cody define and describe human science from Dilthey's perspective. They conclude that Watson's emphasis on the metaphysical, spiritual realm clouds the issue of primacy of the lived experience and, therefore, is inconsistent with human science.

Morse, J. M., Solberg, S. M., Neander, W. L., Bottorff, J. L., & Johnson, J. L. (1990). Concepts of caring and caring as a concept. *Advances in Nursing Science, 13*(1), 1–14.

Morse, J. M., Bottorff, J., Neander, W., & Solberg, S. (1991). Comparative analysis of conceptualizations and theories of caring. *Image: Journal of Nursing Scholarship, 23*, 119–126.
> The authors explain that Watson's perspective of caring reflects a conceptualization of caring as a moral imperative. They point out that Gadow, Fry, and Brody also view caring in that manner. Other conceptualizations of caring are as a human trait, an affect, an interpersonal interaction, and a therapeutic intervention. Their analysis revealed that Watson regards caring as unique to nursing and affecting both nurse and patient. Caring, in Watson's view, is not a behavioral task, and the caring intent does not vary between patients. In their 1990 paper, the authors note that the depth of the nurse-patient relationship required by Watson's theory may be impossible to attain in brief encounters and with unconscious or cognitively impaired patients.

Norris, C. M. (1989). To care or not care. Questions! Questions! *Nursing and Health Care, 10,* 545–550.

Norris explains how the stereotyping of nurses as not caring parallels the increasingly technologic orientation of patient care. The author reflects on the recent care initiative as a defense against the rigor of scientific practice. The human caring value within the context of health care raises social and economical issues. The author expresses concerns about the conceptual and operational definition of care and challenges Leininger's and Watson's assertions that caring is a central focus of the discipline. The marketability of caring and implications for research are presented.

Neil, R. M., & Watts, R. (Eds.). (1991). *Caring and nursing: Explorations in feminist perspectives.* New York: National League for Nursing.

This edited book contains papers presented at a 1988 conference sponsored by the Doctoral Student Group and the Center for Human Caring at the University of Colorado School of Nursing. Chapters by Sharon Horner and Carol Green-Hernandez present their models of caring, which are derived in part from Watson's work.

Ryan, L. G. (1989). A critique of nursing: Human science and human care. In J. P. Riehl-Sisca, *Conceptual models for nursing practice* (3rd ed., pp. 237–244). Norwalk, CT: Appleton & Lange.

Ryan presents a brief critique of Watson's theory, including internal evaluation of its elements and external evaluation of its utility and significance.

Sarter, B. (1988). Philosophical sources of nursing theory. *Nursing Science Quarterly, 1,* 52–59.

Sarter explains that the key philosophical elements of Watson's theory are soul, dualism, harmony, causality and time, spiritual evolution and self-transcendence, actual caring occasion, and self. She then identifies the philosophic sources of those elements.

Smerke, J. M. (1990). Ethical components of caring. *Critical Care Nursing Clinics of North America, 2,* 509–513.

Consistent with Watson's and Leininger's works on caring, Smerke posits that caring is the ethical foundation for nursing. Factors such as specialization and the development of science and technology have eroded the meaning and notion of caring. Using the critical care context, Smerke describes the ethical dilemmas that critical care nurses face and maintains that nursing must bridge advancing technology with human caring.

Smith, M. C. (1991). Existential-phenomenological foundations in nursing: A discussion of differences. *Nursing Science Quarterly, 4,* 5–6.

Smith discusses the existential and phenomenological foundations of several nursing theories. She points out that Watson's theory includes the tenets of freedom, subjectivity, intersubjectivity, and meaning of experience.

Talento, B. (1990). Jean Watson. In J. B. George (Ed.), *Nursing theories: The base for professional nursing practice* (3rd ed., pp. 293–309). Norwalk, CT: Appleton & Lange.

Talento identifies Watson's academic and experiential credentials and describes and analyzes her theory. She also presents a brief application of the theory within the context of the nursing process.

Taylor, R. L., & Watson, J. (Eds.). (1989). *They shall not hurt: Human suffering and human caring.* Boulder, CO: Colorado Associated University Press.

The titles of the chapters in this edited book are: Introduction (by the editors); Compassion, Caring, and Religious Response to Suffering; Compassion: A Critique of Moral Rationalism; Human Suffering in Comparative Perspective; Woman's Answer to Job; Medical-Ethical Perspectives on Human Suffering; The Severely Physically Disabled: A Subjective Account of Suffering; and Human Caring and Suffering: A Subjective Model for Health Sciences (by Watson). In her chapter, Watson explains that human caring and humanities encompass subjectivity and expressivity and that they both approach human existence from a reflective and internal perspective. She claims that there is no hope without shared suffering or joy.

Torres, G. (1986). *Theoretical foundations of nursing.* Norwalk, CT: Appleton-Century-Crofts.

Torres presents a brief description and an evaluation of Watson's theory. She also describes the application of the theory within the context of the nursing process framework of assessment, diagnosis, planning, implementation, and evaluation.

Updike, P. (1991). The other side of the polished doors. In P. L. Chinn (Ed.), *Anthology on caring* (pp. 133–140). New York: National League for Nursing.
Updike explains that the carative factors of sensitivity to self and others and existential-phenomenological-spiritual forces were exemplified in her experience of seeing and attending to a small boy lying on his back on a sidewalk outside the WHO building in Manila.

Vezeau, T. M., & Schroeder, C. (1991). Caring approaches: A critical examination of origin, balance of power, embodiment, time and space, and intended outcome. In P. L. Chinn (Ed.), *Anthology on caring* (pp. 1–16). New York: National League for Nursing.
The authors include brief descriptions of the caring perspectives of Watson, Mayeroff, Noddings, Buber, Jonas, and Audubon.

Watson, J. (1981). The lost art of nursing. *Nursing Forum, 20*, 244–249.
In this article, Watson reflects on nursing practice. A discussion on how nursing science must integrate scientific and artistic/humanistic knowledge follows. Finally, Watson expresses her concerns with nursing's failure to claim its scientific knowledge.

Watson, J. (1981). Nursing's scientific quest. *Nursing Outlook, 29*, 413–416.
Concerned with nursing's scientific progress, Watson presents the historical and philosophical influences on nursing theory development. The scientific assumptions of the Received View are discussed and analyzed. Watson identifies the dichotomies nursing has created in practice, research, and theory development. Several nursing leaders' views about nursing practice, theory, and research are compared. The author suggests the need for a new research tradition in nursing.

Watson, J. (1987). Academic and clinical collaboration: Advancing the art and science of human caring. *Communicating Nursing Research, 20*, 1–16.
Watson provides a multidimensional perspective for advancing the art and science of human caring in the world of academe, the health care system, and in society. She acknowledges pressing epistemic issues facing nursing in science and society. Dimensions affecting the advancement of the art and science of human caring are discussed. Finally, the academic and clinical-research collaborative model developed at the University of Colorado is described. The paper was presented at the 1987 Western Society for Research in Nursing Conference held in Tempe, Arizona.

Watson, J. (1987). Nursing on the caring edge. Metaphorical vignettes. *Advances in Nursing Science, 10*(1), 10–18.
Watson attempts to convey some enduring truths about nursing on the caring edge of evolutionary human consciousness. She uses selected literary and poetic metaphorical vignettes to depict the tacit, expressive elements of caring in nursing that give it an evolutionary edge in the health care system and in society.

Watson, J. (1988). Human caring as moral context for nursing education. *Nursing and Health Care, 9*, 422–425.
Watson proposes that a moral context, based on a contextual human science, should be included in advanced professional education. She describes initiatives taken by the University of Colorado School of Nursing to develop a new health and human caring science model as well as a new educational model for the preparation of professional nurses.

Watson, J. (1990). Caring knowledge and informed moral passion. *Advances in Nursing Science, 13*(1), 15–24.
Watson contends that caring knowledge should be incorporated into the nursing metaparadigm. The paper is based on an address at the 1989 Forum on Doctoral Education in Nursing.

Watson, J. (1990). Human caring: A public agenda. In J. S. Stevenson & T. Tripp-Reimer (Eds.), *Knowledge about care and caring: State of the art and future developments* (pp. 41–48). Kansas City, MO: American Academy of Nursing.
Watson discusses the revolution in health care and maintains that human science and human caring represent a renaissance. She contends that the postmodern era requires a balance between cure and care. The paper was originally presented at a Wingspread Conference held in February 1989.

Watson, J. (1990). The moral failure of the patriarchy. *Nursing Outlook, 38,* 62–66.
    Watson claims that caring is essentially invisible and is regarded as women's work.
    She contends that the failure to recognize the value of caring demands a health care
    revolution that will require society to give up what no longer works. The paper is
    based on Watson's keynote address at the American Academy of Nursing Scientific
    Session in October 1989.

Watson, J. (1992). Notes on nursing. Guidelines for caring then and now. In F. Nightingale,
    Notes on nursing: What it is, and what it is not (Commemorative edition, pp. 80–85).
    Philadelphia: J.B. Lippincott. (Original work published in 1859).
    Watson explains how Nightingale's wisdom is part of nursing's caring theory and
    elaborates on how the carative factors are consistent with Nightingale's call for a val-
    ues-based approach to nursing and the oneness of mindbodyspirit.

Watson, J., & Ray, M. A. (1988). *The ethics of care and the ethics of cure: Synthesis in chro-
    nicity.* New York: National League for Nursing.
    This edited book presents discussions of how advances in technology have pushed
    caring into the background; why caring is an end in itself, rather than a fall-back posi-
    tion; how problems of misdiagnosis and ineffective communication can be handled;
    and the implications of the failure to comprehend the human dimension of what it
    means to have cancer. The papers were presented at a conference co-sponsored by
    the University of Colorado Center for Human Caring and the Hastings Center.

Practice

Aucoin-Gallant, G. (1990). La théorie du caring de Watson. Une approache existentielle-
    phénoménologique et spirituelle des soins infirmiers. *The Canadian Nurse, 86*(11),
    32–35. [English abstract].
    The author describes Watson's carative factors and describes their use in nursing
    practice. She comments that use of the carative factors can help clients and their fam-
    ilies develop a sense of responsibility and control over illness-induced stress, and can
    provide a source of motivation and job satisfaction for nurses.

Jones, S. B. (1991). A caring-based AIDS educational model for preadolescents: Global
    health human caring perspective. *Journal of Advanced Nursing, 16,* 591–596.
    Jones describes a teaching intervention about AIDS for preadolescents based on Wat-
    son's carative factors.

Karns, P. S. (1991). Building a foundation for spiritual care. *Journal of Christian Nursing,
    8*(3), 10–13.
    Karns describes Watson's view of spirituality and presents her own view of interac-
    tional spiritual care.

Lyne, B. A., & Waller, P. R. (1990). The Denver Nursing Project in Human Caring: A model
    for AIDS nursing and professional education. *Family and Community Health, 13,* 78–
    84.
    Based on Watson's work, this article presents a model of care, the Caring Center,
    which provides AIDS care, allows the implementation of nursing theory in practice,
    and fosters a caring environment for educating health care providers. The authors
    describe the client services, professional education, and a graduate student's expe-
    rience at the Denver Nursing Project in Human Caring.

Neil, R. M. (1990). Watson's theory of caring in nursing: The rainbow of and for people
    living with AIDS. In M. E. Parker (Ed.), *Nursing theories in practice* (pp. 289–301). New
    York: National League for Nursing.
    Neil describes the Denver Nursing Project in Human Caring, which is based on Wat-
    son's theory of human caring. The Project is devoted to caring for clients with AIDS
    and those who are HIV positive.

Schroeder, C., & Maeve, M. K. (1992). Nursing care partnerships at the Denver Nursing
    Project in Human Caring: An application and extension of caring theory in practice.
    Advances in Nursing Science, 15(2), 25–38.
    Schroeder and Maeve describe the history and recent advances in the application of
    Watson's theory at the Denver Nursing Project in Human Caring, which is a nurse-
    managed center for people with HIV/AIDS. The nursing care partnership, which is
    defined as a care-enabling method that aims to establish authentic caring relation-

ships between clients and nurses for the goal of mutual empowerment, has recently been implemented. They include narrative accounts of the partnerships from both clients and nurses.

Sithichoke-Rattan, N. (1989). A clinical application of Watson's theory. *Pediatric Nursing, 15,* 458–462.
   The author describes Watson's theory and its application in a pediatric setting. The principles, as reflected in the 10 carative factors, are used to guide the nursing care of premature infants and their parents.

Education

Bevis, E. O., & Watson, J. (1989). *Toward a caring curriculum: A new pedagogy for nursing.* New York: National League for Nursing.
   This edited book contains a chapter by Watson describing her ideas regarding curricula for professional nursing education based on the philosophical foundations of human freedom, self-reflection, and transformative thinking, and another chapter dealing with her theory of human caring.

Bunkers, S. S., Brendtro, M., Holmes, P. K., Howell, J., Johnson, S., Koerner, J., Larson, J., Nelson, J., & Weaver, R. (1992). The healing web. A transformative model for nursing. *Nursing and Health Care, 13,* 68–73.
   The Healing Web is a model designed to integrate nursing education and nursing service and to bring together private and public educational programs for baccalaureate and associate degree nursing. The project involved the Augustana College Department of Nursing, Sioux Valley Hospital Department of Nursing, and the University of South Dakota Department of Nursing and School of Medicine. Watson's theory provided some of the content for the project philosophy, conceptual framework, and outline of the nurse's caring capabilities.

Forsyth, D., Delaney, C., Maloney, N., Kubesh, D., & Story, D. (1989). Can caring behavior be taught? *Nursing Outlook, 37,* 164–166.
   The authors describe the nursing curriculum at Luther College in Decorah, Iowa, which is based in part on Watson's carative factors. The basic curricular concept is caring, which the faculty members believe provides a balance between the art and science of nursing.

Hagell, E. I. (1989). Nursing knowledge: Women's knowledge. A sociological perspective. *Journal of Advanced Nursing, 14,* 226–233.
   The author presents Leininger's contribution to the current perspectives on nursing and Watson's description of nursing knowledge. Several suggestions for change and improvement in nursing education are outlined.

Leininger, M., & Watson, J. (Eds.). (1990). *The caring imperative in education.* New York: National League for Nursing.
   This edited book contains the papers presented at the 11th National/International Caring Conference held in Denver, Colorado, in 1989. The conference themes of education about caring and caring in the educational process are well represented in the 26 chapters.

Roberts, J. E. (1990). Uncovering hidden caring. *Nursing Outlook, 38,* 67–69.
   Roberts contends that the currently hidden characteristics of caring should be uncovered so that they may be recognized, rewarded, and taught to students. She cites Watson with regard to the invisibility of caring. The paper is based on Roberts's presentation at the American Academy of Nursing Scientific Session in October 1989.

Sakalys, J. A., & Watson, J. (1985). New directions in higher education: A review of trends. *Journal of Professional Nursing, 1,* 293–299.
   The authors review six reports on the quality of education in the United States, including Adler's Paideia Proposal on elementary and secondary education, Bok's and the Association of American Medical Colleges' reports on medical education, the National Institute of Education's report on the quality of undergraduate education, the National Endowment for the Humanities' report on the humanities in higher education, and the Association of American Colleges' report on baccalaureate education. Sakalys and Watson conclude that the baccalaureate degree is no longer adequate for

professional education and recommend postbaccalaureate education for the first professional degree in nursing.

Sakalys, J. A., & Watson, J. (1986). Professional education: Postbaccalaureate education for professional nursing. *Journal of Professional Nursing, 2*, 91–97.

The authors claim that professional studies should occur only after the completion of an undergraduate liberal arts curriculum and recommend that the first professional degree in nursing be postbaccalaureate. They also describe the organizational structure of the University of Colorado School of Nursing.

Tanner, C. A. (1990). Caring as a value in nursing education. *Nursing Outlook, 38,* 70–72.

Tanner contends that caring should be a core value in the curriculum. She cites Watson's work as having a major influence on the curriculum revolution resulting in the centrality of caring. The article is based on Tanner's presentation at the American Academy of Nursing Scientific Session in October 1989.

Watson, J. (1982). Traditional vs. tertiary ideological shifts in nursing education. *Australian Nurses' Journal, 12*(2), 44–46, 64.

Since American nursing education has moved from the hospitals to tertiary institutions, nursing has developed a more professional identity. Watson explains how the ideological differences between the traditional hospital-based nursing "training" and tertiary-based nursing education have influenced nursing education and, consequently, nursing practice knowledge. She addresses the effects of such a movement into tertiary-based programs on improving Australian nursing.

Watson, J. (1988). A case study: Curriculum in transition. In *Curriculum revolution: Mandate for change* (pp. 1–8). New York: National League for Nursing.

Watson describes the Doctorate of Nursing (ND) program at the University of Colorado in her presentation at the National League for Nursing's Fourth National Conference on Nursing Education. The conference initiated discussion of the revisions in nursing curricula required for the contemporary and future health care system.

Watson, J. (1988). The professional doctorate in nursing. In *Perspectives in nursing—1987–1989* (pp. 41–47). New York: National League for Nursing.

Watson discusses the plans for the Doctorate of Nursing (ND) program at the University of Colorado in a paper delivered at the National League for Nursing's 1987 Biennial Convention.

Watson, J. (1990). Transformation in nursing: Bringing care back to health care. In *Curriculum revolution: Redefining the student-teacher relationship* (pp. 15–20). New York: National League for Nursing.

Watson maintains that caring must be the central value to guide health care policy. The paper draws from Watson's address at the 1989 American Academy of Nursing Scientific Session (c.f. annotation in Commentary section for Watson, J. [1990]. The moral failure of the patriarchy. *Nursing Outlook, 38,* 62–66) and was presented at the Sixth National Conference on Nursing Education sponsored by the National League for Nursing.

Watson, J., & Bevis, E. O. (1990). Nursing education: Coming of age for a new age. In N. L. Chaska (Ed.), *The nursing profession. Turning points* (pp. 100–106). St Louis: C. V. Mosby.

Watson and Bevis describe postbaccalaureate nursing programs in health and human caring. They recommend that the Doctorate of Nursing (ND) be the first professional degree in nursing.

Watson, J., & Phillips, S. (1992). A call for educational reform: Colorado nursing doctorate model as exemplar. *Nursing Outlook, 40,* 20–26.

Watson and Phillips describe the postbaccalaureate Doctor of Nursing (ND) program currently offered at the University of Colorado School of Nursing.

Research

Burns, P. (1991). Elements of spirituality and Watson's theory of transpersonal caring: Expansion of focus. In P. L. Chinn (Ed.), *Anthology on caring* (pp. 141–153). New York: National League for Nursing.

Burns reports the results of her study on the metaphysical concept of spirituality. She found that the lived experience of spirituality in the well adult is the process of striving for and/or being infused with the reality of the interconnectedness among the self, other human beings, and the Infinite, that occurs during a depth, or crisis, experience. Burns draws parallels between the essential elements of spirituality and Watson's concept of transpersonal caring.

Chipman, Y. (1991). Caring: Its meaning and place in the practice of nursing. *Journal of Nursing Education, 30,* 171–75.

The author is an instructor at St. Francis Medical Center School of Nursing, which has based the curriculum on Watson's Theory of Human Caring. The article is a report of a qualitative study designed to clarify the meaning and value of caring in nursing practice as perceived by second-year diploma nursing students. Giving of self, meeting patients' needs in a timely fashion, and providing comfort measures for patients and their families emerged as the three categories of caring nurse behaviors.

Clayton, G. M. (1989). Research testing Watson's theory: The phenomena of caring in an elderly population. In J. P. Riehl-Sisca, *Conceptual models for nursing practice* (3rd ed., pp. 245–252). Norwark, CT: Appleton & Lange.

Clayton reports the findings of a study of the caring needs of the institutionalized elderly, as identified in interviews with four nurse-elderly person dyads. Data analysis revealed four themes that are consistent with Watson's carative factors: feelings of heightened sensitivity to own feelings prior to and following the caring interaction; the existence of a helping-trusting relationship; a supportive, protective, and permissive environment; and existential forces.

Hegyvary, S. T. (1987). Collaboration in nursing research: Advancing the science of human care. *Communicating Nursing Research, 20,* 17–22.

In her keynote address at the 1987 Western Society for Research in Nursing Conference held in Tempe, Arizona, Hegyvary discusses how nurses can further advance the science of human care and the types of collaboration necessary to promote those advances.

Hinds, P. S. (1984). Inducing a definition of hope through the use of grounded theory methodology. *Journal of Advanced Nursing, 9,* 357–362.

Drawing from the different conceptualizations of hope by Watson, Travelbee, and Roberts, the author describes how the grounded theory methodology has guided the definition of hope. Twenty-five adolescents (both well and hospitalized) participated in the study. The definition of hope was used to demonstrate the rules that have been put forth in the social science literature to guide the formulation of construct definitions. Steps to link the processes of conceptualization with those of measurement were suggested.

Krysl, M., & Watson, J. (1988). Existential moments of caring: Facets of nursing and social support. *Advances in Nursing Science, 10*(2), 12–17.

This paper presents Krysl's work on her subjective experiences about the day-to-day lives of patients and nurses in a cross-section of health care situations and circumstances. Five poems, based on Watson's work on caring, convey existential moments that reflect the art and science of nursing.

Lemmer, C. M. (1991). Parental perceptions of caring following perinatal bereavement. *Western Journal of Nursing Research, 13,* 475–494.

Lemmer reports the results of her study of bereaved parents' perceptions of nurses' and physicians expressions of caring, which was based on Watson's theory of human caring. Two main categories emerged: taking care of and caring for or about. Taking care of refers to activities undertaken by health care providers that were designed to meet the physiological and safety needs of mother and/or baby, and the informational needs of family members. Subcategories were providing expert care and providing information. Caring for or about refers to activities undertaken by care providers that demonstrated to parents a sensitivity to and an empathic awareness of the emotional pain of bereavement and a desire to help them through it. Subcategories were providing direct emotional support, providing individualized, family-centered care, acting as a surrogate parent, facilitating the creation of memories, and respecting the rights of parents.

Martin, L. S. (1991). Using Watson's theory to explore the dimensions of adult polycystic kidney disease. *American Nephrology Nurses' Association Journal, 18,* 493–496.

Martin reports the results of her study of the experiences of persons with adult polycystic kidney disease (APKD) and their at-risk family members, which was based on Watson's theory of human caring. The four major themes identified were: knowledge about APKD and the process through which it is acquired, attitudes toward APKD, attitudes toward genetic testing, and family planning decisions. Martin concludes that, in keeping with Watson's theory, nurses must use sensitivity to assist the clients to explore the desire for information, must assist the clients to understand the meaning of an experience, and must suspend judgment and listen to the clients' words to assist them to make personal decisions.

Smerke, J. M. (1989). *Interdisciplinary guide to the literature for human caring.* New York: National League for Nursing.

This book contains a comprehensive bibliography of the literature on human caring found in the areas of psychoneuroimmunology, sociobehavioral sciences, anthropology, fine arts, philosophy, ethics, theology, and nursing. In the preface, Watson explains that the book is a direct outgrowth of interdisciplinary collaborative projects sponsored by the University of Colorado Center for Human Caring.

Stember, M., & Hester, N. K. (1990). Research strategies for developing nursing as the science of human care. In N. L. Chaska (Ed.), *The nursing profession: Turning points* (pp. 165–172). St Louis: C. V. Mosby.

The authors maintain that the preferred solution to the debate concerning qualitative and quantitative paradigms for research dealing with the science of human care is the transcendent paradigm. They describe that paradigm as viewing the nature of reality as singular and multiple, objective and subjective, and particularistic and holistic; the nature of truth as a stable and dynamic world; and valuing individual uniqueness as well as generalizations across individuals.

Swanson, K. M. (1991). Empirical development of a middle range theory of caring. *Nursing Research, 40,* 161–166.

Swanson describes a middle-range theory of caring that emerged from three phenomenological studies in perinatal contexts. She comments that her findings provide a base for why Watson's carative factors may be perceived as nurturing or helpful by nursing clients.

Watson, J. (1983). Commentary on "The IDIR model for faculty research with students." *Western Journal of Nursing Research, 5,* 310–311.

Watson explains how the Instructor Directed Research Model could facilitate the research demands in the university system. Concerned about nursing attitudes that experimental design is the "top-dog" in research methodology, the author emphasizes the need for nursing to adopt a methodology consistent with a human science perspective.

Watson, J. (1985). Reflections on different methodologies for the future of nursing. In M. M. Leininger (Ed.), *Qualitative research methods in nursing* (pp. 343–349). New York: Grune and Stratton.

In this chapter, Watson presents nurses' dilemma in knowledge discovery about nursing phenomena. The continuation and alternative paths are compared and contrasted. According to the author, the alternative path is congruent with nursing's tradition of human care. New methodological approaches that incorporate features of human care are suggested.

Watson, J. (1988). Response to "Caring and practice: Construction of the nurse's world." *Scholarly Inquiry for Nursing Practice, 2,* 217–221.

Watson responds to an article by David Kahn and Richard Stevens reporting the results of their study of the meaning for nurses of the caring relationship between nurses and patients. She notes that the report is an excellent example of the state-of-the-art approaches to and complexities of caring research. She concludes that further research is needed to answer questions about the extent to which the moral ideal of caring is actually incorporated into nursing practice.

Watson, J. (1990). Response to "Reconceptualizing nursing ethics." *Scholarly Inquiry for Nursing Practice, 4,* 219–221.

Watson responds to Mary Cooper's analysis of the four central concepts of moral theory, including autonomy, moral posture, universal versus particular, and the role of rules and principles. She notes that Cooper's analysis is based on an ethic of care and feminism, with heavy reliance on Gilligan's work.

Watson, J. (1992). Response to "Caring, virtue theory, and a foundation for nursing ethics." *Scholarly Inquiry for Nursing Practice, 6,* 169–171.

Watson responds to Pamela Salsberry's examination of virtue theory as a foundation for a nursing ethic embodied in the ideal of caring. She notes that Salsberry's contention that virtue theory does not offer a viable alternative to ethical theories grounded in duty requires further dialectic discourse. Watson claims that the notion of caring as a moral ideal remains underdeveloped.

Watson, J., Burckhardt, C., Brown, L., Bloch, D., & Hester, N. (1979). A model of caring: An alternative health care model for nursing practice and research. In *American Nurses' Association clinical and scientific sessions* (pp. 32–44). Kansas City: American Nurses' Association.

This article describes a health caring model for nursing based on a philosophy and structure of caring. Basic premises, generalizations, and definitions of caring are presented. Specific components of a professional model are discussed from a caring perspective. Informal empirical findings related to caring confirmed some general theoretical and philosophical notions as well as served to clarify the concept of caring. Implications for further research are discussed.

Doctoral Dissertations

Chen, Y-C. (1989). A Taoist model for human caring: The lived experiences and caring needs of mothers with children suffering from cancer in Taiwan. *Dissertation Abstracts International, 49,* 3101B.

Fazzone, P. A. (1991). Caring for abused and neglected children on inpatient child psychiatric units: A cross-sectional ethnography. *Dissertation Abstracts International, 52,* 1951B.

Leners, D. W. (1990). The deep connection: An echo of transpersonal caring. *Dissertation Abstracts International, 51,* 2818B.

Smerke, J. M. (1989). The discovery and creation of the meanings of human caring through the development of a guide to the caring literature. *Dissertation Abstracts International, 49,* 4236B.

Smith, J. S. (1990). Implications for values education in health care systems: An exploratory study of nurses in practice. *Dissertation Abstracts International, 50,* 3449A.

Stanfield, M. H. (1992). Watson's caring theory and instrument development. *Dissertation Abstracts International, 52,* 412B.

Stiles, M. K. (1989). The shining stranger: A phenomenological investigation of the nurse-family spiritual relationship. *Dissertation Abstracts International, 49,* 4236B–4237B.

Master's Theses

Harrison, B. P. (1988). Development of the caring behaviors assessment based on Watson's theory of caring. *Masters Abstracts International, 27,* 95.

Hutcherson, G. J. (1991). Nurses' perceptions of the use of prayer to instill faith and hope. *Masters Abstracts International, 30,* 299.

Nowicki, M. E. (1991). Knowledge, attitudes, and intervention strategies of nurse managers in dealing with employees who refuse to care for AIDS patients. *Masters Abstracts International, 30,* 300.

Schindel-Martin, L. J. (1990). A phenomenological study of faith-hope in aging clients undergoing long-term hemodialysis. *Masters Abstracts International, 28,* 583.

CHAPTER

9

Testing Nursing Theories

The ultimate goal of theory development in professional disciplines such as nursing is the empirical testing of interventions that are specified in the form of predictive middle-range theories. It is, however, still important to test theories that have not yet reached the precision of interventions. In other words, it is important to test grand theories, descriptive middle-range theories, and explanatory middle-range theories. In this chapter, various approaches to testing grand and all types of middle-range nursing theories are discussed.

The terms associated with theory testing are listed below. Each term is defined and described in this chapter.

KEY TERMS

Theory Testing	Personal Experiences
Grand Theories	Critical Reasoning
Middle-Range Theories	Problem Solving
Approaches to Theory Testing	
Traditional Empiricism	

THEORY TESTING

Theory testing is defined as "one or more processes through which one verifies whether what was purported or experienced is indeed so, or whether what was purported or experienced solves problems of significance in one's discipline or practice" (Silva & Sorrell, 1992, p. 14). That definition indicates that more than one approach can be used to test nursing theories and permits consideration of the different ways to test *grand theories* and *middle-range theories*.

Different approaches are needed to test grand and middle-range theories because the two vary in scope. Recall from Chapter 1 of this book that grand theories are broader in scope than middle-range theories. Grand theories are substantively nonspecific, and their concepts are written at a relatively abstract level of discourse. Middle-range theories, in contrast, are substantively specific, and their concepts are written at a relatively concrete level of discourse.

Even more to the point of this chapter, because of their abstract nature, the concepts of grand theories lack operational definitions, and their propositions are not amenable to direct empirical testing. In contrast, the concepts of middle-range theories typically have operational definitions, and their propositions can be tested empirically.

Inasmuch as grand theories cannot be operationalized, empirical approaches cannot be applied to grand theories in a direct manner. Instead, grand theories can be empirically tested only in an indirect manner, through the testing of middle-range theories that were derived from the grand theories.

APPROACHES TO TESTING NURSING THEORIES

With the foregoing distinctions between grand theories and middle-range theories in mind, attention is turned to formal theory testing. Four **approaches to testing nursing theories** have been identified: *traditional empiricism, descriptions of personal experiences, critical reasoning*, and *problem solving*.

Traditional Empiricism

The most frequently cited approach to theory testing can be called *traditional empiricism*. The goal of traditional empiricism is to determine if what is purported to be so is, in fact, so. Emphasis is, therefore, placed on evaluating the validity or empirical adequacy of the theory.

Traditional empiricism requires the identification of empirical indicators for theory concepts and the conduct of a descriptive, correlational, or experimental study designed to determine if what the theory asserts is empirically demonstrated. The criteria used to evaluate the report of the theory-testing work, which were adapted from criteria identified by Silva (1986) and Fawcett (1989), are as follows:

- Theory testing is an explicit goal of the research.

- The middle-range theory is explicitly identified as the underlying guide for the study.
- The middle-range theory is discussed in sufficient breadth and depth so that the relationship between the theory and the research question(s) is clear.
- The study methodology reflects the middle-range theory:
    The study subjects are drawn from a population that is appropriate for the focus of the theory.
    The instruments are appropriate empirical indicators of the middle-range theory concepts.
    The study design clearly reflects the focus of the middle-range theory.
    The data analysis techniques are in keeping with the focus of the middle-range theory.
- The data are interpreted in terms of evidence regarding the middle-range theory concepts and propositions.
- Discussion of research findings includes explicit conclusions regarding the empirical adequacy of the middle-range theory.

Traditional empiricism is admittedly quantitative and is appropriate only as a direct test of descriptive, explanatory, and predictive middle-range theories. It can be used to test grand theories, but only indirectly. More specifically, traditional empiricism can be used to test middle-range theories that were purposefully derived from the grand theory. Evidence regarding the empirical adequacy of the middle-range theory is then used to draw conclusions about the validity of the grand theory concepts and propositions. If the evidence supports the empirical adequacy of the middle-range theory, it is appropriate to conclude that the grand theory is valid. If, however, the evidence does not support the empirical adequacy of the middle-range theory, the validity of the grand theory must be questioned.

Orlando (1972) used traditional empiricism to determine the empirical adequacy of her theory. That approach has also been applied to Peplau's (1952) theory.

Description of Personal Experiences

A variation of the traditional empiricism approach to theory testing that can be especially effective for grand theories is *description of personal experiences*. Like traditional empiricism, the description of personal experiences approach is an empirical method of theory testing, but it permits a more direct test of the validity of the grand theory than does the traditional empiricism approach. As implied by the label for the approach, emphasis is placed on the analysis of individuals' personal experiences with regard to a phenomenon encompassed by a grand theory. The product is "generalities that constitute the substance of [middle-range] nursing theories" (Silva & Sorrell, 1992, p. 19).

The personal experiences approach employs empirical inductive strategies to generate middle-range theories. More specifically, it requires selection of a phenomenon that is represented by the grand theory content and an inductive, qualitative research methodology that is in keeping with the philosophical claims and content of the grand theory.

The criteria used to draw conclusions regarding the validity of a grand theory using the description of personal experiences approach, which were adapted from criteria proposed by Silva and Sorrell (1992), are:

- The research questions elaborate the grand theory concepts and propositions at the middle-range theory level.
- The research method is qualitative and inductive.
- The research methodology is congruent with the philosophical claims of the grand theory.
- The primary data sources include sufficient in-depth descriptions of personal experiences to capture the essence of the phenomenon under investigation.
- The data may come from multiple personal experiences of an individual and/or similar personal experiences of several individuals.
- The data are analyzed and interpreted in terms of the grand theory concepts and propositions.
- Explicit conclusions are drawn regarding the congruence of the study findings with the concepts and propositions of the grand theory.

Although the description of personal experiences approach provides evidence regarding the validity of grand theories, the potential for circular reasoning exists. In particular, if data are always interpreted in light of the grand theory, it may be difficult to "see" results that are not in keeping with that theory. Indeed, the potential for circular reasoning exists whenever theory testing is limited to the use of an inductive research methodology that is associated with a grand theory. More specifically, if researchers constantly uncover, describe, and interpret personal experiences through the lens of the grand theory, the outcome may be limited to expansion of the grand theory (Ray, 1990). Therefore, unless alternative theories are considered when interpreting data or the data are critically examined for both their fit and nonfit with the grand theory, circular reasoning will occur, and the grand theory will be uncritically perpetuated. Circular reasoning can be avoided if the data are carefully examined to determine the extent of their congruence with the concepts and propositions of the grand theory, as well as from the perspective of alternative grand theories (Platt, 1964).

The description of the personal experiences approach is similar to the research methodologies developed by Leininger (1991), Newman (1990), and Parse (1992). Newman advocated using interviews to elicit descriptions of phenomena that represent patterns of expanding consciousness; Leininger described the qualitative, inductive method of ethnonursing to identify cultural values, meanings, and actions; and Parse described a qualitative, inductive technique to identify lived experiences of health.

Critical Reasoning

Silva and Sorrell (1992) described a nonempirical approach to theory testing that can be used with all kinds of theories. That approach, which they termed *critical reasoning*, is an intellectual activity that emphasizes an internal critique of a theory's strengths and limitations. More specifically, the critical reasoning approach "highlights strengths and exposes problems inherent in a line of reasoning" (Silva & Sorrell, 1992, p. 17).

The result of application of the critical reasoning approach is a descriptive, analytical, and critical commentary that enhances understanding of the theory and can lead to refinements in the theory concepts and propositions (Meleis, 1991). The commentary should address the following criteria, which were adapted from a list given by Silva and Sorrell (1992):

- The explicitly stated purpose of the commentary is to test the theory through a process of critical reasoning.
- The criteria used to guide the commentary are discussed in sufficient breadth and depth so that a comparable critique can be undertaken by other scholars.
- The philosophical claims undergirding the theory are examined.
- The content of the theory is examined and judged with regard to its congruence with the philosophical claims.
- The content of the theory is judged with regard to internal consistency, including clarity of terms, consistency in the use of the meanings for the same terms throughout the discussion of the theory, lack of redundant terms, and a logically connected set of propositions.
- The potential of the theory for further theory development efforts is evaluated.
- The evidence regarding the utility of the theory for such

practical activities as education and clinical practice is examined.
- Explicit conclusions are drawn regarding ambiguities, internal consistency flaws, and the pragmatic adequacy of the theory.

The critical reasoning approach does not address the empirical adequacy of the theory, which makes it especially appropriate for grand theories. When that approach is applied to a grand theory, emphasis may be placed on the potential of the theory to guide the development of middle-range theories. Individuals whose philosophical allegiance is to empiricism could then use the traditional empiricism approach to examine the results of testing the derived middle-range theories and draw conclusions with regard to the indirect evidence of the empirical adequacy of the grand theory.

The critical reasoning approach is reflected in the analysis and evaluation of each theory presented in this book. The approach is also evident in several other books, including those edited by Fitzpatrick and Whall (1989), George (1990), and Marriner-Tomey (1989).

The Problem-Solving Approach

The *problem-solving* approach to theory testing is an evaluation of the outcomes from using a theory in the real world of clinical practice. That approach emphasizes the problem-solving effectiveness of a theory and seeks to determine "whether what is purported or experienced accomplishes its purpose" (Silva & Sorrell, 1992, p. 19).

The problem-solving approach to theory testing is based on the position that theories are developed "to solve human and technical problems and to improve practice" (Kerlinger, 1979, p. 280). Although theory is "the most important source of influence on practice" (Kerlinger, 1979, p. 296), practice can influence theory. Theory and practice are, then, intertwined in an ongoing reciprocal relationship. Figure 9–1 depicts that reciprocal relationship for the professional discipline of nursing. There it can be seen that a professional discipline—nursing in this case—has two primary dimensions: inquiry and practice. The dimension of inquiry, which ranges from thoughtful reflection to empirical evaluation of clinical intervention protocols, is concerned with theory development. The dimension of practice, which encompasses all practical activities, is concerned with theory utilization. A reciprocal relationship is evident in that practical problems catalyze inquiry and the results of inquiry provide solutions for the problems. The reciprocal relationship is also evident at an operational level in that the clinical protocols derived from theories developed through various

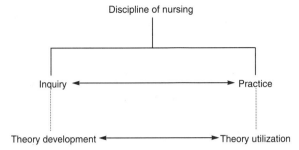

Figure 9-1. The professional discipline of nursing: reciprocal relationships between inquiry and practice and theory development and theory utilization.

forms of inquiry are used in the practice arena and the outcomes of the utilization of the protocols are used to refine the theory.

The reciprocal relationship between theory development and theory utilization is evident in the following comment made by Chinn and Kramer (1991):

> One way that theory challenges existing practice is that it provides new ways to think about problems. Thinking about a problem or a situation in a new or different way makes it possible for practitioners to envision new approaches to practice. Since theories are not sets of rules, but are tentative, practice also challenges theory. . . . People who do research and develop theories learn to think differently about theoretic problems and issues as they perceive the realities of practice. (p. 162)

The problem-solving approach requires what Chinn and Kramer (1991) called a "deliberate application" of a theory. They explained that the application

> involves using research methods to demonstrate how a theory affects nursing practice, . . . places the theory within the context of practice to ensure that it serves the goals of the profession, . . . [and] provides evidence of the theory's usefulness in ensuring quality of care. (p. 167)

The problem-solving approach can be used with all types of theories but is most effective when applied to predictive middle-range theories. In that case, the theory-testing effort seeks to determine the effects of interventions specified in predictive middle-range theories on the health status of the persons who receive the interventions (Hegyvary, 1992). In the case of grand theories, as well as descriptive and explanatory middle-range theories, the focus of the theory-testing effort using the problem-solving approach frequently is "to ascertain if the theory [actually] can be applied in practice" (Chinn & Kramer, 1991, p. 167).

The criteria used to determine the problem-solving effectiveness of nursing theories, which were adapted from criteria identified by Silva and Sorrell (1992), are:

- The theory is applied in the real world of clinical practice.
- The explicitly stated purpose of the application is to demonstrate the problem-solving effectiveness of the theory for nursing practice.
- The theory is explicitly identified as the framework for the application.
- The application is designed so that comparisons can be made between outcomes of use of the theory and outcomes in the same situation when the theory was not used.
- The problems and outcomes addressed are regarded as significant by nurse clinicians.
- Outcomes are measured in terms of the problem-solving effectiveness of the theory.
- Explicit conclusions are drawn with regard to how the theory was instrumental in defining and implementing problem-solving strategies.

The critical examination of the use of a nursing theory in practice represents a very important advance in the clinical scholarship of the professional discipline of nursing. Paraphrasing Speedy (1989), the impact of nursing theories will continue to be limited when the theories are not grounded in the realities of practice. Emphasis should, therefore, be placed on selection of outcomes used to measure the problem-solving effectiveness of a theory that are especially meaningful to nurse clinicians. The outcomes may go beyond those proposed by the theory, such as nursing care recipients' health status and their perceptions of the quality of care received, to encompass such organizational outcomes as continuity and efficiency of nursing care, cost-effectiveness, and nurse satisfaction (Chinn & Kramer, 1991).

Orlando's (1972) clinically based study of the effectiveness of the deliberative nursing process in identifying and meeting the patient's need for help is one outstanding example of the use of the problem-solving approach. Another example, which yielded both positive and negative outcomes, was Bristow and Callaghan's (1991) test of Peplau's (1952) theory in an English psychiatric hospital. Still another example is Lyne and Waller's (1990) description of the use of Watson's (1985) theory at a nurse-managed center.

CONCLUSION

Repeated tests of nursing theories, from the nonempirical method of critical reasoning to the determination of problem-solving effectiveness, is required prior to the widespread adoption of clinical protocols derived from the theories. Thus theory testing is an essential component of theory development. No theory, no matter how appealing it might be, can be considered valid until it is subjected to repeated formal tests by using one or more of the approaches discussed in this chapter. As noted in Chapters 3 through 8, continued testing of the nursing theories included in this book is required before the validity of the theories can be firmly established or the theories can be refuted. Nurses are, therefore, urged to select one or more appropriate methods from among the four approaches to theory testing discussed in this chapter and test the theories in which they have the most interest.

REFERENCES

Bristow, F., & Callaghan, P. (1991). Using Peplau's model in affective disorders. *Nursing Times, 87*(18), 40–41.

Chinn, P. L., & Kramer, M. K. (1991). *Theory and nursing: A systematic approach* (3rd ed.). St. Louis: C. V. Mosby.

Fawcett, J. (1989). *Analysis and evaluation of conceptual models of nursing* (2nd ed.) Philadelphia: F. A. Davis.

Fitzpatrick, J. J., & Whall, A. L. (1989). *Conceptual models of nursing: Analysis and application* (2nd ed.). Norwalk, CT: Appleton and Lange.

Hegyvary, S. T. (1992, June). *From truth to relativism: Paradigms for doctoral education.* Paper presented at the Annual Forum on Doctoral Nursing Education, Baltimore, MD.

George, J. B. (Ed.). (1990). *Nursing theories: The base for professional nursing practice* (3rd ed.). Norwalk, CT: Appleton and Lange.

Kerlinger, F. N. (1979). *Behavioral research: A conceptual approach.* New York: Holt, Rinehart and Winston.

Leininger, M. M. (1991). Ethnonursing: A research method with enablers to study the theory of culture care. In M. M. Leininger (Ed.), *Culture care diversity and universality. A theory of nursing* (pp. 73–117). New York: National League for Nursing.

Lyne, B. A., & Waller, P. R. (1990). The Denver Nursing Project in Human Caring: A model for AIDS nursing and professional education. *Family and Community Health, 13,* 78–84.

Marriner-Tomey, A. (1989). *Nursing theorists and their work* (2nd ed.). St. Louis: C. V. Mosby.

Meleis, A. I. (1991). *Theoretical nursing: Development and progress* (2nd ed.). Philadelphia: J. B. Lippincott.

Newman, M. A. (1990). Newman's theory of health as praxis. *Nursing Science Quarterly, 3,* 37–41.

Orlando, I. J. (1972). *The discipline and teaching of nursing process (An evaluation study).* New York: G. P. Putnam's Sons.

Parse, R. R. (1992). Human becoming. Parse's theory of nursing. *Nursing Science Quarterly, 5,* 35–42.

Peplau, H. E. (1952). *Interpersonal relations in nursing: A conceptual frame of reference for psychodynamic nursing.* New York: G. P. Putnam's Sons.

Platt, J. R. (1964). Strong inference. *Science, 146,* 347–353.

Ray, M. A. (1990). Critical reflective analysis of Parse's and Newman's research methodologies. *Nursing Science Quarterly, 3,* 44–46.

Silva, M. C. (1986). Research testing nursing theory: State of the art. *Advances in Nursing Science, 9*(1), 1–11.

Silva, M. C., & Sorrell, J. M. (1992). Testing of nursing theory: Critique and philosophical expansion. *Advances in Nursing Science, 14*(4), 12–23.

Speedy, S. (1989). Theory-practice debate: Setting the scene. *Australian Journal of Advanced Nursing, 6*(3), 12–20.

Watson, J. (1985). *Nursing: Human science and human care.* Norwalk, CT: Appleton-Century-Crofts.

ANNOTATED BIBLIOGRAPHY

Chinn, P. L., & Kramer, M. K. (1991). *Theory and nursing: A systematic approach* (3rd ed.). St. Louis: C. V. Mosby.
  The authors describe the four processes required to create an empiric theory: creating conceptual meaning, structuring and contextualizing theory, generating and testing theoretic relationships, and deliberative application of the theory to demonstrate how the theory affects nursing practice.
Kerlinger, F. N. (1979). *Behavioral research: A conceptual approach.* New York: Holt, Rinehart, and Winston.
  Kerlinger contends that the purpose of basic research is to develop theory, whereas the purpose of applied research is to solve particular human and technical problems or to improve practice. He explains that research findings never tell clinicians what to do but rather may influence their ways of thinking, perceiving, and reacting. He also explains that basic research typically is not directly applicable to practical problems, and that although applied research is applicable, the findings rarely have a lasting impact because such studies are driven by specific and relatively narrow goals that change as new problems arise.
Lindsay, B. (1990). The gap between theory and practice. *Nursing Standard, 5*(4), 34–35.
  Lindsay contends that the gap between theory and practice is unavoidable, but not undesirable, because a gap can be regarded as an indication of growth, development, and progression. He explains that the gap exists because theory constantly sets new goals for practice through the development of new concepts and ideas intended for health care improvements.
Meleis, A. I. (1991). *Theoretical nursing: Development and progress* (2nd ed.). Philadelphia: J. B. Lippincott.
  Meleis contends that nursing science requires a close relationship between theory, research, and practice and that theoreticians, researchers, and clinicians all share the goal of understanding the health care needs of clients. She then identifies and describes five strategies for theory development: theory-practice-theory, practice-theory, research-theory, theory-research-theory, and practice-theory-research-theory.
Platt, J. R. (1964). Strong inference. *Science, 146,* 347–353.
  Platt describes the pitfalls of the single hypothesis approach to theory testing and urges scientists to generate and test multiple competing hypotheses derived from different theories in every study. He contends that that approach eliminates errors in interpreting research findings that might be due to the investigator's intellectual or emotional commitment to a particular theory.
Silva, M. C. (1986). Research testing nursing theory: State of the art. *Advances in Nursing Science, 9*(1), 1–11.
  Silva reports the results of her analysis of 62 studies based on nursing models or theories, including the works of Johnson, Roy, Orem, Rogers, and Newman. She identifies three ways in which researchers have used conceptual models or theories to guide their studies: minimal, insufficient, or adequate. Silva reported that 24 of the 62 studies reflected minimal use; 29, insufficient use; and 9, adequate use. She concluded that the impediments to adequate use of a model or theory to guide research include lack of investigator commitment to explicitly test a nursing model or theory, lack of tolerance of such methodological imperfections in the model or theory as abstractness and imprecision, and lack of systematic retrieval strategies to locate relevant studies due to the failure of investigators to identify the nursing model or theory in the study title or abstract.
Silva, M. C., & Sorrell, J. M. (1992). Testing of nursing theory: Critique and philosophical expansion. *Advances in Nursing Science, 14*(4), 12–23.
  Silva and Sorrell critique Silva's 1986 article, with emphasis on her criteria for ade-

quate use of nursing models or theories to guide nursing research. Following a discussion of the correspondence, coherence, and pragmatic philosophic theories of truth, they offer criteria for three alternative approaches to testing nursing models and theories: critical reasoning, description of personal experiences, and application to nursing practice. The three approaches provide alternatives to the more traditional empirical testing of models and theories.

Speedy, S. (1989). Theory-practice debate: Setting the scene. *Australian Journal of Advanced Nursing, 6*(3), 12–20.

Speedy explains the relationship between theory and practice and examines the meaning of the statement that "theory informs and transforms practice by informing and transforming the ways in which practice is experienced and understood."

Appendix_____

AUDIO PRODUCTIONS

The Second Annual Nurse Educator Conference

Audio tapes available from Teach 'em, Inc., 160 E. Illinois Street, Chicago, IL 60611. [Tapes are no longer available from the distributor.]

Audio tapes of the papers presented at the Nurse Educator Conference held in New York, New York, in December 1978. Presentations are by Leininger; Newman; Johnson; King; Levine; Orem; Paterson and Zderad; Rogers; and Roy. A presentation by Dickoff and James was also taped.

Nurse Theorist Conference

Audio tapes available from Kennedy Recordings, RR5, Edmonton, Alberta, Canada T5P 4B7

Audio tapes of the papers presented at the Nurse Theorist Conference held in Edmonton, Alberta, Canada, in August 1984. Presenters include Newman, King, Levine, Rogers, and Roy.

Nursing Theory in Action

Audio tapes available from Kennedy Recordings, RR5, Edmonton, Alberta, Canada T5P 4B7

Audio tapes of the papers and concurrent sessions on applications to practice, research, and education presented at the Nursing Theory in Action Conference held in Edmonton, Alberta, Canada, in August 1985. Presenters include Newman, Parse, King, Levine, Neuman, Orem (pre-

263

sented by S. Taylor), Rogers, and Roy. In addition, a presentation on the Roper/Logan Tierney Framework also is available.

Nursing Theory Congress, 1986

Audio tapes available from Audio Archives International, 100 West Beaver Creek, Unit 18, Richmond Hill, Ontario, Canada L4B 1H4

Audio tapes of the papers and concurrent sessions on applications to practice, research, and education presented at the Nursing Theory Congress, "Theoretical Pluralism: Direction for a Practice Discipline," held in Toronto, Ontario, Canada, in August 1986. Presentations are by Parse; King; Levine; Neuman; Rogers; Roy; Holaday (Johnson's model); Taylor (Orem's framework); Allen (a developmental health model); Kritek (nursing diagnosis); Dickoff and James (theoretical pluralism); and McGee (criteria for selection and use of a nursing model for practice).

Nursing Theory Congress, 1988

Audio tapes available from Audio Archives International, 100 West Beaver Creek, Unit 18, Richmond Hill, Ontario, Canada, L4B 1H4

Audio tapes of the papers presented at the Nursing Theory Congress, "From Theory to Practice," held in Toronto, Ontario, Canada, in August 1988. Presentations are by Parse (nursing science as a basis for research and practice); Watson (one or many models); Henderson (historical perspective); Lindeman (elitism or realism of nursing theory); Moccia (emerging world views); Gordon (nursing diagnosis); and Kritek (agendas for the future). In addition, a panel presentation on the impact of nursing theory on the profession is moderated by Kritek. Concurrent sessions focus on the application of nursing models and theories to practice, education, research, and quality assurance and administration.

Research Seminar: Research Related to Man-Living-Health: An Emerging Methodology

Audio tapes available from Meetings Internationale, Ltd., 1200 Delor Avenue, Louisville, KY 40217

Audio tapes from a research seminar sponsored by Discovery International, Inc., with a paper by Parse describing her research methodology, papers by Sklar and M. J. Smith reporting research results, and a panel discussion moderated by M. Smith.

Research Seminar: Research and Practice Related to Parse's Theory of Nursing

Audio tapes available from Meetings Internationale, Ltd., 1200 Delor Avenue, Louisville, KY 40217

Audio tapes from a research seminar sponsored by Discovery International, Inc. Parse describes her research and practice methodologies; Cody, Beauchamp, and M. Smith report results of their research; and Menke critiques the research reports. In addition, Mitchell and Santopinto discuss their experiences using Parse's theory in practice, and Menke moderates a panel discussion.

Research Seminar: Guided Practice in Qualitative Research

Audio tapes available from Meetings Internationale, Ltd., 1200 Delor Avenue, Louisville, KY 40217

Audio tapes from a research seminar sponsored by Discovery International, Inc., with four papers by Parse describing qualitative and quantitative research methodology, the phenomenological method (two parts), and the ethnographic method; and two papers by M. J. Smith describing the descriptive method and other qualitative methods.

Research Seminar: General Topics

Audio tape available from Meetings Internationale, Ltd., 1200 Delor Avenue, Louisville, KY 40217

Audio tape of a paper by Parse discussing nursing education in the 21st century.

VIDEO PRODUCTIONS

The Nurse Theorists: Portraits of Excellence

Video tapes available from Fuld Institute for Technology in Nursing Education, 28 Station Street, Athens, OH 45701

A series of video tapes, funded by the Helene Fuld Health Trust and produced by Studio Three of Samuel Merritt College of Nursing in Oakland, California, depicting the major events and incidents in the lives of 16 nurse theorists. Interviews are conducted by Jacqueline Fawcett. The series includes separate video tapes of Leininger, Newman, Orlando, Parse, Peplau, Watson, Rubin, Johnson, King, Levine, Neuman, Orem, Rogers, Roy, Henderson, and Nightingale.

Nursing Theory: A Circle of Knowledge

Video tape available from National League for Nursing, 350 Hudson Street, New York, NY 10014

Patricia Moccia interviews several nurse theorists, including Watson, Henderson, Orem, Rogers, Roy, and Benner. The discussion emphasizes philosophy of science.

Theories at Work

Video tape available from National League for Nursing, 350 Hudson Street, New York, NY 10014

Video tape of innovative applications of nursing theory in actual practice settings. Patricia Moccia interviews Jean Watson, Janet Quinn, Dorothy Powell, Bernadine Lacey, Sunny Sutton, and Maria Mitchell. Coverage includes the work with the homeless spearheaded by Powell and Lacey at Howard University College of Nursing and the Center for Human Caring (Watson and Quinn). Sutton and Mitchell discuss the importance of home care, which they contend will be the major health care delivery system of the future.

A Conversation on Caring with Jean Watson and Janet Quinn

Video tape available from National League of Nursing, 350 Hudson Street, New York, NY 10014

Video tape of Patricia Moccia's interviews with Jean Watson and Janet Quinn. Watson and Quinn discuss their views of human caring and health. Coverage includes the Denver Nursing Project in Human Caring, which focuses on individuals with AIDS, and Quinn's Senior Citizen's Therapeutic Touch Education Program.

AUDIO AND VIDEO PRODUCTIONS

Nurse Theorist Conference, 1985

Audio and video tapes available from Meetings Internationale, Ltd., 1200 Delor Avenue, Louisville, KY 40217

Audio and video tapes from the 1985 Nurse Theorist Conference sponsored by Discovery International, Inc. Audio-taped presentations are by Parse, King, Orem, Rogers, and Roy, followed by critiques of each model or theory. In addition, Peplau presents an historical overview of nursing science, and a panel presentation features all conference speakers. Video tapes are available for the presentations by Orem and Peplau, as well as for the panel presentation.

Nurse Theorist Conference, 1987

Audio and video tapes available from Meetings Internationale, Ltd., 1200 Delor Avenue, Louisville, KY 40217

Audio and video tapes from the 1987 Nurse Theorist Conference sponsored by Discovery International, Inc. Presentations are by Parse, Watson, King, Rogers, and Roy. In addition, Peplau presents a paper on the art and science of nursing, Schlotfeldt presents a paper on nursing science in the 21st century, and a panel presentation features all conference speakers. Audio tapes are also available of the small group sessions led by Parse, Watson, King, Rogers, and Roy.

Nurse Theorist Conference, 1989

Audio and video tapes available from Meetings Internationale, Ltd., 1200 Delor Avenue, Louisville, KY 40217

Audio and video tapes from the 1989 Nurse Theorist Conference sponsored by Discovery International, Inc. Presentations are by Parse, King, Neuman, and Rogers. In addition, Meleis presents a paper on being and becoming healthy, Pender presents a paper on expression of health through beliefs and actions, and a panel presentation features all conference speakers.

COMPUTER SEARCH STRATEGIES

Cumulative Index to Nursing and Allied Health Literature (CINAHL)

CINAHL may be accessed via on-line BRS Colleague, CD-ROMs available at libraries, and other databases. The following headings yield the most relevant citations for *nursing theories* when searching CINAHL:

Leininger Transcultural Model
Newman Health Model
Orlando's Nursing Theory
Parse's Theory of Human Becoming
Peplau Interpersonal Relations Model
Watson's Theory of Caring

Before 1988, the most relevant citations for specific nursing theories in the CINAHL database can be located by using the subject headings listed below. The same subject headings can be used to locate citations of general materials about nursing models and theories.

Models, Theoretical
Nursing Theory

MEDLINE

MEDLINE may be accessed via on-line Grateful Med, BRS Colleague, CD-ROMs available at libraries, and other databases. The following subject headings yield the most relevant citations for *nursing theories* when searching MEDLINE:

Nursing Models
Nursing Theories

Dissertation Abstracts International (DAI)

DAI, which also includes Master's Abstracts, may be accessed via on-line BRS Colleague, CD-ROMs available at libraries, and other databases. The following subject headings yield the most relevant citations for *nursing theories* when searching DAI:

Leininger
Transcultural Nursing
Newman and Health
Orlando
Parse
Man Living Health
Peplau
Watson and Caring
Human Caring

Sigma Theta Tau International Directory of Nurse Researchers

The Sigma Theta Tau International Directory of Nurse Researchers is available on-line via the Virginia Henderson International Nursing Library. The Directory and other research-oriented databases provided by the library contain information on both completed and ongoing research.

Contact Sigma Theta Tau International, 550 W. North Street, Indianapolis, IN 46209-0209, (317) 634-8171 for instructions on access to the on-line databases.

The subject headings for *nursing theories* are:

Leininger-Transcultural
Newman Health
Orlando
Parse Man-Living-Health
Peplau Interpersonal Relations
Watson Human Caring

Index_____

A "T" following a page number indicates a table; an "F" following a page number indicates a figure.

Cultural care, concept of, in Leininger's
Theory of Culture Care Diversity
and Universality, 57
Cultural care accommodation, defined,
58
Cultural care diversity, defined, 57
Cultural care maintenance, defined, 58
Cultural care negotiation, defined, 58
Cultural care preservation, defined, 58
Cultural care repatterning, defined, 58
Cultural care restructuring, defined, 58
Cultural care universality, defined, 57
Cultural-congruent nursing care, in
Leininger's Theory of Culture Care
Diversity and Universality, 58
care systems and, 59
nursing practice and, 74–75
Culture, concept of, in Leininger's Theory
of Culture Care Diversity and
Universality, 56
Culture care, Leininger's philosophy of,
52. *See also* Leininger's Theory of
Culture Care Diversity and
Universality
Cumulative Index to Nursing and Allied
Health Literature (CINAHL), 267

DAI (Dissertation Abstracts International),
268
Data collection. *See also* Research
ethnonursing research and, 65–66
Newman's Theory of Health as
Expanding Consciousness and, 99–
100
Orlando's Theory of the Deliberative
Nursing Process and, 132
Data organization, Peplau's Theory of
Interpersonal Relations and, 198
Definitional propositions, 18
Definitions
constitutive, 18
operational
empirical indicators in, 23
Orlando's Theory of the Deliberative
Nursing Process and, 131T
theoretical, 18
Deliberative nursing process, 123, 124,
126. *See also* Orlando's Theory of
the Deliberative Nursing Process
Denver Nursing Project in Human Caring
(DNPHC), 238
Descriptive theories, 19–20
Deterministic-particulate paradigm, 10,
10T
Diagnoses, nursing, taxonomy of, 19–20
pattern identification and, 103, 103T
Dialogical engagement, Parse's Theory of
Human Becoming and, 163
Direct observations, 135

Disciplinary matrices. *See* Conceptual
models
Disciplines, adjunctive, theory context
and, 39
Dissertation Abstracts International (DAI),
268
Diversity, universality and. *See*
Leininger's Theory of Culture Care
Diversity and Universality
DNPHC (Denver Nursing Project in
Human Caring), 238

Economic factors, culture and, 56
Educational factors. *See also* Nursing
education
culture and, 56
Emotions. *See* Feeling(s)
Empirical adequacy
critical reasoning approach and, 256
in theory evaluation, 42–43
Leininger's Theory of Culture Care
Diversity and Universality and, 68–
73, 69T–71T
Newman's Theory of Health as
Expanding Consciousness and,
100–101
Orlando's Theory of the Deliberative
Nursing Process and, 132–133
Peplau's Theory of Interpersonal
Relations and, 199–200
Watson's Theory of Human Caring
and, 235–236
Empirical indicators
middle-range theories and, 23, 23F
theory testability and, 41–42, 252–253
Empirical testing, indirect, in theory
evaluation, 42
Empirically observable concepts, theory
testability and, 41
Empiricism, traditional, theory testing
and, 252–253
Enablers, in Leininger's research, 65–
66
Enabling-limiting, rhythmicity and, in
Parse's Theory of Human
Becoming, 156
Environment
human relationship to, philosophies of,
8–11, 9T–12T
Leininger's Theory of Culture Care
Diversity and Universality and, 54
metaparadigm concept of, 2–3
proposed exclusion of, 4, 6
Watson's Theory of Human Caring and,
228
Environmental contexts, concept of
in Leininger's Theory of Culture Care
Diversity and Universality, 57, 61
metaparadigm of nursing and, 5

in Peplau's Theory of Interpersonal Relations, 192–193
in Watson's Theory of Human Caring, 228–231
Nonverbal behavior, in Orlando's Theory of the Deliberative Nursing Process, 122
North American Nursing Diagnosis Association (NANDA), taxonomy of nursing diagnoses of, 20
pattern identification and, 103, 103T
Nurse-patient relationship
Orlando's Theory of the Deliberative Nursing Process and, 136
Peplau's Theory of Interpersonal Relations and, 188–193, 189F, 190F. See also Peplau's Theory of Interpersonal Relations
transpersonal caring and. See Watson's Theory of Human Caring
Nurse Theorist Conference, 263
Nurse Theorist Conference, 1985, 266
Nurse Theorist Conference, 1986, 266
Nurse Theorist Conference, 1989, 266–267
Nurse Theorists: Portraits of Excellence, 265
Nurse's activity, in Orlando's Theory of the Deliberative Nursing Process, 123–125, 125T
relational propositions and, 126–128
Nurse's reaction, in Orlando's Theory of the Deliberative Nursing Process, 122–123
relational propositions and, 126–127
Nursing
Leininger's concept of, 52, 54
medicine distinguished from, Orlando's Theory of the Deliberative Nursing Process and, 119–120
metaparadigm concept of, 3
Orlando's Theory of the Deliberative Nursing Process and, 117
Peplau's Theory of Interpersonal Relations and, 185
proposed elimination of, 3–4
Peplau's definition of, 187
purpose of, in Orlando's Theory of the Deliberative Nursing Process, 120
Nursing actions. See also Nurse's activity; Practice
theory-based. See also Theories
pragmatic adequacy of theory and, 43–44
Nursing care. See Care
Nursing diagnoses, taxonomy of, 19–20
pattern identification and, 103, 103T
Nursing education
Newman's Theory of Health as Expanding Consciousness and, 101–102

Orlando's Theory of the Deliberative Nursing Process and, 133–135
Parse's Theory of Human Becoming and, 165–167
Peplau's Theory of Interpersonal Relations and, 200–201
transcultural, Leininger's Theory of Culture Care Diversity and Universality and, 73–74
Watson's Theory of Human Caring and, 236–237
Nursing interventions. See also Practice
Leininger's view of term, 75
Nursing knowledge. See also Nursing education
components of, 2F. See also specific components
conceptual models, 12–13, 14T–17T, 18F
empirical indicators, 23, 23F
metaparadigm of nursing, 2–8
philosophies, 8–11, 9T–12T
theories, 13, 14T–17T, 18F, 18–23, 21F, 22F
influencing Leininger's Theory of Culture Care Diversity and Universality, 54–56
influencing Newman's Theory of Health as Expanding Consciousness, 92–93
influencing Parse's Theory of Human Becoming, 154–155
influencing Peplau's Theory of Interpersonal Relations, 188
influencing Watson's Theory of Human Caring, 225
literature about, 27–33
terminology and, 24
Nursing practice. See Practice
Nursing process theory. See Orlando's Theory of the Deliberative Nursing Process
Nursing theories. See Theories; specific theories
Nursing Theory: A Circle of Knowledge, 265
Nursing Theory Congress, 1986, 264
Nursing Theory Congress, 1988, 264
Nursing Theory in Action, 263–264

Observable action, of nurse, in Orlando's Theory of the Deliberative Nursing Process, 123–125, 125T
Observation
in nurse-patient relationship, Peplau's Theory of Interpersonal Relations and, 197
in nursing practice, Orlando's Theory of the Deliberative Nursing Process and, 135–136

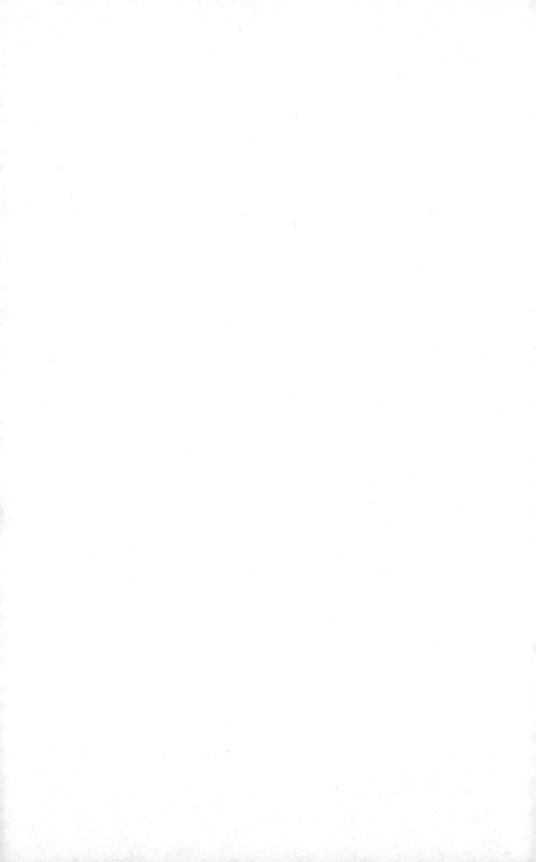